W9-DEN-862

MID-LIFE
BODY
SIGNALS

3721 4942

RA
777.5
L68
1995c

DISCARDED

MID-LIFE
BODY
SIGNALS

THE OVER-40 GUIDE TO HEALTH SYMPTOMS
AND WHAT THEY MEAN

Bruce K. Lowell, M.D.

WITH LISA ANGOWSKI ROGAK

Produced by the Philip Lief Group Inc.

NORMANDALE COMMUNITY COLLEGE
9700 FRANCE AVENUE SOUTH
BLOOMINGTON MN 55431-4399

HarperPerennial
A Division of HarperCollinsPublishers

NOV 0 9 1999

A hardcover edition of this book was published in 1995 by HarperCollins Publishers, Inc. under the title *Body Signals*.

BODY SIGNALS. Copyright © 1995 by The Philip Lief Group Inc. and Bruce K. Lowell, M.D. All rights reserved. Printed in the United States of America. No part of this book may be used or reproduced in any manner whatsoever without written permission except in the case of brief quotations embodied in critical articles and reviews. For information address HarperCollins Publishers, Inc., 10 East 53rd Street, New York, New York 10022.

HarperCollins books may be purchased for educational, business, or sales promotional use. For information please write to: Special Markets Department, HarperCollins Publishers, Inc., 10 East 53rd Street, New York, New York 10022.

First HarperPerennial edition published 1997.

Book design by Maura Fadden Rosenthal

The Library of Congress has catalogued the hardcover edition as follows:

Lowell, Bruce K., 1946–
    Body signals / Bruce K. Lowell.
      p. cm.
    Includes index.
    ISBN 0-06-270111-8 (hc)
    1. Middle aged persons—Health and hygiene.   2. Symptomatology.
  I. Title.
  RA777.5.L68 1995
  613'.0434—dc20   95-9673

ISBN 0-06-273477-6 (pbk.)

97 98 99 00 01 ❖/RRD 10 9 8 7 6 5 4 3 2 1

To my wife, Diane; my children, Jennifer and Matt;
my mother, Goldy, a true example of how to age successfully;
and my ever supportive in-laws, Marie and Frank

CONTENTS

I would like to thank my family for their support during this time-consuming project and my wife, Diane, for tolerating my difficult and hectic schedule. I also appreciate the hard work and patience put forth by Lisa Angowski Rogak, who helped make sense of the material, and Judy Linden, my editor at the Philip Lief Group and friend, who had the foresight and fortitude to make this book a reality.

This book has been made possible by the many years of joy I've had from practicing primary care and providing care to all my special patients. The final acknowledgment goes to my physician colleagues at New York Primary Care, who help shine the beacon into the future.

This book contains advice and information relating to health care for people approaching or in mid-life. It is not intended to replace medical advice and should be used to supplement rather than replace regular care by your physician. Since every individual is different, you should consult your physician regarding any questions specific to your own health.

Produced by the Philip Lief Group Inc.

PART I

WHY THIS BOOK NOW?

Chapter 1

THE DOCTOR INSIDE US ALL

I remember the conversation quite clearly. A woman in her early 50s, who was a regular patient, called my office to make an appointment, and she insisted on speaking to me. The receptionist offered to have me return her call later that day, but no, she said, she had to talk to me right now.

My receptionist pulled me out of an examination room where I was with a patient and told me about the situation. To my knowledge, this patient hadn't had any serious health problems before, and I felt she wouldn't be so insistent if it was something minor. So I picked up the phone and braced myself for the worst.

Here's how the conversation went:

"Oh, Doctor Lowell, I don't feel so good," she said in a voice verging on panic. "And I don't know why!"

I asked her to describe her symptoms.

"I just feel weak, Doctor, I don't feel like myself and I'm belching a lot—"

I interrupted her. "Do you have a headache, or has your stomach been upset lately?"

"No."

I kept going. "Have you been tired lately? Do you feel short of breath?"

"Yes, and I have no energy. And this morning I started to sweat heavily when I tried to clean up the house."

I then proceeded to run down a list of general symptoms. When some of them appear together, they make for an easy diagnosis, while others point to the need for further testing to narrow down the possible causes. Her negative replies to most symptoms became more frenzied with each answer. I started to become concerned as well.

"Well, then, exactly what is it that doesn't feel well?"

"I just don't know," she blurted out. "I hate to say it, Doctor Lowell, but I think I'm going to die. Please help me."

I tried to calm her down and focused more on her belching and upset stomach. I asked her if she was taking aspirin or eating spicy foods; she said no. She had said that the belching had appeared suddenly that morning and that she couldn't stop. Since she had also said that she was sweating heavily and lacked energy, I asked her what she had eaten recently, and she replied that she had eaten her usual dinner. Though she told me she did not have any chest pains or palpitations, I told her to call 911 immediately and go to the emergency room. She became a little panicked, but she said she would meet me there.

When she described all of her symptoms, I knew she was having a heart attack, since belching and sweating are typical symptoms of a heart attack in a woman who's 50 years or older. The symptoms of a heart attack aren't always chest pain and pain down the left arm. The doctor inside her told her that her life was in jeopardy, even though she wasn't sure what was wrong. This is what had prompted her to make that very important phone call to me. The doctor inside her was telling this woman, who usually doesn't call physicians, that she had to contact me immediately. Listening to the doctor inside her saved her life.

Her experience is not unusual. Many of my patients tell me that they don't know when they need to call me and when to deal with a health problem themselves. Sometimes they wait until it passes and they feel better; at other times they call me like this patient did, their voices filled with anxiety and confusion. They also want to know what their symptoms mean so they'll know exactly what is wrong with them and what they can do about it. However, as my experience with my 50-something patient showed, many men and women are unable to articulate the signals their bodies are sending them due to fear, embarrassment, and the physiological changes that normally occur with age. In addition, the symptoms don't necessarily match what they've heard about or have seen on television and in the media, which could add to their hesitation. Of course, in an emergency situation, the ability to describe your symptoms accurately can become a matter of life or death. In some cases, however, we immediately know what a series of particular symptoms means: for instance, many of us are familiar with the signs of a stroke, and diabetics are taught about how their bodies will react if they get too much or too little insulin.

The main reason I wrote this book is to help men and women in midlife learn how to interpret the signals their bodies are sending them, their Body Signals. When I talk about a Body Signal, I am referring to a symptom, a sign your body is sending you to let you know when something is wrong. Midlife adults especially need to heed their Body Signals because frequently the symptoms in a person who's 50 may indicate a totally different problem than for someone in her 20s. For example, in a 25-year-old, a sore throat is usually just a sore throat. In someone who's 40 or older, however, it could be a sign of a hiatal hernia, a condition causing a reflux of stomach acid. Obviously, the treatment for each problem would differ dramatically. In addition, men and women who are just entering their 40s may find that their bodies are changing in ways they don't expect. Usually, these changes are not as drastic as those that occur during puberty; they're more subtle and so can be more frustrating because people don't know what's happening. In fact, many people confuse these changes with signs of disease. For this reason, many of my midlife patients frequently tell me that they don't feel quite right but can't articulate how they feel. Because of this, I've addressed many of these signs of aging in this book as Body Signals. Finally, there are many illnesses common to midlife adults that a person in her 20s never has to worry about, like gastrointestinal cancer and heart disease.

Being able to describe your Body Signals accurately is important, since 95% of all diagnoses are made through how a patient is able to describe his symptoms. Based on your descriptions, your physician will be able to plan the course of treatment that's best for you.

As I mentioned, in terms of listening to your Body Signals, we all have a doctor inside us who knows when we're sick and when we're not. In order to assist this personal, internal doctor, you should ask yourself several questions whenever you're feeling unwell:

- Do I need to call the doctor even though it's 2 A.M.?

- Do I see or feel something I know shouldn't be happening to me?

- Do I feel doom or fear?

- Do I have the worst pain I have ever felt in my life?

- Do I feel it can wait until the morning? Do I feel I can go to my job and worry about it this weekend or after work?

- Have I had this symptom before, and is it usually something that goes away very quickly?

Answering these questions can help the doctor inside you to differentiate between a very serious problem and one that probably isn't serious at all.

My advice to all of my patients is to always trust that internal doctor. Listen to that voice just as you would listen to a best friend. After all, you know what you feel like when you're feeling fine, and how that compares with when you're feeling under the weather. Keep in mind that this "inside doctor" may be you, or it may be a friend or family member who is also able to notice the subtle changes in your health if you're unable to.

I've always felt that if you think there is something seriously wrong with your health, you should err on the side of common sense and call your doctor or go to the emergency room. The worst thing that can happen is that you turn out to be in perfect health because you have misread a Body Signal; you may also be a little embarrassed. The best thing is that your quick action—for you or for someone else—could save a life. For instance, here's a story about the father of one of my patients. One day, he was standing on line at the bank and he passed out. This had never happened to him before, and he refused to go to the hospital. When his family found out what had happened, he assured them he would be okay. They, of course, felt otherwise. My patient, who was the man's daughter, called to tell me about her father, and I told her to bring him in to the emergency room immediately. Again he refused, but after extensive negotiations he finally agreed. While he was in the emergency room, he passed out again. It turned out that he had been taking large quantities of antiarthritis medication and as a result had developed a bleeding ulcer. After a blood transfusion, intravenous antiulcer medication, and a few days in the hospital, he was able to go home. If his daughter had ignored his Body Signals and hadn't forced him to go to the hospital, his significant loss of blood could have led to a stroke or heart attack, since his bleeding ulcer was preventing enough blood from reaching his heart and brain.

THE DOCTOR INSIDE YOU HELPS
YOUR DOCTOR, TOO

Whenever you're evaluating your own or somebody else's symptoms, rely on the instincts of the doctor inside you and put yourself behind the doctor's desk: ask yourself what information you would need to know if you were the doctor.

Along with your Body Signals, your doctor needs your past medical history to make the correct diagnosis and offer the right treatment. An illness you had five years ago is important if it pertains to the symptoms you're experiencing now or if it has affected your health since you were sick; you and your doctor can disregard it if it's unrelated to your present symptoms. For example, if you've come in to see the doctor about your malaise, it's not important for him to know that you fractured your foot in summer camp 25 years ago; however, you should let him know about the diabetes you've had for most of your life.

To help your doctor diagnose your illness, you should also try to be as specific about your symptoms as you can. The phrase "I just don't feel well" can be frustrating for your doctor to hear, because it doesn't tell him anything. A few ways in which you can be more specific about your symptoms is to ask yourself the following questions:

- Have I recently lost or gained weight?

- Do I feel more tired than usual?

- Do I feel a pain somewhere in my body? Is it sharp or dull? Is it constant, or does it appear after a particular activity?

- Is my temperature over normal?

- Has my appetite changed?

- Do I feel short of breath?

- Have I noticed a change in my personal hygiene?

The amount of time you've had your symptoms is also important. If you have had a number of different symptoms for more than a few days, you should be sure to tell your doctor how many days, weeks, months, or years you've had that particular symptom. And if you're trying to read the Body Signals of a family member or close friend, ask him or her these same questions as they pertain to his or her condition.

Remember, relying on the doctor inside you will speed up your own physician's diagnosis and treatment plan and ultimately your own recovery as well.

HOW TO USE THIS BOOK

Flip through *Mid-Life Body Signals* freely in order to familiarize yourself with the organization and the language I've used to describe specific symptoms. The information in each entry is presented in an easy-to-use format that's designed to put information at your fingertips so you can quickly arrive at a conclusion and know what your next step should be. What you'll see are the most common types of health problems that I treat in my patients over 40. Reading this book will help you to determine when you're seriously ill and when you're not. It will also help you learn how to describe your symptoms in detail the next time you feel something is wrong. And if you use these same terms to describe your symptoms when you seek medical treatment, your doctor will be able to diagnose and treat you much faster than if you aren't able to articulate what you're feeling.

Chapters 3 through 18 detail the body's symptoms from head to toe. Each chapter is devoted to a specific region of the body and provides concise descriptions of approximately 300 symptoms, explanations of possible illnesses and treatments, and illustrative case studies.

Each chapter begins with a Body Signal Alert section that briefly tells you which particular symptoms indicate the possibility that there is an emergency situation and you should call your doctor or head for the emergency room right away.

After the Body Signal Alert chart is a section that explains how aging affects the body system or group of organs that I cover in that chapter. With this information, you will be able to understand how the mature body functions and also how it responds to illness. This is followed by the Body Signals themselves, which are arranged alphabetically within each chapter. Each Body Signal is divided into two main sections: "Description and Possible Medical Problems" and "Treatment." From symptoms that show up in the head ("Fainting"; "Headache, Occasional") to the skin ("Dry, Scaly Patches That Itch") through the chest ("Chest Pain Worsened by Movement") and on down to the legs and feet ("Toenail, Painful"), *Mid-Life Body Signals* covers a whole lot more than the average number of aches, pains, and illnesses you, your friends, and your family—fortunately—will ever face.

SPECIAL THOUGHTS FOR SPECIAL PEOPLE AND SITUATIONS

Some of the Body Signals in the book address special health problems and concerns for readers over the age of 75 under the section "Special Mention for the Elderly". This section follows the "Treatment" section and includes specific warnings about medications, treatments, and illnesses to which they may be especially prone. For instance, in Chapter 6, "Ears and Nose," readers will learn that when an older person is affected with Ramsay Hunt syndrome, a form of shingles, an extremely painful condition called postherpetic neuralgia can sometimes occur. Readers are then provided with special information about the symptoms of this illness as well as how to minimize their discomfort.

Another section I've included in some of the entries is called "Tips and Precautions." This section includes self-help treatments you can try at home before you see your doctor as well as certain preventive measures you can take to lower your chances of having the condition recur.

READERS, TAKE NOTE

While many Body Signals can be monitored or even treated at home, some require professional attention even if they aren't listed in the Body Signal Alert chart. Most often your doctor will prescribe medication to treat your illness, and in this book I do, too. However, whenever I recommend medications and their dosages in a particular entry, I'm including them as examples only. There are hundreds of brands and generic substitutes that are available, and I have used these interchangeably throughout the book, concentrating on the ones that are most commonly prescribed. As far as dosages are concerned, these can vary greatly depending upon a person's weight, age, sex, and general health. Always follow the exact directions of your physician or pharmacist.

Another thing you should understand is that this book is not a textbook of medicine. It is not meant to be all-inclusive, and it is not meant to substitute for a physician. The approximately 300 Body Signals I detail are the most common symptoms I've seen in my 20 years as a primary care physician, the term used to describe the doctor a patient visits before being referred to a specialist. A primary care physician is also known as a general practitioner, family medicine specialist, or internist. I'll tell you more about how a primary care physician functions in Chapter 2.

Speaking of Chapter 2, "Health Care Today: It's Radically Different Than You Think," you may wonder about the connection between your Body Signals and the way health care is changing in our country. Actually, as you will read, it is this new era of "managed" care, as indicated by the rapid growth and expansion of HMOs and other group practices, that mandates consumers to become active participants in the way they are treated for illness and disease. I know. In addition to caring for my patients, I have long been involved in the New York City health care industry to help both patients and doctors better understand the shifting medical climate. In addition, as a board member and advisor to New York Hospital–Queens Medical Center in its efforts to develop a hospitalwide HMO, I have personally established one of the largest groupings of primary care physicians in New York State who are committed to delivering quality care by getting people more involved in their own health care. Clearly, this "involvement" begins with a solid understanding of your body's signs and symptoms. By training yourself to hear what your body tells you, you'll be able to provide your doctors with all the information they need to choose the correct diagnostic path and best course of treatment.

I sincerely hope you will turn to *Mid-Life Body Signals* again and again for reassurance, guidance, and a true sense of empowerment.

Bruce K. Lowell, M.D.

Chapter 2

HEALTH CARE TODAY: IT'S RADICALLY DIFFERENT THAN YOU THINK

TERMS YOU NEED TO KNOW
ABOUT HEALTH CARE TODAY

Accept assignment: This is an agreement between the health care provider, i.e., the physician, and the insurance company in which the provider agrees to accept the agreed-upon fee for each service as it's set by the insurance company. Patients are often required to pay a small copayment or deductible per their contract with their insurance company. Sometimes an accept assignment means that the physician participates with the given insurance plan.

Capitation payment: This is an arrangement in which the health care provider is paid a specific amount that is set in advance by the insurance company and the health care provider as a fair payment for a particular service. This payment, which is made in a lump sum once a month, is paid to the health care provider for services; the figure is based on a specific number of patients treated each month. The insurance company pays this fee to the health care provider whether or not an actual service has been performed. Usually only primary care physicians (PCPs) are "capitated," since they are the gatekeepers of the first line of care; they are responsible for large numbers of patients, and it's more cost-effective for the insurance company to have primary care physicians on a capitation program. The advantage of capitation payments is that the health care provider receives a guaranteed income each month, with almost no billing hassles; the insurance

11

carrier benefits because it can retain better control over its costs by monitoring its panel of providers. The patient chooses a primary care physician from a selected group of physicians that is established by the insurance carrier.

Copayment: When an insurance company pays only a certain percentage of a medical bill, the copayment is the amount of the difference that the patient is responsible for paying. For example, if the insurance company pays for 80% of the fee for a surgical procedure, the patient will pay 20%, which doesn't include the deductible. A copayment can be a fixed amount for each visit, such as $10, regardless of the service that is delivered.

Deductible: This is an amount of money that must be paid by the patient before the insurance company will start paying for the total fee or a portion of it. Many deductibles range from $100 to $500, though some can be up to $10,000 or more.

EOMB: This is the acronym for "Explanation of Medicare Benefits." An EOMB is the statement that's sent by Medicare to the patient to inform him or her of the amount that has been paid by Medicare, as well as any balance the Medicare recipient is legally obligated to pay the health care provider.

Fee for service: With a fee-for-service arrangement, a health care provider is paid based on the particular service he or she performs. This service can be either an office visit or an ancillary service like a lab test or an X ray. The fee for service is usually paid to the health care provider by the patient or the patient's insurance company, which is usually paid at a discounted rate if the provider participates with the insurance company. If the insurance company pays for less than the doctor's actual fee, in most cases the patient is required to pay for the difference out of pocket if the provider does not participate. This is known as conventional insurance or indemnity insurance. Today, insurance companies frequently ask to preapprove a certain medical procedure before they will pay for it. Because some medical procedures will automatically drive up the cost of an insurance premium, or because a patient may have a lifetime cap on benefits he or she receives, a patient may prefer to pay the fee for service without prior approval from the insurance carrier and without submitting the claim to the insurance carrier.

Many specialists are on a fee-for-service basis at a discounted rate, whereas a primary care physician might be on a capitated payment plan if he participates with an insurance company where the doctor's fee is in essence set by the insurance company.

Health care provider: This is any person who provides care to a patient, from a physician to a bedside aide. In the eyes of an insurance company, a health care provider can also be an institution, like an HMO or a hospital.

HMO: This is the acronym for "health maintenance organization." An HMO is a group that provides health care under the definition of managed care. An HMO can consist of doctors in their own private practices who are spread out over a city or region, or it can be one general office where all the health care providers are in one location. The HMO can be owned and operated by an insurance company, hospital, union, private corporation, or other group.

Managed care: This is a system in which the people and companies that pay for health care—the patients and the insurance companies—and the providers of health care—doctors, nurses, and the hospital—cooperate to provide quality care while working to keep medical costs down.

Point of service (POS): This is any service that's provided in a physician's private office.

Preferred physician organization (PPO): This is a group of private physicians who agree to participate with a given insurance company. They are usually on a fee-for-service basis. A PPO is frequently established by a hospital to link its entire staff of physicians with one insurance carrier.

Primary care physician (PCP): A primary care physician can be a generalist, internist, family practitioner, pediatrician, and, in some cases, an OB/GYN. In other words, a primary care physician is a health care provider who is the first person a patient will see before being referred to a specialist.

If you haven't been living in a cave for the last few years, you know by now that one of the buzzwords of the 1990s is health care reform—whether it's instituted by the government or by private industry—and not a day goes by where we don't hear about it on the TV, on the radio, in the newspapers, or from our neighbors. The problem with health care reform at this point in time is that both health care providers and the public don't fully understand what health care reform means and how it will affect each of them.

Why do we need health care reform? Here are a few good reasons:

• The inflation rate in the medical field averages 11% each year.

• There are 40 million Americans without health insurance.

• Medicare and Medicaid cost the taxpayers $200 billion a year.

• Middle-class men and women frequently find they have to choose between leaving a job and keeping their health insurance. As a result, many hang on to their job, even if they would rather leave it, so that they'll be covered.

A new era of health care in the United States has arrived. The ascent of managed care and the prevalence of health maintenance organizations (HMOs) is quickly phasing out the familiar fee-for-service system. In the old system, a consumer could choose both his general practitioner and his subspecialists freely, regardless of whether he really needed the medical services or not. The physician was then paid directly by the patient's insurance company or by the patient, who would then be reimbursed by his insurance company.

Under health care reform, which is already quickly growing in many parts of the country, insurance companies will essentially assign patients to see a primary care physician, who will then decide if the patient needs to see a specialist. However, there's a big problem with this new, efficient method: only 20% of the doctors in the United States are trained as primary care physicians, while the remaining 80% are specialists. This means that as health care reform takes hold, 20% of the country's physicians will be responsible for seeing 100% of the health care consumers. Unfortunately, with this amount of work, physicians will have even less time to devote to individual patients than they do now. For this reason, physician assistants and nurse practitioners will become essential parts of any health care organization, working with patients who require minor medical attention, while physicians concentrate on patients who need more specialized care.

In addition to the change in medical responsibilities, many insurance plans will require physicians to be paid on a capitation basis, under which a physician is paid a monthly service fee by the insurance company for all the patients the HMO assigns to him or her, regardless of the number of visits each patient makes. For instance, Dr. Smith, a primary care physician, may be assigned a caseload of 220 patients per month and receive $10 per patient no matter how many times each patient visits. However, to prevent the possibility of abuse by both patients and physicians, financial incentives are built into this type of plan to encourage the primary care physician to limit repeat visits, utilize the support of fewer specialists, and order fewer tests. So while this will result in improved medical access for patients, it also means they will need to become more familiar with their Body Signals and to learn why certain medical tests they had under the old method of health care are now not appropriate.

Clearly, the way we receive our medical care is changing. In this decade, we may pay less for treatment, but we will also see fewer sub-specialists and will undergo fewer unnecessary diagnostic tests than before. Patients may find that their doctors are reluctant to schedule appointments, especially if they're being paid so much less for each patient encounter. In addition, examinations may seem shorter and more focused on the specific health problem, and the doctor may appear to be more rushed. Your new insurance plan may actually force you to switch to a new primary care physician who is unfamiliar with your medical history or face paying higher premiums to see a physician who's not in the HMO. As a result, most people will make the switch whether they like it or not. Without a doubt, the health care consumer of the 1990s and beyond will have to learn to make the most of each office visit.

Since patients will need to accept more of the burden of their own health care, from being screened by a nurse practitioner before ganing access to a physician to paying a larger share of medical expenses, it's imperative that you learn how to recognize the signals your body is sending you and how to relay this information to your doctor in an efficient manner.

THE NEW ERA OF AMERICAN HEALTH CARE

When I first began to kick around the idea for this book, I started to see that one of the most important things *Mid-Life Body Signals* could do would be to help the reader function better within the complex world of a rapidly changing health care system. We're years away from instituting an ideal model of health care reform, though in some areas it's already here. When it makes its appearance in all facets of American medicine, it will affect every American. Midlife adults will be affected even more, since they are reaching the stage of life when they need to access the health care system a little more each year. As health care reform begins to take shape over the course of this decade, it's a good idea to know why it has become so necessary. To understand that, you'll need to know how the medical establishment progressed in its treatment of disease from leeches to X rays to sophisticated MRIs and CAT scans.

Therefore, the first thing you must do to understand the complexities of our current health care system is learn how medicine developed and expanded in the United States after World War II. For centuries before the war, the physician's role in maintaining the health of a community was actually quite limited. In this country, medical training was almost nonexistent until the late 1700s. To make a diagnosis, doctors were mostly limited to the use of elementary medical tools like the stethoscope, neurological hammer, and tongue depressor. A physician's role was first to diagnose an illness and then to prescribe various medications, many of which would be considered to be homeopathic today, like herbs. The diagnostic skills of a physician were limited to what his five senses were able to detect, and a diagnosis often required surgery that many times was more dangerous than the illness itself.

In those days, however, the relationship between the doctor and the patient was quite close, and many times was itself the primary form of treatment, since comfort and supportive care were frequently all a physician could offer in the case of a terminal illness like cancer or heart disease. The price of medical care was also relatively low. In the early part of this century, office visits and house calls often cost only a few dollars, depending on the region of the country and the doctor. Most of the time, a patient paid for the doctor's fee and any tests, medications, and hospital stays out of pocket. The family doctor was a generalist, caring for pregnant women and their babies, sick children, and adults as well as elderly members of the family. In this situation, a doctor couldn't help but develop close relationships with each family he cared for over the years. On the rare occasion when it became necessary to refer a patient to a specialist, many patients refused, feeling that "Doc" could do as well as any fancy-pants specialist. Then, in the early part of this century, medicine began to change.

Medical advances like the development of anesthesia, the electrocardiogram, and the first crude X rays entered in the wake of indoor plumbing and sewage waste management; these two benchmarks of civilization directly resulted in a drop in the number of infectious diseases that were usually fatal.

After World War II, the way medicine was practiced in the United States continued to change. Surgeons developed new, sophisticated techniques during the war, and new specialties also began to develop. The fields of biology, genetics, biomechanics, electronics, and pharmaceuticals began to change due to new technology, and, as a result, both new and experienced doctors began to use these new techniques to practice medicine. This increased reliance on technology, however, began to change the cornerstone of medicine in years past: the one-to-one relationship a patient shared with his family doctor. It seemed that both physicians and patients were so distracted by these new and exciting medical advances that they almost didn't notice that the degree of personal attention began to change as well, especially as new doctors entered medicine better trained in technology than in patient relations. Patients also became more educated about medicine and their health as a result of media reports about the new advances, and they began to expect more tests and newer medications.

With all these new medical techniques, however, the cost of medical care began to go up. People who had health insurance through their employers didn't mind at first, but older Americans who got by on limited funds did. As the price of an office visit, necessary tests, and prescription medications began to climb, the government began to see that many older Americans needed some help with their medical bills, especially since they tended to visit doctors more than younger Americans; they were also unlikely to carry any kind of health insurance. The result was Medicare, established in 1965 as a government-run health insurance program to help Americans 65 years old and over to get the care they need. Medicare consists of two programs: Part A, which covers inpatient care in a hospital or a skilled nursing facility, rehabilitation services, physician visits, and home health care or hospice care where the guidance of a physician is necessary. Part B requires a deductible and copayment and will pay for only a portion of the physician's fee, outpatient hospital care, outpatient physical therapy and speech therapy, and certain ancillary tests done on an outpatient basis, like X rays, as well as flu vaccine.

When Medicare was started, no one could have envisioned the route medical technology would take. And Medicare had the unseen benefit of allowing medical technology to advance even more in this country than it would have without the program, since it meant more money for research.

Another government program, Medicaid, is a state-run program that receives federal money to meet the health care expenses of poor people, including the elderly, blind, and disabled people and poor families with dependent children. There is also Medigap, which is offered by private insurance companies and covers the deductible and copayments in Part B of Medicaid.

In the 1960s and '70s, the medical profession began to develop into the research-oriented high-tech industry it is today. The logical next step was to involve computer technology, and today new advances in computers as well as in medicine have fueled every big medical break-through. Needless to say, hospitals and medical schools have flourished in this new environment. Physicians can use a vast array of tests that are designed to make diagnosis easier and more precise, and, amazingly, there are a number of medications that can be genetically engineered to provide the best treatment for a particular person and his or her condition.

High-tech medicine has also made it possible for specialties to form within the existing specialties. Even to me, it sometimes seems as though there is a specialist for each different cell in the body. For example, the specialties in the ophthalmological field include retinal specialists, corneal specialists, and so on. Surgery has also become extremely focused, so that each organ now has its own superspecialists. Even a radiologist who used to just look at X rays now performs delicate needle biopsies guided by a computer attached to CAT scan equipment.

Alongside this technological explosion in medicine, the amount of medical information Americans receive every day has grown proportion-ately. As a result, the American population has developed an insatiable thirst for medical knowledge. No matter where you go, to a supermarket or cocktail party, it seems that the talk always seems to turn to the lat-est news in medicine, from acne treatments to face-lifts. Women from all walks of life are able to talk knowledgeably about the pros and cons of using hormonal therapy to ease the symptoms of menopause, and newspapers, magazines, and TV and radio shows offer constant updates on the newest high-tech diagnostic tools and treatments that some-times were only invented the previous week. Along with all of this information, I see a lot of misinformation making its way out onto the airwaves and into print. The proliferation of medical trauma shows that appear each night on television only adds to the public's faulty perceptions about medicine, frequently giving the impression that the practice of medicine is quite simple—a cause, an effect, and subsequent treatment—and that the outcome will always be a happy one for patients and doctors alike.

HIGH TECH MEANS HIGH COSTS

Even though modern medicine has enhanced the health and extended the lives of people who would have otherwise perished without it, the advances have come at a price: the amount of money that is required to research and develop these new techniques is enormous, amounting to billions of dollars each year. Someone has to pay for high-tech medicine, and it eventually filters down to the point where it's paid for by the consumer. And since research must continue so that we can improve on the type of medicine we currently practice, the cost will continue to rise. It is for precisely this reason that the price of medical insurance has gone through the roof since the 1970s and '80s and it has become impossible for working poor, middle-class, and even upper-middle-class Americans to take advantage of these incredible advances. Only people who are on welfare and receive Medicaid or are elderly and benefit from Medicare are able to benefit directly from the system—that is, besides people who have employer- or self-funded health insurance. Even then, people who have private health insurance are frequently shocked to discover that their insurance sometimes doesn't cover everything they think it does. Of course, we hear about the great numbers of Americans without health insurance, which is estimated to be 37 to 40 million people. These Americans learn to keep their fingers crossed and maintain their own health; in the case of an injury or major illness affecting themselves or a family member, they either draw on their savings or go into massive debt.

As if all these changes weren't enough to influence health care in America and point out the need for reform, it is also important for you to realize that even as the medical technology has made significant advances, the type of physician who graduates from medical school has also changed. When I finished medical school in 1975, everyone in my class chose a specialty like plastic surgery, ophthalmologic reconstruction, or another extremely narrow field of medicine. Back then, graduating physicians quickly realized that the glamour and financial rewards of medicine were primarily in doing specialty work, not in general practice. Even those physicians who chose to go into general medicine became specialists in family practice or primary internal medicine. Most physicians also opted for private practice, many times in partnership with another doctor who was in a complementary specialty, like an OB/GYN who shared an office with a pediatrician. And specialists also earned more money than generalists, which undoubtedly helped many new med school graduates with hundreds of thousands of dollars of student loans staring them in the face to decide their destinies.

When doctors begin to practice, they soon realize that they will have to purchase specialized equipment that will allow them to perform tests right in the office instead of sending them to a lab. This not only increases doctors' revenue but also makes them appear to be more high tech than the doctor next door, helping them to attract new patients. Of course, if the office next door already has all the same high-tech equipment, the new kid on the block usually has to go one better, purchasing either more expensive equipment or simply more of it.

As many medical practices evolved into high-tech profit centers, the old American image of the physician naturally began to erode. The friendly family doctor who made house calls became the high-tech whiz-kid specialist who used CAT scans, MRIs, and other high-tech devices to help make a diagnosis. It became clear that the public was torn: they still wanted the old family doctor, but they were also very attracted to the exciting high-tech aspects of medicine. Access to this new wave of medical care also began to expand to many parts of the country, especially in major metropolitan areas, where the physician population has normally been more concentrated. In essence, it became almost impossible for patients to decline to have a certain test done, since they could choose from a number of conveniently located testing centers where the test could be performed. In this way, patients could seek the opinion of several specialists, who would give them numerous tests in order to offer second and third opinions on the previous doctor's diagnosis. The more patients who walked through the door and the more procedures performed by a physician, clinic, hospital, or diagnostic test center, the more money everyone would make.

In many cases, patients would pick and choose which tests they wanted to take, as recommended by their doctors. Frequently, patients would have every test performed, even the same one several times. In this way, they would feel they were benefiting from the latest in medical technology, in addition to knowing that they were participating in something really new and different. And doctors would suggest a whole battery of tests not only because they stood to benefit from them financially but also because they feared making a misdiagnosis, which might result in a malpractice lawsuit. Therefore, most physicians preferred to perform tests sooner, rather than later, to cover all the bases.

Everyone was thrilled with this arrangement: doctors received their fees, the patients were reimbursed by their insurance companies. Everyone, that is, except the insurance industry.

ENTER THE INSURANCE INDUSTRY

In time, the Medicare system and private insurance companies began to feel the financial pinch of the multitude of tests and procedures that were ordered by all the specialists. Not only did the sheer numbers of tests that were performed raise insurance premiums across the board, the insurance companies also began to ask to have final approval before any test was administered.

When I first began my medical practice, I could clearly see the abuses of the system. I remember one patient in particular who came to me complaining of severe headaches. According to her description, they fit the definition of a classic migraine. She was taking medications that had been prescribed for her by five different neurologists. When she arrived for her appointment, she pulled out a total of five different CAT scans of the head, all of which were negative. When I asked her why she had so many different scans, she told me she wanted to make sure she didn't have a brain tumor. I asked her why, since all five were negative, she hadn't told each of the neurologists about the previous neurologist's tests. She replied that she wanted each doctor to come to his own conclusion. "After all," she concluded, "my insurance company was paying for all the tests, so what's the big deal?"

I have also seen patients who have had complete medical workups a month before they saw me who wanted me to repeat all of the same tests so they would get the results quickly and not have to wait for the records to be released from their previous physicians. Are you beginning to get the picture? It's pretty clear why doctors' fees as well as health insurance premiums have rocketed skyward in the last decade.

WHAT TO EXPECT UNDER THE NEW AMERICAN MODEL OF HEALTH CARE PROVISION

Given these rising costs, it's not surprising that something had to happen. Because the practice of medicine has changed so radically in the last 50 years, I like to think that today's health care reform is not a revolution but a natural evolution in the history of health care in America. The purpose of health care reform is to provide the best possible care for all Americans and to guarantee everyone equal access to care without driving our nation into bankruptcy from the expense. Right now, I and many other doctors think the current system provides too much care. In other words, most of us agree it needs an overhaul.

Any reform plan must be fair to the three groups that are involved in health care. They are:

1. *Purchasers of health care.* This includes the government, the insurance industry, and you and me. Within this group, there are direct purchasers, like insurance companies, who pay for health care directly; uninsured people who must pay health care providers themselves; and indirect purchasers, who pay premiums to the insurance company.

2. *Providers of health care.* This includes doctors, nurses, hospital workers, and nonprofessionals in the health care system, as well as the insurance companies that administer the system.

3. *Consumers of health care.* This consists of the people who use health care in this country—which includes every American—and who expect their care to be of top quality.

Needless to say, there is some overlap among all the groups; for instance, the health care consumer may also be a direct or indirect purchaser and may even help to provide the care.

You also should realize, however, that many of the changes I discuss below are already taking place in various parts of the country without benefit of federal legislation. Many individual states as well as local health care markets are dictating the needed changes because they see them as something that will benefit all three groups in the health care system.

Here's how I envision the way health care provision will change and how it will affect each group:

The first group, the purchasers of health care, will expect to be able to choose their doctors, either in an HMO or outside. A health care purchaser who agrees to pay for the deluxe version of traditional, conventional indemnity insurance, will be able to pick any health care provider he wants. But this will be the exception. The majority of health care consumers will participate in an HMO or other group practice plan. The employers and governments that pay for the plan will want to make sure that the doctors, hospitals, and ancillary services provide quality health care. They might also want a plan with an HMO or group practice that emphasizes child care and prenatal and obstetrical care if they have a lot of employees with families. On the other hand, if the company is in an industry that's particularly stressful, it will want to make sure the plan provides psychological care benefits. The plan the purchaser ultimately selects will depend on cost, quality of care, and availability of service.

The aim here is to assign each patient in the HMO to one primary care physician—who is usually a generalist, a primary care internist, a family practitioner, a primary care pediatrician for those with children, and an OB/GYN for women, which some insurance plans will cover. This physician will serve as the captain of the patient's health care, and the patient will see this physician before any testing or further specialists are ordered. The purpose is to establish a close relationship between the physician and the patient and to use only tests and/or specialists that are absolutely necessary, which will help to eliminate duplicate and unnecessary tests. This will help save money for the purchasers of health care—both the employer and the insurance company. In turn, the primary care physician will be monitored by the insurance company to make sure she is providing good care at a reasonable price. The insurance company may also look, for instance, at the number of patients in the HMO who have diabetes and suggest that this group be referred for nutritional counseling or perhaps for eye exams. This will cut down on future medical costs and also maintain current expense levels.

With this new model, the primary care physician will be paid less for the services he provides for each patient, as compared to his old fee-for-service days. But the advantage of this plan is that the doctor serves as the gatekeeper, which ensures improved care, and that medical costs across the board are controlled. Quality is also maintained because the insurance company may institute a plan in which it will issue a periodic report card for each health care provider that will show how each professional in the group is performing.

You'll recall that the second group, health care providers, includes both the hospital and the professional and nonprofessional employees in the health care system. In some ways, the goals of the health care provider run counter to those of the first group, the purchasers of health care. The hospitals want to keep their beds full, and the doctors and other providers want to have a full appointment book, while the insurance companies will tell them they can, but only if the visits are absolutely necessary—and they'll ask for proof. In many cases, in fact, the insurance companies will have the final say. Then again, the development of high-tech surgical procedures that can be performed on an outpatient basis, noninvasive testing, and potent new antibiotics that are given by mouth, not intravenously, has drastically reduced the length of the average hospital stay. The insurance companies have also begun to reward hospitals for encouraging shorter hospital stays by making the longer stays less profitable for them than shorter ones are. The hospitals have also begun to attract their own loyal market by forming their own HMOs—either an on-site staff group or a group of primary care physicians and specialists in private practice who refer their patients to a specific hospital when necessary. Hospital networks will also begin to develop: one hospital in the network will specialize in high-risk pediatric care, for instance, while another hospital will focus on state-of-the-art cancer therapies. This benefits patients who join the hospital-based HMOs, since they can easily be moved to the network hospital that specializes in their particular problem.

But while hospitals will quickly snap into action, many of the physicians in this country will have a dilemma: there are too many specialists in this country, and in the age of health care reform it's the primary care physicians who will be in demand. As a result, many specialists will either have to incorporate primary care into their practices or else eliminate their specialty altogether. In addition, U.S. medical schools will need to make primary care an attractive option for medical students.

Another way in which the services of health care providers will change is that a routine visit for a simple complaint may be handled not by a physician but by a nurse practitioner or physician's assistant, who will report back to the physician about the patient's complaint as well as the type of care that was given. Again, to cut costs and maintain efficiency in the HMO, a routine physical, advice about lifestyle concerns, and screening tests of all types will probably be made available by a provider who works with the physician. Assigning these basic responsibilities to other skilled health care providers will free the physician to care for patients who have a more complicated problem and need more care and time.

Though this arrangement may not make everyone happy, I see it as a way of creating a fair system that will allow all health care providers to give the best possible care to their patients in a timely fashion.

Now, for the third and most important group: the consumers of health care. Even though I've described how health care providers and health care purchasers will function differently under health care reform, the whole of health care actually concerns this group the most.

Under the increase in managed care systems, the availability of medical care will be more tightly controlled by the first two groups, yet each patient will be able to receive the amount and type of medical care that he or she needs. Just as a company will need to choose an effective, adequate health care plan for its employees, an employee will also usually be able to pick from several options within that plan. Plan A, for example, might offer excellent pediatric care, but Plan B might have a provision to offer care for children who are in college. If some of these options are more expensive than others, the employer may decide to pass the cost along to the employee or else absorb the cost into the company budget. Either way, the choice of options will be up to the consumer.

By far the greatest benefit of the new system for the consumer will be the emergence of the primary care physician as the overseer of health. Having one, trusted individual to turn to for every health care need, the current confusion many patients now face when deciding "what" type of doctor to see for a particular condition will be minimized. For instance, should a person suffering from conjunctivitis see an ophthalmologist or a general practitioner? Should a woman experiencing a urinary tract infection call her gynecologist or internist? In our new era of health care, your primary care physician will lead you through the medical maze and pinpoint the most appropriate treatment.

Another advantage for the consumer is having all family and individual medical histories centrally located with the primary care physician. In the past, how often have you or another family member seen specialist after specialist, only to go home with a prescription for a medication that interacted with a drug you were already taking or with an order for yet another blood test or chest X ray? How often has one specialist changed the dosage of a medication prescribed by another, only to have you fill the prescription—again! Under the new system, the primary care physician will coordinate and monitor second and third referrals, thereby eliminating conflicting medications and duplicate medical tests. Your doctor will also keep a "master" medical chart and history for immediate and easy reference.

Preventive medicine will also be practiced more widely. This will be a boon to the consumer as well as helping to keep medical costs manageable. Preventive medicine not only helps a health care provider detect and treat an illness in its early stages, it also involves established ongoing patient education programs, which gets the patient more involved in his health care and therefore more likely to follow the instructions of his health care provider.

To give you an example, consider one of my female patients, who is at risk for developing diabetes, since her mother was diabetic. She schedules regular checkups with me during which we monitor her blood sugar level and I provide nutritional counseling so she can prevent the disease from developing. If she did have the disease, we would then continue to keep tabs on her condition on a regular basis in order to prevent some of the more severe complications of the disease from developing.

For instance, if she had diabetes, not only would she be seen by her primary care physician, we would recommend she have routine eye care and checkups done by an ophthalmologist in our HMO. She'd also visit with a nutritional counselor, who could advise her about diet and exercise methods that would help keep her disease from progressing. We might also want her to regularly check in with a nurse practitioner, who could help her with her medications and answer any questions she might have. All these health care providers will be part of a local health care network in which they'll be integrated between outpatient care and the hospital. Clearly, patients will benefit greatly from this new system of total care.

Again, I want to reassure you that even though the way medical care is provided will change under ongoing health reform plans, it will result in better, more focused care for everybody. Of course, you may no longer be able to see a physician for a routine complaint, but you will receive better-quality, more coordinated treatment when a more serious illness or condition strikes. That's where *Mid-Life Body Signals* comes in. By showing you how to recognize your body's classic symptoms of distress, you'll be in a strong position to work within this new system, discern when professional attention is required, and convey this need to those in charge of your health care.

WHY YOU NEED THIS BOOK

More than ever, you need to become familiar with your Body Signals to receive the best care possible. Some of the changes in health care are already being implemented, while others are just beginning to appear on the horizon. You can use this book to help keep up with what will eventually be your greatest responsibility: taking care of your health and tuning in to the changes in your body to enable you to become an equal partner in your own health care. The patient who is able to recognize his Body Signals and articulate his symptoms to his health care provider will help to ensure that he receives the right care from the right care-giver. As mentioned previously, when you first call your doctor's office to schedule a visit, the person who takes the call and makes your appointment will usually decide who you will see—a nurse practitioner, a physician's assistant, or your own primary care physician—based on how you describe your symptoms.

As mentioned earlier, people entering midlife and beyond will be the most active users of our health care system. Given the subtle ways their bodies change, however, they may also may be the last able to articulate their symptoms with clarity and confidence. I hope this book remedies this situation. Designed to empower patients in this new, complex system, it should provide the tools men and women need to understand their Body Signals and to communicate them quickly and accurately to whichever health care professional they see.

I sincerely believe this new health care system evolution will result in better medical care for everyone. Although the days of your friendly family doctor making house calls are in the past, the level of care is superior and will continue to improve even as the medical industry reduces its dependency on specialists and relies more on primary care physicians.

As we go through the process of this transition, I believe the golden days of American medicine are just around the corner. My own hope is eventually to see some form of universal health care coverage for the entire country so that every health care consumer receives the care he or she needs. Oh yes, I must tell you that I wasn't totally truthful about one aspect of your future health care. There will still be house calls, but this time around, you will be visited by a nurse practitioner or physician's assistant, who will use a video computer linkup that is hooked up into the central office at the HMO, where she can consult with your doctor in order to deliver cost-effective health care right in your own home.

In the coming years, the numbers of dedicated health professionals who are delivering the finest care we have ever seen will increase; this is my dream. And using this book will help you to greatly benefit from this new, more personalized high-tech evolution in American medicine.

PART II

HEAD-TO-TOE GUIDE TO YOUR BODY SIGNALS

Chapter 3

HEAD AND NEUROLOGICAL SYSTEM

BODY SIGNAL ALERT

Call your doctor immediately if you experience any of the following symptoms:

SYMPTOM	POSSIBLE MEDICAL CONDITION
You or someone close to you suddenly appears to be confused	*Stroke, medication extremes in temperature*
You have thoughts of suicide	*Depression, loss of spouse, financial insecurity*
You are hallucinating	*Drug or alcohol withdrawal, medication interaction*
You feel dizzy, are vomiting, and have a headache	*Stroke, brain tumor*
You feel faint	*Heart failure, stroke, epilepsy*
You have a severe headache and a change in your mental state	*Intracerebral hemorrhage*
You have a headache that usually appears in the morning and is brought on by a cough or a sneeze	*Brain tumor*
You have a headache, and you feel nauseous and notice a change in one of your pupils	*Aneurysm*
You suddenly lose the ability to talk	*Stroke*
You are having seizures	*Drugs, epilepsy*

HOW THE BRAIN AND
NEUROLOGICAL SYSTEM AGE

From the day we're born, the motor skills and psychological development each of us is given vary to some degree. Though children can be expected to develop at more or less the same rate when it comes to acquiring skills such as walking and talking, when we reach our 50s, a gap begins to form. Among people over 65, the differences in ability between people of the same age can be quite striking. For instance, on the one hand, there was George Burns, who was active for so long that he was compared to the Duracell bunny: he just kept going. On the other hand, there are thousands of beds in nursing homes that contain men and women twenty and thirty years younger than Mr. Burns was when he passed away.

However, the vast majority of seniors are able to function at high levels of ability, due in part to the dramatic increase of 25 years in life expectancy in the United States since 1900. And as a result, the numbers of Americans over the age of 65 over the next 50 years will increase as well; today, there are nearly 3 million Americans 85 years of age or older; less than a quarter of them are living in nursing homes. In fact, contrary to popular belief, only 5% of Americans over the age of 65 are in nursing homes. Your golden years can be active, happy ones if you stay healthy and follow good habits—like proper diet and exercise. Genetics can help, but you can improve your chances for living well into your 90s if you take care of your health when you're still in your 40s.

The brain and its associated neurological functions do begin to show early effects of aging, usually starting in the 60s, but the changes are gradual and, for most people, very subtle. As a result, your reflexes may not be as quick as they once were, and you may have minor short-term memory lapses like misplacing the car keys or forgetting the name of a person you were introduced to five minutes ago. However, in our sped-up society, memory lapses are common even in people in their 20s, so you should consider this to be a relatively minor problem.

One change that many of us start to experience in our 40s is that we start to become more resistant to change. Habits, friends, and skills have been so deeply imprinted into our neurons and daily life that unless we're confronted by a change that's forced on us by external circumstances, some people may get into a rut and stay there, because it's easier to stay the same than it is to change. Yes, these people may be miserable, but they seem to be more interested in being stuck and being right than being happy, so miserable they remain.

Also, as we grow older, along with this resistance to change, we begin to look back fondly on our youth, comparing it favorably to what is happening today, of course colored through the filter of several decades. We'll still be listening to the Beatles in our 70s and 80s while our grandchildren will scoff.

People in their 70s and above will find that projects and tasks that involve repetition are easier for both the mind and the fingers to handle. Needlepoint, model shipbuilding, and other crafts are among the most popular classes at senior citizen centers.

Whether the elderly people you know spend their time knitting blankets and booties for their grandbabies, volunteering at the local hospital five days a week, or even continuing to work, it seems that we're slowly beginning to change our attitudes about the elderly: the majority are not frail and in nursing homes, they're out being active and productive and, yes, even sexual.

CONFUSION

As with any kind of personality change, the way in which confusion takes hold of an elderly parent or relative lies in the eyes of the beholder—and the beholden. Many times, even though your elderly mother may realize that she has become more forgetful and confused lately, she may resist mentioning it to you and her other children. Of course, you probably already have noticed it, but you may not want to admit the fact that since your mother is getting older, it means that you are too.

Confusion can develop slowly, or it can seemingly appear from nowhere, within a matter of days or even hours. When this happens, it's usually a sign of a change in a person's physical health. When confusion develops more slowly, it is those people who are close to the elderly person who notice—or choose to ignore—the subtle changes. A physician or somebody who sees that person on a more occasional basis probably won't notice the changes.

What is confusion, anyway? And when does it start to become a problem where it becomes necessary for a doctor to become involved?

Above all, the single most important factor that indicates that you should seek outside help for your relative is the speed at which the person has changed from being a person who is coherent and stable to someone who is confused and unable to understand even simple terms and explanations. The quicker the transformation, the more important it is to call a doctor.

If you notice that an elderly relative has recently become confused and disoriented, it will help if you ask yourself the following questions about his or her condition. Be sure to communicate the answers to his or her doctor.

- Has she suddenly become confused in the last week, for instance, or has she changed more gradually, over a period of several months?

- Has he always been confused to some degree?

- If he refuses to seek medical attention, do you feel it would be best to override his wishes?

- Ask the person for the time or her address. You can also ask her to add up a simple series of numbers. Don't be embarrassed to ask these questions.

- Does he have any other signs of physical and/or emotional deterioration, such as loss of the ability to speak or to form full sentences, loss of the use of an arm or leg, loss of consciousness, or loss of bladder or bowel function? Does he sweat heavily or have a high fever? Has he recently been exposed to extreme heat or cold?

- Has she recently begun to take a new medication?

- Is he abusing alcohol or controlled drugs, either on purpose or by accident?

- Has she been falling a lot lately?

- Has he undergone any sudden personality changes?

- If she has a history of dementia in the past, have you noticed any acute changes recently?

ANXIETY, DIFFICULTY BREATHING, NUMBNESS IN HANDS, PANIC

Description and Possible Medical Problems

If a patient tells me that he's never had an anxious moment in his life, I tell him that either he's not human or he's lying.

We all know the physical signs of anxiety—sweaty palms, increased heartbeat, and a feeling of panic. Usually, the anxiety passes in time. For some people, however, anxiety can become overwhelming, even crippling. A person who is having a panic attack can develop heart palpitations and start to hyperventilate. His hands might become numb as a result of the hyperventilation. In rare cases, the hyperventiliation becomes so severe that he heads for the emergency room because he's positive that he's having a heart attack. Once I was on a plane over the Atlantic when a fellow passenger developed a panic attack so acute that he was absolutely convinced that the plane was going to crash before we landed.

Treatment

If you feel anxious and begin to hyperventilate, breathing into a paper bag will calm you and help you to breathe normally again. For some people, however, the anxiety can become so crippling that it can make it impossible for them to cope with even small problems. These people can benefit greatly from psychiatric intervention with regular therapy sessions and medications such as BuSpar, Xanax, and Valium. Relaxation and exercise can also have a soothing effect on people who are prone to anxiety attacks.

BODY SIGNAL ALERT

CONFUSION, ACUTE

Description and Possible Medical Problems

The story of Dr. Jekyll and Mr. Hyde may or may not have been true, but to watch a relative change from a self-assured, coherent person into a confused, insecure person can be scary for everyone involved. When an elderly relative sometimes calls you by your sister's name, it's certainly annoying and troubling, but most people consider it as part of the process of growing older.

On the other hand, if you've recently witnessed an elderly relative become confused and incoherent within a matter of days or even hours, it's a sign that she needs immediate medical attention. Acute confusion tends to be accompanied by serious physical symptoms that usually point to a direct cause of the confusion.

For instance, when acute confusion is coupled with other Body Signals such as losing control of the bladder, losing the use of a limb, or slurring words, it can be a sign of a stroke, which is caused when the blood supply to a part of the brain is interrupted by a blockage or clot. Typically, a stroke affects only one side of the body, like one arm, or an arm and leg on the same side, or even the face, arm, and leg. A person who has a stroke may also lose consciousness for a while, and her breathing may have also been altered by the stroke, since a stroke can affect the area of the brain that controls breathing.

Confusion can also be caused by a new medication or a combination of medications. Elderly adults are especially prone to medication-induced confusion because of the tendency to mix sleeping medications and antidepressants or other medications, either prescribed or those purchased over the counter.

Have you ever seen an elderly man or woman in the park wearing a sweater when it's 90 degrees out? One commonly overlooked cause of confusion in the elderly is the temperature inside and out. Many times, when an older person is exposed to extreme heat in the summer, she may get heatstroke; confusion is a common symptom.

Similarly, in the wintertime, extremely cold temperatures can cause a person to become confused, as the body sends most of its blood to the torso and away from the brain and extremities. Unfortunately, this scenario has become more common because the increasing number of elderly people on fixed incomes need to save money, and they often do so by cutting back on their heating costs, even in the extreme northern parts of the country.

Sometimes, however, a person who suddenly becomes confused will have no other symptoms. He will still need help, however, even though the cause is not clear, which is why it's still important to get immediate medical attention even if nothing seems wrong.

If you have a relative with Alzheimer's disease or other type of dementia who suddenly becomes more confused than usual or is more difficult to cope with, it's possible that he has a physical problem that is making his condition worse.

Sudden confusion can also be caused by a heart attack, a rapid or slow heart rate, a urinary tract infection, pneumonia, meningitis, or a blood infection called sepsis.

Treatment

Fortunately, regardless of the cause of your relative's confusion, in most cases she will return to normal with proper treatment. Immediate medical attention is the key; when medical care is delayed, a person will sometimes recover fully, but her short-term memory may be permanently affected; it seems that the area of the brain that controls short-term memory is extremely fragile and can easily be altered by any physical changes.

If an elderly relative has suddenly become confused, her doctor will do a complete medical history and physical exam and run some blood tests to check for problems that are easy to treat. These include blood sugar that is too high or too low, coronary disease, a sodium-potassium imbalance in the body, which frequently occurs in people who take diuretics, and certain medications, especially Digoxin, which is used to treat cardiac disease, and Dilantin, which is often prescribed to treat seizures. An infection can also cause a person to be confused, whether it is the result of pneumonia, a urinary tract infection, or a skin infection. Your doctor may also take a few X rays and conduct other tests according to the particular symptoms. The diagnosis will dictate the treatment, whether it's discontinuing a medication, treating an infection, or even buying an air conditioner or filling the oil tank.

CONFUSION THAT DEVELOPS SLOWLY

Description and Possible Medical Problems

When an elderly relative begins to show signs of confusion and memory loss and the incidents are few and far between, both you and your relative are likely to chalk it up to the aging process and its insidious, mysterious ways. Most of the time, this is exactly what it is.

However, as with what happens when an elderly person suddenly becomes confused (see "Confusion, Acute" above), when other symptoms appear in addition to the confusion, an underlying disease may be responsible.

Some of these other symptoms may include difficulty in doing tasks that were once considered to be simple; frequently becoming lost and disoriented; a failing memory; and poor hygiene. The elderly person may also undergo personality changes and become increasingly aggressive and/or depressed.

When a parent or other elderly relative becomes increasingly confused over a period of time, many people automatically jump to the conclusion that Alzheimer's disease is setting in. Contrary to popular belief, Alzheimer's disease is actually a rare illness, and when it does occur, it's not always severe. In fact, many Alzheimer's patients have just a mild case of the disease with some memory loss, or else they may just have some trouble working with numbers and figuring out their checkbook balances. As the disease becomes more severe, however, a person with Alzheimer's disease will start to have trouble with her daily routine. At this point, the family will need to consult a doctor and local health agencies to place companions and workers in the home, since the person's safety becomes an issue. However, no matter whether the disease is mild or severe, people with Alzheimer's disease are very aware of their problem and are usually very depressed. Many work hard to hide their confusion and memory loss from their doctor and family. In the advanced stages of Alzheimer's disease, the person will need total care, and placement in a nursing home is usually necessary.

Unfortunately, at this time, there is no known cause and no cure for Alzheimer's disease. Some researchers speculate that it might be due to genetics, while others feel that the environment and the food we eat may play a role. Before making a positive diagnosis of Alzheimer's disease, however, a doctor will first look for an underlying disease, such as a vitamin deficiency or thyroid disorder, that might be causing the confusion and memory loss.

Treatment

If an adult child brings in an elderly parent and complains that the parent has been confused and forgetful lately, I ask the parent to draw a clock face, to both diagnose the adult and reassure the child. If the parent can draw a clock and hands and place the numbers in their proper place, I tell the parent and child that there's nothing to worry about. With normal aging, an elderly person's concepts of space and time gradually become more difficult for them to grasp; I feel that as long as they include all of the numbers as well as the hands, they are okay. If, however, you notice that an elderly relative has become increasingly confused over a long period of time and that it's beginning to affect the quality of her life, the first step is for her to see her physician, who will probably conduct blood tests to check for vitamin deficiencies, thyroid disease, or another underlying treatable illness. If, however, the doctor determines that your relative does have Alzheimer's disease, treatment will depend on the severity of the disease.

If placement in a nursing home is not necessary, many people with Alzheimer's disease will thrive in a day program at a specialized center. The daily activity, as well as regular treatment, can help ease the underlying depression that is a common problem for many people with Alzheimer's.

Recently a new medication called Cognex or Tacrine has been shown to help some people with Alzheimer's. These medications seem to slow and even reverse some of the cognitive changes in these patients by improving the response of the neurotransmitters. In the beginning, the doctor will start a patient out on a low dose of the medication and slowly increase it over a period of several weeks. But the effects are usually not dramatic; slowing the speed at which Alzheimer's progresses can take months to occur. Cognex or Tacrine can also be highly toxic to the liver, so a patient needs to be monitored regularly with blood tests to check the degree of toxicity. Even though these medications are a bright light on the horizon for Alzheimer's patients, I don't consider them to be a panacea, as I've seen them work well in some of my patients while they've had no effect on others.

MINI MENTAL EXAM[1]

Many physicians and hospital personnel find the Mini Mental Exam shown below to be a useful screening tool for cognitive disorders. Scores less than 24 are usually a sign that there's a problem. Obviously, dozens of factors ranging from medical illness to depression to educational levels can influence scores, but whatever the reason, such results should be looked at by a qualified doctor.

MINI MENTAL EXAM

Maximum Score	Score	
		Orientation
5	( )	What is the (year) (season) (date) (day) (month)?
5	( )	Where are we: (state) (county) (town) (hospital) (floor)?
		Registration
3	( )	Name 3 objects: 1 second to say each. Then ask the patient all 3 after you have said them.
		Give 1 point for each correct answer. Then repeat them until he learns all 3. Count trials and record.
		Trials
		Attention and calculation
5	( )	Serial 7s. 1 point for each correct answer. Stop after 5 answers. Alternatively, spell "world" backwards.
		Recall
3	( )	Ask for 3 objects repeated above. Give 1 point for each correct answer.
		Language
9	( )	Name a pencil and watch. (2 points)
		Repeat the following: "No ifs, ands, or buts." (1 point)
		Follow a 3-stage command: "Take a paper in your right hand, fold it in half, and put it on the floor." (3 points)
		Read and obey the following: "Close your eyes." (1 point)
		Write a sentence. (1 point)
		Copy design. (1 point)
		ASSESS level of consciousness along a continuum.
Total Score		Alert Drowsy Stupor Coma

[1]Mini Mental State Examination form. (Reprinted with permission from *Journal of Psychiatric Research*, Vol. 12, M. F. Folstein, S. E. Folstein, P. McHugh. "Mini-mental state: A practical method for grading the cognitive state of patients for the clinician," copyright 1975, Elsevier Science Ltd., Pergamon Imprint, Oxford, England.

BODY SIGNAL ALERT

DEPRESSION

Description and Possible Medical Problems

Depression is probably the most underdiagnosed and misdiagnosed disease in America today. As a result, it is vastly undertreated. Part of the problem stems from the stigma against mental illness that exists in all segments of society. Particularly among the elderly, depression is extremely common and many times goes unrecognized. Depression is also a side effect of many chronic diseases, and it frequently develops after a person is hospitalized for a heart attack, small stroke, or another illness.

If you answer yes to one or more of the following questions about yourself or a loved one, chances are that depression is the cause.

1. Have you noticed a change in your sleeping habits? Are you sleeping more or less lately?

2. Do you lack motivation and energy?

3. Do you have difficulty concentrating for long periods of time?

4. Are you eating more than usual? Or have you lost your appetite?

5. Have you felt suicidal lately?

Depression is often the result of lifestyle changes that we are ill prepared to accept. For example, it's very common for a man to become depressed after he retires, since his role as employee as well as his status within the company probably served as his primary identity for many years. Once that position is taken away, many people have an identity crisis and can become very depressed.

In younger people in their late 40s or early 50s, a midlife crisis can spark a lengthy depression; premenopausal women who are leaving their childbearing years behind are also at risk for depression.

In my practice, I once saw a police captain who had retired after many years of service. He had taken a job as a security guard so he'd have something to do. However, he had become very depressed over the change in status in his life and job, and he had attempted suicide. After he failed, he sought help and learned that the change in his life hadn't changed who he was as a person. As a result, he began to enjoy life again.

Occasionally, depression can be a sign of a serious illness that has not yet manifested itself. This is especially true in any cancer of the gastrointestinal system, such as pancreatic or colon cancer. Though we don't know the exact reason for this, some speculate that it may be a result of the body's inability to process food and nutrients properly once the cancer begins to grow. And in elderly people, depression is a major cause of suicide.

Treatment

Depression is a serious disorder; however, the vast majority of people who seek help for it are treated successfully.

If you have been depressed, it's a good idea to contact your family physician. His first task will be to eliminate any underlying disease that might be causing your depression by taking your medical history, doing a physical exam, and possibly taking a blood test. He will also do a depression screening test, which consists of asking questions similar to the ones you've just answered. If your doctor determines that there is no physical condition that is causing you to be depressed, he may suggest that you visit a therapist or a support group to begin working on the psychological problems that may be responsible for your depression. Many times, I've seen regular exercise work wonders on my depressed patients.

Medication is also a major part of treating depression. The tricyclic medications such as Amitryptyline and Elavil that were popular in the 80s are effective, but they also have many potential side effects, such as an irregular heart rate and low blood pressure, which are particularly dangerous for a person over 50 who has a history of cardiac problems. If you are taking Elavil, you will need to be monitored first with an electrocardiogram followed by blood pressure checks every few months.

The newer medications such as Prozac and Zoloft are very effective in stopping depression, and they're also relatively safe.

If you're being treated by a therapist with or without medication, you need to stick with it. A big problem that I see in my patients is that they prematurely end treatment because they're feeling better. As with the use of antibiotics, any treatment for depression should continue past the point when the person simply starts to feel good again.

DIZZINESS UPON CHANGE IN BODY OR HEAD POSITION

Description and Possible Medical Problems

Do you feel dizzy whenever you change the position of your body or your head? Does this happen regardless of whether you're sitting, standing, or lying down? Does the room feel as though it's spinning? If you've answered yes to these questions, you should see your doctor.

The most common cause of dizziness is a condition called labyrinthitis, which is a viral infection of the inner ear. You might also be nauseated and vomiting.

Treatment

If your doctor suspects that you have labyrinthitis, she will make sure by inducing dizziness by having you change your position or rapidly turn your head. She will also visually check your ears for signs of infection and perform a physical exam to rule out any other underlying neurological illness, such as a small stroke or a benign tumor. If you have an inner ear infection, bedrest and a medication called Antivert, taken three times a day for a week, will ease your dizziness. If you are dizzy for more than a week, however, or if the dizziness becomes worse over the course of a few days, your doctor will refer you to an ear, nose, and throat specialist for more tests, including a CAT scan to check for a neurological cause such as a stroke or tumor.

DIZZINESS AND FEELING FAINT
WHEN STANDING UP

Description and Possible Medical Problems

The movie *Vertigo* is everyone's nightmare of a world that won't stop spinning no matter what you do. If you feel dizzy and faint whenever you stand up from a lying or sitting position, it's likely that the cause is a temporary one and easy to fix. Most often, a high emotional state, certain medications that lower your blood pressure—most often cardiac and psychiatric drugs—and even prolonged bed rest can make you feel dizzy and faint. Sometimes, even quickly changing positions can bring on this feeling of vertigo.

In rare cases, however, dizziness and a faint feeling can occur in a person who has a bleeding ulcer or severe anemia, which lowers the blood pressure. Any change in blood pressure that results from these illnesses is called orthostatic hypotension.

Treatment

If you think your dizziness is caused by changing positions quickly, try moving around less abruptly to see if that's all that is necessary. And if you've recently been upset or have spent a lot of time lying down and resting, the dizziness should disappear when you return to your previous state. If you've recently changed or added a new medication, see your doctor about switching to a medication without these side effects.

If these suggestions don't help, you should see your doctor, who will do a complete medical history and physical and take your blood pressure when you're both standing and lying down to check for any significant change. If you have anemia or a bleeding ulcer, your doctor will prescribe a regimen to treat these conditions, which will include medication, diet, and exercise.

DIZZINESS WITH VOMITING, HEADACHE, NUMBNESS AROUND THE MOUTH

Description and Possible Medical Problems

If you feel dizzy no matter if you're moving around or sitting still and the dizziness is accompanied by vomiting, headache, loss of speech, numbness around the mouth, and/or loss of the use of one of your limbs, you should see your doctor immediately. Your dizziness may be caused by a problem in the brain, not your inner ear. In addition to the dizziness and other symptoms, you may have trouble walking.

These are all signs of a small stroke or a tumor. Arteriosclerosis, or narrowing of the arteries, often reduces the amount of blood that reaches the brain, which can cause these symptoms. A tumor can grow to the point where it begins to press on an artery, which cuts off the blood going to the brain.

Treatment

Your doctor will take your complete health history and do a complete physical, which will include an evaluation of your neurological system with a CAT scan or MRI scan to check for a possible old or new stroke, an echocardiogram to check for any heart irregularities or clots, or a carotid Doppler test, which measures the flow of blood from the neck to the brain.

If your doctor thinks you've had a stroke, he will prescribe treatment that includes a low-fat diet that is also low in sodium if your blood pressure is elevated, and one baby aspirin taken daily, which seems to inhibit the blood's ability to clot, meaning that no obstructions to the flow of blood to the brain will develop. If your doctor believes you've had a series of persistent small strokes as shown by an MRI but that you may have not noticed, he may prescribe a medication called Ticlid, taken three times a day, which also helps keep the blood from clotting but is stronger than baby aspirin. If you are taking Ticlid, your doctor will want to monitor you with periodic blood tests, since the medication can sometimes cause your white blood cell count to decrease.

Another medication is Coumadin, which actually thins the blood and is only used in severe cases when aspirin and Ticlid are not strong enough to prevent the blood from clotting. If you are taking Coumadin and you also have an ulcer, you may need to take an antiulcer medication such as Carafate or Zantac to coat your stomach in order to protect it from the Coumadin. Also, you need to make sure your doctor monitors your health closely when you are taking Coumadin and call your doctor immediately if you notice that you are bleeding excessively from a small cut or notice blood in your stool or urine. All of these symptoms can be a sign of internal bleeding, which can be caused by the Coumadin.

If your doctor thinks you may have a brain tumor, see "Headache in the Morning, Made Worse by Sneezing, Coughing," below, for a description of the condition and your treatment options.

FALLS

Even though we don't like to admit it, most of us fall at least once during the course of a year. Falls come as a result of losing our balance or tripping over something, and they're actually very common among adults of all ages. Of course, toddlers who are just learning to walk fall at least a couple of times a day, but because they have flexible bones to absorb the shock, serious injury from a fall by a two- or three-year-old is rare.

In my own practice, I've seen that most adults will fall once or twice a year. Usually, it's not a serious problem. However, as we get older, falls can become more serious, primarily because our bones are more brittle and we have less fat to cushion the fall. In fact, there's a definite link between an older person's activity level and the number of times she falls over the course of a year; the more active you are, the more you'll fall. Since older people tend to fall over rugs, slip in bathtubs, and fall down the stairs, it's important that just as you'd do for a child, you should look around the home to eliminate anything that may cause an older person to fall.

Falls are responsible not only for physical injuries but for emotional ones as well. The most common physical injuries that come as a result of a fall are fractured hips and wrists. The emotional problems that develop from a serious fall can be devastating, since a person can become afraid to walk. She may therefore become more housebound, especially in the winter.

If you or an elderly relative appears to be falling more frequently, there are several things you can check for:

1. Any safety hazards in and around the home

2. Any physical changes that might make her more prone to a fall, such as a change in her eyesight or hearing, as well as a decrease in mobility due to arthritis

3. Proper-fitting shoes

With the help of your doctor, you can also look for any medical reasons for an increase in falls. These can include a medication like an antihypertensive or antipsychotic medication that might cause a change in blood pressure and make her more prone to falls. A urinary tract infection may cause her to fall out of bed in her rush to get to the bathroom.

It's important that just because someone has a tendency to fall down frequently does not mean she should be restrained, especially in a nursing home. An elderly relative's ability to move around is very important to maintaining her physical and emotional health. If she has trouble walking, she needs the help of a physical therapist to learn how to walk without falling.

EXHAUSTION WITH LACK OF INTEREST

Description and Possible Medical Problems

If you always feel tired, no matter how much sleep you get, and find it hard to become interested in doing anything new, chances are you may be suffering from a condition that's more psychological than physiological.

The go-go lifestyle that is typical for many Americans today has caused a lot of people to burn out. We simply put too much on our plate and don't know how to say no to more. Considering the long hours we

spend at work, family and social obligations, and leisure time that frequently resembles a competition, anyone would feel burned out after a
while.

Treatment

The best way to treat burnout is by taking time out. An occasional day
off or a day with nothing scheduled, a brief vacation, or indulging in
hobbies and exercise will give you some perspective on your jam-packed
life. It will also refresh you and possibly make you feel so good that you
make it a point to take some time off at least once a week.

For some people, however, it's not enough to take a vacation or start
a new hobby. When burnout is particularly severe, a person may need to
quit his job and move to another part of the country, where he won't be
tempted to resume his previous lifestyle. Though this is rare, I've seen
it happen.

FACE RESEMBLES A MASK, DROOLING, CHANGE IN VOICE, DIFFICULTY WALKING, TREMBLING HANDS

Description and Possible Medical Problems

If an elderly relative shows any of the above symptoms, it's likely that
she has Parkinson's disease, which is a relatively rare condition that usually affects people in their late 60s or older. Typical characteristics of
the disease include a tremor in the hands that occurs primarily during
periods of inactivity; the tremor will usually cease during even slight
physical movement. This tremor—called a resting tremor—usually
looks as though a person is rolling a pill between her fingers, over and
over again.

Another sign of Parkinson's disease is that the muscles become rigid;
a third is that the facial muscles will also become rigid and fixed, resulting in a masklike expression. A fourth common symptom of Parkinson's
is that when the person starts to walk, she has to start slowly because of
her inflexible muscles, and she has to take small, shuffling steps; her
torso is also probably bent forward.

The first thing to say about Parkinson's is that we don't know what causes it. Although a virus that caused an influenza epidemic in the early 1900s is sometimes identified as the cause of Parkinson's disease, not everyone who has the disease today had that particular flu. In some cases, medication that is prescribed to treat psychiatric problems can cause symptoms that mimic Parkinson's disease, especially antipsychotic medications like Haldol, which is commonly used in nursing homes. In some advanced cases of the disease, dementia can develop; however, some of my Parkinson's patients who are in their 90s have no change in their mental state at all.

Treatment

If you suspect that an elderly relative has Parkinson's, the physician will do a complete medical history and physical exam and run some routine tests to check for thyroid disease, liver abnormalities, and a blood count to make sure that she can tolerate any medications she is taking. First, he will check to see if medication is causing the symptoms. Once he rules that out, treatment for Parkinson's will begin.

Medications that are commonly prescribed to treat Parkinson's disease not only control the tremors of the illness but also slow down its disability. Sinemet is a drug commonly used to treat the disease. Your relative may find support groups helpful, but the truth is that most Parkinson's patients can successfully manage their households for many years without additional help.

FACIAL PARALYSIS ON ONE SIDE, WITH AN INABILITY TO CLOSE ONE EYE

Description and Possible Medical Problems

A patient recently told me what happened the morning he first saw the signs of Bell's palsy staring back at him in the mirror.

"I had just gotten up and was getting ready to go to work," he said. "I was in the bathroom and just about to shave my face when I noticed that the right side of my face was distorted and drooping. I was also drooling a little. At first I thought that I'd had a stroke, but then I noticed that my arms, legs, and speech were all fine."

My patient had the classic symptoms of Bell's palsy, which is not a stroke, as is commonly thought, but the inflammation of a facial nerve in the brain, called the fifth nerve or the trigeminal nerve, which is responsible for neurological sensations in the mouth, the nasal cavity, the eyes, and the front of the scalp. In most cases it is caused by a virus and the symptoms will totally disappear after a few weeks. The most serious problem with Bell's palsy is that the eye tends to dry out at night because it won't stay closed.

Treatment

In order to confirm the diagnosis of Bell's palsy, you should see your physician, but beyond that nothing else is needed since the condition is viral and the symptoms and the nerve inflammation disappear eventually.

Some physicians prescribe steroids such as prednisone to hasten the recovery, starting at about 40 milligrams a day and then tapering down the dosage after about four days. If one of my patients has Bell's palsy, I will send him to an ophthalmologist so that he can receive proper eye care, which may include artificial tears or a special bandage to protect the eye during sleep.

BODY SIGNAL ALERT

FAINTING

Description and Possible Medical Problems

Most people have experienced what it's like to faint. Although the cause is not always known, fainting should always be taken seriously, whether the person recovers immediately or remains unconscious for several minutes or longer.

If a person faints in front of you, you should ask yourself the following questions while you call 911. Be sure to tell the answers to the medical person who responds to your call.

1. Is the person breathing?

2. Does she have a pulse?

3. Is he conscious?

4. Has she lost control of his bladder or bowels?

5. Is he wearing a special ID bracelet or dog tag that indicates allergies, diabetes, or heart disease?

Fainting may result from any one of a number of medical problems. Often, a person will faint when a small amount of food gets stuck in her windpipe. Heart failure can also cause a person to faint. Some people faint when they become highly emotional, while others faint when they're having blood drawn. Epilepsy and other neurological seizures can also cause fainting; a clue is if one part of the body or all of it is twitching while the person is still unconscious.

After a person has fainted, when she comes to, you should look for other signs of neurological problems such as slurred speech or loss of the use of a limb; these symptoms can be a sign of a stroke. If, however, a person suddenly faints and temporarily loses consciousness but shows no sign of neurological distress, she may be having a transient ischemic attack, or TIA, a kind of ministroke. And if she's sweating heavily, it may be a sign of low blood sugar or a cardiac problem.

Treatment

If you see a person who has fainted, you should call 911. The dispatcher will ask you some of the questions above and advise you to attend to the person while the paramedics are on their way. The most important factor in determining treatment will be to have the patient and/or the observers tell the doctor or paramedics what caused the person to faint, along with describing any other symptoms she may have. If the dispatcher thinks the person has suffered heart failure due to your description, he may instruct you to start CPR and talk you through the procedure.

FOREHEAD PAIN RUNNING
ALONG BLOOD VESSEL

See "Eye Pain with Headache and Neck Pain" in Chapter 5.

HALLUCINATIONS

Description and Possible Medical Problems

Remember Ray Milland in the movie *The Lost Weekend?* Toward the end of the movie, as he was withdrawing from alcohol, he began to hallucinate, seeing rats climb out of a hole in the wall and bats swoop down on him.

Frequently, we think of hallucinations in tandem with stories about bad drug experiences or withdrawal from alcohol. And whether this is accidental or deliberate, the truth is that these factors are the major cause of hallucinations.

What people don't know about hallucinations is that mixing over-the-counter preparations or prescription medications with certain kinds of sleeping pills can also cause hallucinations. People who have long-term psychiatric illnesses may hallucinate, and hallucinations are not an uncommon occurrence in people with infections, fever, or Alzheimer's disease. In fact, any acute illness, from an infection of the central nervous system or the urinary tract to high or low abnormalities in blood sugar levels can cause hallucinations. Patients with lung disease may also hallucinate since their carbon dioxide level may increase while their oxygen level decreases. In addition, any fever that measures above 100 degrees F. can also cause hallucinations.

Treatment

The treatment for hallucinations depends on the underlying cause, whether it's a physical illness or an emotional one. If the hallucinations are caused by an infection or a fever, these conditions will need to be brought under control with medication, either aspirin or antibiotics. If the hallucinations are the result of drug or alcohol withdrawal, a person may need to be hospitalized and/or sedated. For people with a long-term psychiatric illness or Alzheimer's disease, ongoing treatment that includes therapy, medication, and support will be necessary.

The family of a person who is having hallucinations faces special problems; some don't know whether to force the person into treatment or to agree with the hallucinations, like saying that you "see the rats, too." I'd say that your criterion for deciding what to do should be based on keeping the person from hurting herself. The important thing to keep in mind is that not only does the person with the hallucinations need support, but you and the other caregivers need support in order to learn how to cope with the situation. Ask your relative's doctor for advice.

WHAT IS CAUSING YOUR HEADACHE?

The location of the headache also points to its cause. Ask yourself the following questions; I've provided the possible causes after each question.

1. Does the pain start in my neck and radiate up through my head? Do my headaches tend to appear when I'm stressed? The headache is probably due to tension.

2. Do I have a pain in my forehead that's accompanied by sinuses that feel blocked? It's probably a sinus headache.

3. Does the top of my head feel as though it's pounding? Elevated blood pressure may be the cause, but this is also a sign of tension.

4. In addition to a headache all over the head, do I feel numb in the arms or legs, am I vomiting, and/or has my vision changed? It's probably a migraine.

5. Is this the worst headache I've ever had, and am I vomiting as well? The cause may be a brain aneurysm—call the doctor immediately.

6. Do I have a fever, and am I experiencing seizures? The cause may be an infection of or tumor in the brain.

BODY SIGNAL ALERT

HEADACHE IN THE MORNING, MADE WORSE BY SNEEZING, COUGHING

Description and Possible Medical Problems

Some people get their headaches most often in the late afternoon or evening, after the stress of the day finally hits them.

Other people, however, are prone to headaches in the morning, and though the pain might be just barely there, the headache is often brought on by a cough or sneeze. Though brain tumors rarely occur, your doctor will probably want to check for evidence of one, especially if you have a history of either breast or lung cancer. A headache that appears in the morning will raise the possibility that the cancer has spread to the brain.

Treatment

If you regularly have headaches in the morning that start when you cough or sneeze, see your doctor, especially if you've fought cancer in the past. Your doctor will first perform a complete neurological evaluation to determine if you have a brain tumor. This will include taking your complete medical history, doing a physical exam, and performing routine lab tests, including an electrocardiogram and an electroencephelogram to check for any seizure activity. A neurological exam will include a pinprick test, a hammer reflex test in which the doctor hits just below your knee with a rubber hammer, and a check of your visual fields as well as your muscular strength. He will also probably perform a CAT scan of your brain or an MRI, which will show any signs of a tumor, hemorrhaging, or an enlarged blood vessel, which is a sign of an aneurysm.

If your doctor strongly suspects that you have a tumor or an infection of the brain, he may want to perform a spinal tap or a lumbar puncture, which will help confirm or rule out either of these diseases. First he will give you a local anesthetic. Then a small needle is placed at the base of the spine in order to withdraw a small amount of fluid so that it can be analyzed by a lab for signs of an infection or tumor. After the test, you will be advised to stay in bed for at least 12 hours, and you might have a headache for a day or two following the procedure.

If the headache turns out to be caused by a tumor, it may be either malignant or benign. If it's benign, your doctor may decide to leave it alone. A malignant brain tumor may be treated with surgery or radiation, especially if it's detected at an early stage. If the tumor is isolated in one spot, a new technique called stereotaxic surgery can be used. Stereotaxic surgery is less risky than traditional surgery; special microscopes and new imaging techniques have made it possible for surgeons to work in areas of the brain that contain critical and risky neurological pathways.

HEADACHE, OCCASIONAL

Description and Possible Medical Problems

All of us get headaches from time to time. Sometimes they're mild, while at other times it's impossible to do much more except lie down in a dark room until it passes. A simple headache with no other symptoms—like vomiting or vision changes—is usually not serious. Most headaches are triggered by stress, from working too long at a computer screen to having a trying day at work. Missing a meal is also a common cause. Unlike many health problems, we usually know why we have a headache when it first appears.

Treatment

Fortunately, we also know the solutions. Most often, a headache is treated with an over-the-counter medication such as Tylenol, Advil, or aspirin, two tablets or capsules every four hours until the headache disappears. Our individual perceptions of pain have a lot to do with how we respond to a headache. Some people take nothing for the pain, while others load up on anything that promises to make it disappear.

Massage and physical exercise have been found to reduce the frequency of headaches in people who get them more than once or twice a week.

BODY SIGNAL ALERT

HEADACHE WITH CHANGE IN THE SIZE OF ONE PUPIL, NAUSEA, DOUBLE VISION, SEVERE PAIN BEHIND THE EYE, AND CONFUSION

Description and Possible Medical Problems

If you get severe headaches from time to time or even a migraine, which is a severe headache coupled with sensitivity to light, nausea, and vomiting (see also "Headache with Sensitivity to Light, Nausea, and

Vomiting" below), you may find that because your eyes become more sensitive to light during the headache, whenever you do manage to open them all the way, the pupils in both eyes are dilated, or enlarged. Usually, the pupils return to their normal size after your headache goes away.

If, however, you have a headache and only one pupil is dilated, you're confused, and you also feel nauseous and a have stabbing pain behind this same eye, call your doctor immediately.

Though the condition is rare and usually appears in men and women under 50, these body signals are signs of internal bleeding of the brain, known as an intracerebral hemorrhage. This condition is usually caused by a weakened blood vessel or an aneurysm in the section of the brain called the circle of Willis, which is located at the base of the brain and controls the blood supply to the brain. A tumor in the brain or meningitis can also cause a severe headache with a change in mental state, but an intracerebral hemorrhage is frequently brought on by an extreme physical activity like weight lifting or hanging upside down; there seems to be a genetic aspect to developing an intracerebral hemorrhage. It can be life-threatening, so immediate medical attention is necessary.

Treatment

Twenty years ago, when a person was diagnosed with an intracerebral hemorrhage, many doctors often opted against treatment since the condition almost always meant certain death. Today, if the intracerebral hemorrhage is caught early and treated with microsurgery, the person can be saved. Once in the emergency room, the doctor will examine you for signs of an intracerebral hemorrhage with a CAT scan and maybe do a lumbar puncture (see treatment under "Headache in the Morning, Made Worse by Sneezing, Coughing" above, for more information about this procedure). Once the diagnosis is confirmed, surgery can begin to repair the blood vessel or aneurysm. If the aneurysm is caught early, you will recover fully.

I have a 52-year-old patient who experienced a severe headache on a subway platform one morning. She also felt weak, and she passed out. She later told me that she had had a constant headache for several days before she passed out, and she had never suffered from headaches before.

She was rushed from the subway platform to a large New York hospital where the doctors were able to quickly diagnose that she had a brain aneurysm that was bleeding; her different-sized pupils gave her condition away. The doctors performed emergency surgery to clip the bleeding vessel and stop the hemorrhage. Since the surgery, she has had no residual side effects and has been carrying on with her life as usual. After surgery, she spent two weeks in the hospital, and after two months she returned to work. A year later she shows no signs of the aneurysm.

HEADACHE WITH MUSCLE TENSION

See "Headache, Occasional" above.

HEADACHE WITH SENSITIVITY TO LIGHT, NAUSEA, AND VOMITING

Description and Possible Medical Problems

If you have a headache, feel nauseous, and are vomiting and your eyes are sensitive to light, you should see your doctor. Headaches with these three additional symptoms fall into migraine territory, and at times the pain can be quite severe, almost incapacitating.

In some people, migraines make their first appearance in childhood. For others, often women in their 30s, migraines make their debut in midlife and continue for ten years or more, usually disappearing at the onset of menopause.

Treatment

If you think you have a migraine headache, you need to be evaluated by your doctor. He will take your medical history, do a physical exam, and run some lab tests, including a blood test. He might also order a CAT scan to rule out the possibility of a brain tumor, but in my experience I've found that most worry about tumors of the brain is needless, since they are so rare.

The first step in treating migraines is to eliminate certain foods that may be causing the headaches, commonly cheese, chocolate, and dairy products. Over-the-counter medications for pain work well for some people, but others will need to use a strong prescription medication such as Fiorinal three or four times a day from the time the migraine starts until it clears up. Antidepressant medications such as Elavil and beta-blockers such as Inderal have also been used with some success to treat migraines, as has biofeedback.

There is a new medication used to treat migraines called Imitrex, or Sumatriptan. It comes in a kit that provides the patient with everything she needs to adminster the medication through self-injection. The medication is injected at the first signs of a migraine, when nausea and spots before the eyes begin to appear and the head begins to hurt. If the symptoms have not begun to subside after an hour, another injection can be given; this is usually effective. However, people with heart disease shouldn't use Imitrex, since the medication can cause spasm in the coronary arteries.

Ergotamine is another medication that should be taken at the beginning of a migraine, except it is taken orally or sublingually and can be repeated at 30-minute intervals, or as often as necessary until the symptoms subside. If you want to take ergotamine, your doctor will want to monitor your health, since the medication can be habit forming and a rare disorder called ergotism can develop. Since ergotamine helps decrease the pain of a migraine through a process known as vasoconstriction, in which the blood vessels become narrow and the pain is reduced, some of the side effects of the medication include rapid heart rate, muscular aches and pains, coldness in the hands and feet, depression, and seizures, which explains why ergotamine is not a medication to be taken lightly.

A migraine headache doesn't necessarily have to immobilize a person. The most important part of treatment is to recognize the onset of a migraine and treat it with medication immediately, as well as to eliminate foods that tend to trigger a migraine.

HEADACHE WITH STIFF NECK, FEVER, NAUSEA, AND BODY ACHES

Description and Possible Medical Problems

The last time you spent the night away from home and without the pillow it's taken you years to mold just right, you may have woken up with a stiff neck and maybe even a headache. The stiffness may have subsided as the day proceeded, but you were bound to be greeted by the same discomfort when you woke up the next morning, until you got back home and back to your pillow.

One kind of neck stiffness isn't so easy to fix, and, in fact, is a sign of a serious problem. If your neck is stiff when you try to move your head up and down and you have a headache and fever and feel nauseous, you may have meningitis, which is an inflammation of the lining of the brain. If the stiffness occurs when you try to move your head from side to side and you also feel achy, you may have a variation of meningitis called meningismus. This condition differs from meningitis in that it appears to originate from spasms in the muscles of the neck, not from an infection in the brain. Also, while one sign of meningitis is stiffness when you try to touch your chest with your chin, the primary characteristic of meningismus is overall aches and pains.

Though meningitis is usually caused by a virus, it can also be caused by bacteria. Bacterial meningitis tends to be more severe and therefore more serious than meningitis that is caused by a virus. While the symptoms of bacterial meningitis and viral meningitis are initially similar, with bacterial meningitis you'll eventually appear more confused and have a higher fever than with viral meningitis. In addition to the other symptoms, it's possible that you may also have encephalitis, which is an inflammation of the brain itself.

Treatment

To diagnose meningitis, your doctor will need to perform a spinal tap and sometimes will also order a CAT scan (for a description of the procedure, see the treatment under "Headache in the Morning, Made Worse by Sneezing, Coughing," above). If the cause is due to bacteria, the treatment will be with antibiotics, and you may need to be hospitalized. If the meningitis is viral in origin even though it may not be severe, you may need to be hospitalized anyway to make sure that you are properly hydrated and treated with an antiviral medication. With proper rest, lots of liquids, and proper medication, recovery usually takes two to three weeks. If you are also diagnosed with encephalitis, the treatments prescribed for meningitis will also help ease the symptoms of encephalitis. Your doctor may also prescribe a corticosteroid preparation like prednisone to reduce the inflammation.

INSOMNIA

Description and Possible Medical Problems

If you're like most Americans, you probably don't get enough sleep. Your schedule is crammed to the hilt with work and family responsibilities that make you tired just to think about them. But then, when bedtime does roll around, you're so stressed out by your life that you can't shut it off enough to fall asleep. And so you may end up staring wide-eyed at the numbers on the clock as the hours drag by.

Besides stress, the aging process also affects our sleep; the older we get, the easier it is to wake up out of a deep sleep. As we age, we don't necessarily need less sleep, but starting in our 40s and 50s, we do need less rapid eye movement (REM) sleep, the stage in which dreams occur.

If you have trouble falling asleep or staying asleep on a regular basis, ask yourself the following questions:

1. Am I napping during the day?

2. Do I try to go to sleep when I'm not tired?

3. How many hours of sleep would it take for me to awake fully rested?

4. Am I drinking coffee or caffeinated drinks during the day or evening?

5. Have I been anxious or worried lately?

6. Am I getting up to urinate during the night? Do I find it hard to get back to sleep?

Treatment

If your insomnia is due to a temporary stress in your life, your sleep habits will return to normal once it ends. In the meantime, try to take catnaps during the day whenever you feel tired. The traditional advice for insomnia—warm milk before going to bed and using your bed only for sleeping—may work for you. It may help if you stay busy during the day and eliminate eating late at night and drinking caffeinated beverages past midafternoon. Staying up later until you're really tired some-times helps. And if you're getting up in the middle of the night to uri-nate and find that it's hard to fall back asleep, don't drink liquids after 8 P.M. If your insomnia lasts longer than a week, however, and these sug-gestions haven't worked, you should see your doctor. When I complete the examination and conclude that a patient's inability to sleep is due to stress, he or she often asks me for a prescription to induce sleep. I try to discourage them, since most sleeping medications are extremely habit forming, and the effects usually only last for a few days before they begin to lose their effectiveness. Certain sleep-inducing medica-tions may also cause short-term memory loss.

Medications to help you sleep should be used for only a short period of time to help you get over a temporary period of stress and worry.

The effects of over-the-counter sleeping medications are of a very lim-ited duration. These preparations typically consist of a natural sedative called tryptophan, which is the same substance that makes us feel sleepy after a turkey dinner. Use them only once in a great while, if you must.

MEMORY LOSS

See "Confusion, Acute" above.

NERVOUSNESS

Description and Possible Medical Problems

Even though it's an old-fashioned term, you may have recently heard someone refer to someone as a "nervous Nellie." As is the case with anxiety, everyone gets nervous at some point, but there are always those who take it to extremes.

Also like anxiety, nervousness can get to the point where it prevents people from functioning normally and begins to interfere with their interpersonal relationships. In fact, nervousness is often linked with anxiety. In most cases, nervousness is a manifestation of stress, prob-lems at home or work, or simply the travails of modern life. It can also result from working too hard and feeling overwhelmed.

In a few cases, however, if you are chronically nervous and also begin to lose weight unintentionally, you may have a thyroid disease.

Treatment

Once your doctor rules out the possibility of thyroid disease, she will suggest that you try some behavioral changes to reduce your nervousness, including exercise, cutting out or down on caffeine, and/or counseling. Sometimes a short vacation or day off is all that's needed.

If your nervousness is interfering with your life and these methods don't work, your doctor may prescribe an antianxiety medication or sedative such as Valium, Xanax, or BuSpar. Your doctor will determine your dosage based on factors such as your age, weight, and sex and will lean towards giving you a smaller dose than is customary to help prevent the medication from becoming habit forming. In the case of BuSpar, it takes a week or two of daily doses until it starts to work, and it doesn't seem to cause dependency like the other antianxiety medications and sedatives.

NIGHTMARES

Description and Possible Medical Problems

It seems as though every TV sitcom that has at least one little kid in the cast runs at least one episode each year where the child wakes up the entire household when he has a nightmare.

Everyone—child and adult—has experienced nightmares. Some people dream about being chased, others about falling. As a rule, however, if you have an occasional nightmare, it's a sign that your imagination is alive and kicking, even during sleep.

If nightmares occur on a regular basis, however, they can be a sign of pulmonary disease or may be due to a lack of oxygen during sleep, which often happens in a person with a severe case of emphysema. Nightmares can also be a side effect of certain medications such as beta-blockers.

Treatment

If you have nightmares only once in awhile, you have nothing to worry about. If, however, they seem to be occurring regularly—at least a couple of times a week—you should see your doctor, who will check you for pulmonary disease or emphysema. If she determines that medication is causing your nightmares, she will change your prescription to another medication that will provide the same benefits without the side effects.

BODY SIGNAL ALERT

SEIZURES WITH LOSS OF CONSCIOUSNESS

Description and Possible Medical Problems

When a person is having convulsions or seizures, our tendency is to jump to one of two conclusions: either the person is going through drug withdrawal, or he is having an epileptic seizure.

Though drug-related seizures are by far more common, epilepsy remains one of the most misunderstood diseases around.

An epileptic seizure is the result of the electrical discharge of neurons from deep within the brain. Seizures are greatest during infancy and gradually decrease in adults, but their activity starts to increase again in people over age 60. Primary epilepsy is when the illness first appears in childhood. If the seizures have begun to appear only in adulthood, it's called secondary epilepsy. Secondary epilepsy is usually caused by an underlying disease that must be treated if future seizures are to be prevented. The most common causes of secondary epilepsy are conditions that change the composition of the blood, such as alcoholism, abrupt withdrawal from sedative or hypnotic medications, and low blood sugar.

When secondary epilepsy appears in an elderly person, the most common causes are a stroke, a brain tumor, or an old head injury.

There are two major types of epileptic seizures. One is called a partial seizure; this occurs in a small area of the brain. The other is a generalized seizure, which involves one or both of the large hemispheres of the brain. A partial seizure may or may not cause a person to lose consciousness; this is commonly referred to as a simple seizure, and it usually occurs in the frontal or temporal areas of the brain. A partial seizure can spread to a generalized seizure if the person loses consciousness. A partial seizure may involve only the shaking of a hand or foot, or it can progress to a series of full-body convulsions.

A generalized seizure can be either convulsive or nonconvulsive. Both of the cerebral hemispheres are affected, resulting in a loss of consciousness and uncontrolled movements that appear all over the body. After a generalized seizure, the person will usually fall into a deep sleep for several hours.

Treatment

If you think a person is having an epileptic seizure, you should call 911 or his doctor, if you know who it is. Don't fight the person, and make sure he has an adequate airway. Hold his tongue down with your fingers so that he is unable to swallow it. This is important, since during an epileptic seizure the tongue loses its muscle tone and can fall back toward the throat and block the airway.

If you don't know the person, check for a medical ID bracelet. Instead of epilepsy, his seizure may be due to low blood sugar.

If you or a family member has experienced seizure for the first time, you must see your physician, who will do a complete medical history and physical exam in addition to a CAT scan of the brain and and an electroencephalogram (EEG), which is used to detect abnormal electrical activity in the brain. The patterns the neurologist will detect in the brain-wave activity will help him select the best possible treatment. Though during most of the test you will be lying still with your eyes closed with electrodes attached to your scalp, your neurologist may choose to stimulate seizure activity in the brain with flashing strobe lights. This explains why flashing lights at a nightclub or rock concert, or even a light that flashes through tree branches as you drive under them in a car, can trigger a seizure in people who are prone to them.

Magnetic resonance imaging, frequently referred to as MRI, is a technique that allows your doctor to get a very detailed X ray of your brain-wave activity on a computer; an MRI may also be done with secondary epilepsy to find the exact location of a tumor that may be responsible for altering the brain waves. The doctor's main task is to find the underlying cause of the seizure, which will lead to proper treatment.

Phenobarbital and phenytoin are two medications commonly used to treat secondary epilepsy; other antiepileptic medications include primidone, carbamazepine, and valproate. The dosage for each medication will depend on your sex, age, and weight. Once you begin taking the medication, your doctor will monitor you regularly to make sure you receive the correct dosage.

Since antiepileptic medications can produce a number of side effects, you will need to visit your doctor regularly. For instance, when the drug Dilantin (phenytoin) accumulates in the bloodstream, you may have walking disturbances and lethargy. That's why it's important for your doctor to closely monitor your blood level as well as your health.

SLEEP, DISTURBED

Description and Possible Medical Problems

While most people who have sleep disorders complain of not being able to fall asleep at night, some people wake up in the middle of the night at least several times a week or even every night. Most of them get up because they have to urinate. Frequently, this is caused by drinking liquids too close to going to sleep, but a urinary tract infection may also be the reason. If you've started taking a new medication or have changed the time when you're taking an old medication, this can cause you to wake up in the middle of the night. Diuretics can also wake you from a sound sleep.

If pain is causing you to wake up, if it occurs in the upper part of your abdomen, you may have an ulcer; frequently, waking in the middle of the night with this pain is the first sign of trouble.

Treatment

If you wake up in the middle of the night because you need to urinate, try eliminating drinking fluids after 8 P.M. If this doesn't help, a change in a medication you're taking might be necessary. Some medications are stimulants; sometimes just taking your medications—especially diuretics—earlier in the day will guarantee nights of uninterrupted sleep. And if you have an ulcer, your doctor will treat you with a combination of medication and diet.

If you still wake up, you should see your doctor, who will consider your health history, take a physical exam, and conduct routine blood and urine tests.

SNORING, CONSTANT FATIGUE, FALLING ASLEEP TOO EASILY

Description and Possible Medical Problems

If an elbow in your partner's side isn't enough to stop him from snoring, and if he can fall asleep at the most inopportune moments, he probably has a condition called sleep apnea, a condition in which a person can actually wake up hundreds of times a night, even though he may not be fully aware of it. Sleep apnea occurs when the weight of the belly pushes on the diaphragm, which can make the passage of air into the lungs difficult. The result is the typical earth-shattering snore. Changes in the position of the neck can also be a cause of sleep apnea. Sometimes a blockage in the lung is the culprit, but this tends to be rare.

The almost total lack of deep sleep in people with sleep apnea results in constant fatigue during the day. The majority of people who have sleep apnea are more than 10% overweight; many of them could be considered obese.

Treatment

If your doctor suspects that a lung problem is causing your sleep apnea, he will suggest that you visit a pulmonary specialist, who will run some tests. If he thinks the problem is in your throat, he will refer you to an ear, nose, and throat specialist, who will examine your throat with a laryngoscope to check the status of the air passages and the vocal cords for polyps or other growths. Most of the time, however, obesity is the most common cause of sleep apnea, and losing weight will usually solve the problem.

If your sleep apnea is particularly severe and your doctor is not sure of the reason, you might be referred to a sleep center, where you will be monitored as you sleep to help determine the cause and therefore the treatment.

BODY SIGNAL ALERT

SPEECH LOSS OR GARBLED SPEECH WITH LOSS OF MOVEMENT ON ONE SIDE OF BODY

Description and Possible Medical Problems

Though we usually think of arteriosclerosis, or hardening of the arteries, as affecting mostly the health of the heart, the same factors that can lead to a heart attack—a diet that is high in fat and sodium, lack of exercise, and lots of stress—are also a major cause of stroke.

Garbled speech or the loss of speech entirely, and weakness or numbness on one side of the body, are classic signs of a stroke. Technically, a stroke occurs when the blood flow to a portion of the brain is interrupted. Though arteriosclerosis—or the narrowing of one of the major blood vessels serving the brain—is the most common cause of stroke, the blood supply to the brain can also be interrupted by a bleeding aneurysm or a cerebral hemorrhage.

Treatment

Sometimes a person will have a minor stroke and recover fully. Other strokes can be quite severe and can cause permanent damage. Hospitalization, neurological testing, and a complete general medical evaluation are necessary for anyone who is suspected to have had a stroke. Your doctor will first try to stop the stroke from progressing any further and to stabilize the person's condition.

For this reason, treatment in the first few days following the stroke is crucial to a person's long-term health. If the stroke patient shows an irregular heartbeat, this may have been the reason why the blood flow to the brain had stopped. People with the condition known as atrial fibrillation are especially prone to stroke, since the major symptom of this cardiac disease is an irregular heartbeat. When a person has mitral valve heart disease, where the valve that lets blood flow from the left atrium of the heart into the left ventricle sometimes allows the blood to back up into the atrium, it is likely that blood clots may form in the heart. These blood clots can then migrate to other parts of the body, including the brain or even the intestine.

In this case, treatment may include therapy with anticoagulant medication like Coumadin or heparin, which will help thin the blood, making it easier for it to pass through narrowed arteries. Coumadin is usually taken by mouth, while heparin is usually administered intravenously in the hospital. After a stroke, you may be given both Coumadin and heparin; however, since Coumadin usually takes several days until it starts to work, once it does, the heparin will be discontinued. Coumadin is a long-term medication used to ensure that the blood remains thin, thus protecting you against future strokes. Because you may be taking the medication for years, you will need to be monitored regularly by your physician with blood tests.

If the stroke has made it difficult for the person to swallow and she cannot eat, a feeding tube may have to be used temporarily. However, within a few days after a stroke, most people fully regain their ability to swallow.

To help prevent future strokes, your doctor will prescribe medication to control your cholesterol level, high blood pressure, and diabetes, if you have that disease.

A common side effect of a stroke that appears even after a person has fully recovered is depression. If this happens, a combination of therapy, exercise, and antidepressants can be effective. The support of the person's family will also be necessary to help the stroke patient make a full recovery.

SPEECH LOSS WITH LOSS OF USE OF ARM OR LEG, TOTAL RECOVERY IN LESS THAN ONE DAY

Description and Possible Medical Problems

If you temporarily lose the ability to talk and are unable to use one of your arms and/or legs, you may think you've had a stroke. The truth is that you've probably had a transient ischemic attack, also called a TIA or a ministroke. While these symptoms may be disturbing to you and your family, the good news is that if you have had a ministroke, the symptoms will completely clear up in less than a day.

A TIA can be caused by an irregular heartbeat or a heart valve problem. More frequently, however, it is the result of a reduced blood supply due to a severe narrowing in the blood vessel that feeds the brain.

Treatment

If you think that you or a family member has had a TIA, you will need to see your doctor for proper diagnosis and treatment. He will do a complete neurological evaluation and may suggest that you be hospitalized so that your heart rate can be checked for a prolonged period of time with an EKG, or echocardiogram, which will check for any abnormalities in your heart valves. He may also decide to hook you up to a Holtor monitor to measure your heartbeat for a full 24 hours. The Holtor monitor is used when you don't need to be hospitalized. Most often, this will be done if you have heart palpitations with no other symptoms, or if you have vague chest pain or discomfort or unexplained shortness of breath. Your doctor may also hook you up to a Holtor monitor if you're taking an antiarrhythmia medication so that he can determine how the medication is affecting your heartbeat. No matter the reason for the test, your doctor may also ask you to keep a log of your activity and symptoms over the 24 hours to see if they correspond with or even cause your irregular heartbeat.

Treatment for a TIA will include a low-fat, low-sodium diet, exercise, and medications such as Coumadin and heparin (see "Speech Loss or Garbled Speech with Loss of Movement on One Side of Body" above for more information about these medications) that will thin the blood and lower your blood pressure.

Even though a TIA is less serious than a stroke, it's important that you follow your doctor's orders—because if you don't take care of your health, you may well have a full-blown stroke sometime in the future.

BODY SIGNAL ALERT

SUICIDAL GESTURES

Description and Possible Medical Problems

In our society, suicide is most often talked about in context of a teenager or a middle-aged man who's become despondent because he's lost his job or his spouse. More common than people think, however, is the high rate of suicide among elderly people. Chronic illness, the loss of a spouse, and financial insecurities can all spark thoughts of suicide in an elderly person.

There are two classifications of suicide: active and passive. An active suicide is when a person attempts suicide by herself, sometimes through physical harm, such as hanging or electrocution. In the elderly, active suicide often involves either stopping medication or taking too much or abusing alcohol, often in combination with an overdose of medication. Passive suicide seems to be in the news every day, since this kind of suicide involves having someone else take responsibility for the act.

Signs of suicide include not only the actual attempt but complaints of severe pain, both physical and emotional. Frequently, a person who is considering suicide feels isolated and lonely and believes her family doesn't care about her. Other signs may include making sure her affairs are in order by making out a will and paying all her bills. I had one patient who had her cat put to sleep right before she made a suicide attempt. In fact, once all of her arrangements are made and everything is cleared up, a person who is thinking about suicide may find that her loneliness will change to euphoria since she may feel that now she has a way out.

Treatment

Be aware of the signals that indicate that a person is thinking about suicide. If a close friend or family member complains of feeling hopeless, is depressed about the future, and starts talking about suicide, even in an offhand manner, she needs immediate medical attention. If she won't seek it out for herself, you'll have to do it for her.

Don't wait. Get help now. Call 911 if the person is threatening to kill herself, or call one of the suicide hot lines in the community. Then, after the crisis has passed, work with the person to get psychiatric counseling on either a private or an individual basis; I've found that even joining a church or other social group can help a person become less depressed.

Chapter 4

HAIR AND FACE

BODY SIGNAL ALERT

Call your doctor if you experience any of the following symptoms:

SYMPTOM	POSSIBLE MEDICAL CONDITION
You are rapidly losing your hair	*Stress, illness, chemotherapy*
You have a group of painful pimples on one side of your face (see Chapter 9)	*Shingles*

HOW THE HAIR AND FACE AGE

From the moment we hit adulthood—which, as children, we wanted desperately to reach—most people begin to look for signs that they're aging. And the first place they usually look is their face. The second is their hair.

Because the hair and face spend so much time exposed to the elements, whether it's sunlight, the cold, or pollution, it's inevitable that they show the first signs of aging. And because they are so visible, in essence broadcasting our age to a society that still largely prefers the bloom of youth, thousands of people are employed and hundreds of substances have been invented to help hide what many people perceive as the ravages of age.

Facial wrinkles, of course, are the first thing that come to mind when we speak of the way the face ages. But they are just one way in which the face grows older, and you can learn more about wrinkles in Chapter 9, "Skin."

The bones in the face also begin to atrophy slowly with age, resulting in a loss of bone mass in the jaw and skull. The cartilage of the nose may also lose some of its definition, and the nasal passages may become smaller (see Chapter 6, "Ears and Nose"). The loss of muscle mass in the face eventually leads to the sunken, drooping look that's common in elderly people.

The hair on our heads and elsewhere on our bodies unfortunately don't escape the aging process, either. Though the hair on your head may become thin and turn grey, excess hair may grow in other parts of the body where it didn't appear before. Men may notice that the hair in their nose and on the outside of their ears has increased in volume, while women may find that the decreased level of estrogen that accompanies menopause causes hair to grow in unexpected places, especially on the face.

The skin of the scalp begins to thicken with age, and the scalp also secretes less oil. As a result, the hair may become more brittle.

The signs of aging on the hair and face are irreversible, though advertisers would have you believe that cosmetic and surgical procedures exist that can turn back the clock. The use of cosmetics and surgery is up to an individual preference or desire. The aging process itself is dictated by the biological clock and one's own genetics. Some people just age faster than others.

BALDNESS

Description and Possible Medical Problems

I remember having a microbiology professor in medical school who refused to admit he was going bald. Memorizing all those elements was bad enough, but the teacher refused to admit that he was going bald. So he combed the few remaining strands over the top of his shiny pate and hoped we wouldn't notice. We did, of course, but at least it kept us entertained during the eternity of that class.

Some men and women lose their hair temporarily as a reaction to physical and/or mental stress such as chemotherapy, emotional upset, or even dieting. This results in a condition called alopecia areata. However, when a man in midlife—or earlier—starts to lose his hair, it's pretty much a permanent sign of aging, especially if his father was bald, since significant hair loss tends to be hereditary.

Men typically begin to lose their hair at the temples and above the forehead. If the hair loss is progressive, the baldness then continues over the top of the head. Women begin to notice thinning hair after menopause because of hormonal changes, but their loss tends to occur all over the head.

Unless the hair loss is sudden and significant, you should consider it a normal part of aging. Whether or not you decide to do anything about it is up to you.

Treatment

In the past, the only possible recourse for men and women who were losing their hair and weren't happy about it was to wear ill-fitting, poorly designed wigs and hairpieces. Most opted to grin and bear it.

Today, things are different. Some men opt for transplants, a procedure in which a patch of skin with hair still growing from it is grafted onto the area that is balding. Hair transplants, however, are painful, and the grafts do not always "take."

In recent years, the drug minoxidil has received a lot of attention for its ability to grow hair, but, as with transplants, the results have been mixed. Some people have also experienced unpleasant side effects from taking the drug, such as an upset stomach, elevated heart rate, and water retention.

Other treatments that are used to induce hair growth include the application of certain chemicals or cortisone preparations to the scalp. The theory behind the chemicals is that if the skin is irritated enough, it may produce hair where there is currently none. Regular use of cortisone has been shown to grow hair in some people as a side effect. But, again, these methods don't always work, and the side effects can be unpleasant.

Sometimes, after trying everything that is rumored to "cure" baldness and having had no success, a person may simply decide to give in to the hair loss and accept it.

See also "Hair Loss, Sudden" below.

DANDRUFF

Description and Possible Medical Problems

Though dandruff can appear at any age, it seems to affect midlife adults more frequently.

Dandruff is caused by one of two genetic skin conditions: seborrheic dermatitis, or eczema; or psoriasis. Eczema is a skin problem in which certain parts of the skin—including the scalp—turn red and flaky; they may also itch. Psoriasis is a condition in which the skin cells that are normally shed by the body build up because the skin can't rid itself of the shed cells fast enough. The unshed cells then accumulate on the skin and form white, flaky areas, which eventually shed themselves in the big white flakes that we know as dandruff. Eczema appears as a red patch that may itch, while psoriasis is characterized by raised, red patches on the skin that are topped with white flaky scales. Psoriasis, however, usually doesn't hurt or itch.

Sometimes, however, what looks like a case of dandruff is actually shampoo that hasn't been totally rinsed from your hair. The soapy residue dries on your hair and scalp and then flakes off.

Treatment

Dandruff that is a result of eczema is more common than dandruff that is caused by psoriasis. To treat either form of dandruff, you should first try shampooing regularly with an over-the-counter dandruff preparation. Some people with psoriasis-based dandruff also find that a moderate amount of sun exposure help, alleviate the problem.

If initial self-treatment has no effect on your dandruff, you should visit a dermatologist, who may prescribe a stronger prescription dandruff shampoo. If that has no effect, he may recommend a topical corticosteroid ointment you can apply to your scalp. This should then clear it up.

FLAT YELLOW GROWTHS UNDER EYELIDS

See "Eyelids, Flat Yellow Growths Under" in Chapter 5.

FACE, PAIN IN, AT TEMPLE, RUNNING TO CHEEK OR JAW

Description and Possible Medical Problems

A sudden sharp, stabbing pain in your face that begins at your temple and radiates to your cheek or jaw can be frightening. But when the pain arrives for no apparent reason, occurs intermittently for up to several weeks, and then disappears completely for anywhere from a day to several months before striking again, you probably have a condition called trigeminal neuralgia.

Trigeminal neuralgia is characterized by its unpredictability and its sharp, sometimes brief ashes of pain. Men and women over the age of 50 tend to have the condition, and the frequency of attacks increases significantly over the age of 70.

The cause of trigeminal neuralgia is unknown. Though some studies point to a brain tumor or a blood vessel pressing on the nerve as the culprit, the exact cause cannot be determined.

Treatment

If the pain recurs with regularity and makes it difficult for you to function, your doctor may recommend you take phenytoin or carbamazepine, anticonvulsant medications that may help reduce the number of attacks. You may need to take the medication for a number of weeks after the initial attack.

For severe cases of trigeminal neuralgia that don't respond to anticonvulsants, your doctor may suggest you undergo an operation that either destroys the trigeminal nerve or reduces its sensitivity, though the final outcome of the operation is difficult to predict and may lead to permanent paralysis of one side of your face. However, in the entire time I've spent working as a physician, I have never seen this surgery performed. In addition to the anticonvulsant medications I've mentioned, some people with trigeminal neuralgia can also take the antidepressant Elavil to control their pain.

FACE, SWELLING IN SIDE OF

See "Chin, Swollen Area Under or at Jaw or Temple" in Chapter 8.
See "Pimples, Painful, on One Side of the Face" in Chapter 9.

FOREHEAD, PAIN IN, FOREHEAD, WITH A CHANGE IN VISION

See "Eye Pain with Tenderness in Forehead and Temples and/or Sudden Blindness" in Chapter 5.

HAIR, GRAYING AND THINNING OF, WITH SOME LOSS

Description and Possible Medical Problems

Most of us accept the fact that, in one way or another, the aging process is going to affect the hair on our heads, whether it becomes thinner or grayer or we begin to lose some of it and it doesn't grow back. For some people, the process began in their 20s; others still have a full head of hair into their 60s, though the color is probably gray or white to some degreee.

The fact is that 50% of men and women will see some significant changes in their hair by the time they turn 50.

Treatment

The effect that aging has on our hair is biologically not reversible, though by using hair color, a body wave or permanent, or even a new hairstyle, these effects can be minimized.

You can either color or perm your hair yourself or go to a professional salon. One caveat about doing it yourself: when coloring or perming hair, many people have a tendency to leave the preparation on too long. This can lead to dryness, breakage, and loss of even more hair. Many of the chemicals that are used in hair color or permanent solution can cause the scalp to become irritated. This may also be more of a problem in elderly men and women, since their scalps produce less of the protective oils than younger people's do. Besides the professional attention you get, it's a good idea to go to a salon because the coloring and perming preparations used in salons tend to be gentler on the hair and scalp than over-the-counter preparations are. To play it safe, you may want to have a professional stylist care for your hair.

BODY SIGNAL ALERT

HAIR LOSS, SUDDEN

Description and Possible Medical Problems

Gradual hair loss is a normal sign of aging. But if your hair begins to fall out in clumps, a serious health condition is probably causing it and you need to seek medical attention immediately.

Frequently, during an illness that is serious enough to require hospitalization, hair growth will cease altogether for a few months. After the initial onset of the illness, the hair will fall out and then begin to grow back when the illness has disappeared. Though everything from emotional stress to surgery can cause this type of baldness, called telogen efuvium, the hair loss is temporary. Some diseases that can cause telogen efuvium include kidney disease, diabetes, and certain skin diseases. And a low-calorie diet can cause temporary hair loss. In rare instances, when the illness is particularly severe, a person can lose all the hair on her body, including the eyebrows and eyelashes and even the pubic hair.

Chemotherapy for cancer will often cause a person to lose all of her hair over the course of several days. Then, when the therapy is over, the hair will usually begin to grow back.

Alopecia areata is the term for when hair falls out in clumps all over the head. It is frequently used to refer to women who have a severe, sudden hair loss that is due to a serious illness and for which there is no other apparent cause.

Treatment

Hair loss due to aging is basically irreversible, hair loss caused by a disease is almost always temporary. Though this is the good news, the bad news is that you need to treat the underlying disease before your hair can grow back. Since one of the causes, kidney disease is life-threatening without proper treatment, if your hair is suddenly falling out in clumps, you need to see your doctor to determine the cause right away.

PIMPLES

See "Pimples" in Chapter 9.

BODY SIGNAL ALERT

PIMPLES, PAINFUL, ON ONE SIDE OF THE FACE

See "Pimples, Painful, on One Side of the Face" in Chapter 9.

SCALP, ITCHY

Description and Possible Medical Problems

If your scalp is itchy and frequent shampooing has no effect, you may have either head lice or dermatitis, an inammation of the scalp that may or may not be accompanied by flaky dandruff. Though it's commonly believed that only children get head lice, adults can get them, too, though the experiences that most adults have with lice are restricted to those in the pubic area.

Head lice are very contagious and are spread through physical contact and clothing. Though it is hard to see a louse itself, you will be able to see lice nits, or eggs, which resemble small grains of rice, in your hair.

If you have contact dermatitis, your scalp will be red, swollen, and itchy. You may also experience blistering and/or flaking if the condition becomes chronic. Dermatitis may appear for a variety of reasons, from contact with a chemical irritant to an allergic reaction to hair sprays or gels, shampoos, or coloring products.

Treatment

If you have head lice, you should see your physician, who will prescribe a special shampoo for you to use along with a special comb to remove any remaining nits. It's a good idea to throw out and/or burn any hat or headgear you might have been wearing during the period of infestation. You should also make sure that all bed linens are thoroughly washed in hot water.

If you have dermatitis, the treatment depends on the specific cause. The best treatment and preventative are avoidance of the particular irritant or allergen. Your dermatologist may recommend the use of a special corticosteroid cream or ointment to reduce the swelling and redness. In most cases, you'll feel better in a day or so.

SMALL, RED SPIDER VEINS

Description and Possible Medical Problems

If small, red spiderlike veins suddenly appear on your face or neck, you have a condition called spider angioma, or spider telangiectasia. Named for the resemblance these veins bear to spiders, with a round, raised patch in the middle and thin legs that branch out from it, spider angioma is usually caused by excessive alcohol intake or medication. It is most often a condition that occurs in tandem with cirrhosis of the liver, a deterioration of the organ common to alcoholics. Spider angioma can also be caused by the elevated estrogen levels that occur during pregnancy or postmenopausal estrogen therapy.

Treatment

Sometimes a spider angioma will appear and disappear for no apparent reason. It does not present a danger to your health; the only reason to remove it is for cosmetic purposes. Since spider angiomas commonly appear on the face, many people do opt for surgical treatment. If you have been taking estrogen and the spider angioma has appeared as a result, you should consult with your doctor about reducing the dosage or eliminating it completely.

A spider angioma may be treated with either cryotherapy or cauterization. The recuperation time is short, but you should stay out of the sun until the area is completely healed.

Chapter 5

EYES

HOW THE EYE AGES

Remember your Uncle Charlie and the problems he used to have reading the newspaper? It seemed as though he had trouble focusing, so he first tried his bifocals. When that didn't work, he held the paper out at arms length. Then, with his arms fully outstretched, he was finally able to settle into his reading.

But you couldn't understand why he ended up that way. "Bring it closer, Uncle Charlie, not farther away," you informed him with the naïveté of youth. Or you may have handed him your father's glasses to try. But while you may have been nearsighted as a child, presbyopia, a form of farsightedness, which is what Uncle Charlie had, is much more common among midlife adults. In fact, as you age, and if you wear glasses or contacts, you may find that your prescription has gone from one extreme to another, from nearsightedness to farsightedness.

Presbyopia is only one characteristic of the aging eye. If you know a man or woman over the age of 50 who has never worn glasses or contact lenses, you should consider yourself to be in rare company. Besides the possibility of having presbyopia as you grow older, you may find that you need to rely on your reading glasses more, whereas before you only needed them for reading or night driving. You may also find that it takes longer for your eyes to adjust to the dark, and even once you've become used to the poor light you may not be able to make out certain objects as clearly as you once did. Your eyes may not water as easily as when you were younger, something that is especially true for post-menopausal women.

There's not much you can do to prevent the effects that each additional year has on your sense of vision. Some ophthalmologists believe that if you work at a computer or a craft where you frequently need to focus on objects up close, your vision will deteriorate less rapidly if you wear regular eyeglasses instead of contact lenses. And remember what your mother told you about reading under poor light? It's true that the less you strain your eyes, the longer you'll keep your eyesight intact.

The chances of getting certain ophthalmologic diseases—such as glaucoma, cataracts, and retinal detachment—increase with age, but the good news is that after about the age of 50, your eyesight will stabilize and may even improve significantly. Overall, if you try to stay aware of any changes in vision you experience and visit your eye doctor at the early signs of change, you'll improve your chances of having healthy eyes well into your 70s, 80s, and beyond.

BULGING, BOTH EYES

Description and Possible Medical Problems

If both of your eyes appear to bulge from their sockets, causing a pop-eyed appearance, you may already be aware that you have a thyroid problem known as Graves' disease, a kind of hyperthyroidism. If only one eye is bulging, it may be due to a tumor behind the eye (see "Bulging, One Eye" below for more information). Hyperthyroidism is a condition in which the thyroid gland produces too much thyroxine, a hormone that helps to regulate growth in the body; the condition often results in weight loss and nervousness, and it primarily affects women in midlife. Graves' disease occurs when an excessively large amount of the hormone is produced; this may cause some parts of the body to grow, including the tissue behind the eyes, causing the eyes to bulge out. In addition to bulging eyes, your eyes may also water frequently and be extrasensitive to light, and your eyesight may be blurry and distorted.

If your eyes start to bulge and you are not aware that you have a thyroid problem, your doctor will probably suggest the possibility when she takes a look at your eyes. Though bulging eyes by themselves are not harmful to your health, the underlying thyroid condition can decrease your quality of life. Fortunately, however, if you begin to treat Graves' disease when you first notice that your eyes begin to bulge, both your eye condition and your thyroid condition will clear up completely.

Treatment

For most people, simple self-care remedies are all you'll need to treat the bulging eyes caused by Graves' disease, in addition to taking medication that will bring your Graves' disease under control. Try sleeping with your head on an extra pillow, which will help reduce the swelling of your eyes. Bulging eyes may become irritated because more of their surface area is exposed, and eyedrops can sometimes help soothe the discomfort.

However, if the condition has been untreated for a long period of time, these treatments may not be effective. In this case, surgery will help. The surgeon will open up a space in a sinus cavity behind the eyes in order to allow the expanded tissues more room. This will reduce some of the pressure the swollen tissue is placing on the eyeballs. At the same time, since the pressure of the tissues can hamper your vision by pressing on the optic nerve, your doctor may repair any damage to the nerve. In addition, your doctor may perform minor cosmetic surgery to return the lower and upper eyelids, which frequently become pulled back in Graves' disease, to their normal appearance.

After surgery, it's important that you follow your doctor's instructions to treat your Graves' disease with hormonal therapy so that your bulging eyes will not recur.

BODY SIGNAL ALERT

BULGING, ONE EYE

Description and Possible Medical Problems

If you notice that one of your eyes is bulging slightly more than the other, possibly accompanied by redness, pain, impaired vision, and a change in the appearance or color of the iris, you should see your doctor immediately. These are all signs of retinoblastoma, which is a tumor that develops behind the eye. In addition to the bulging eye, the tumor may actually be visible in the form of a white object that can be seen through the pupil.

Though retinoblastoma is a form of cancer that usually appears in children under the age of 4, it can also affect midlife adults. In fact, retinoblastoma tends to be hereditary, so if one of your parents had the condition, it's a good idea for you to stay alert to any slight changes in your eye. If your bulging eye is accompanied by a chronic, intense headache, you may have a brain tumor near the eye socket that is causing the eye to bulge.

Treatment

Tumors that appear in or near an eye and cause it to bulge out are usually treated with surgery and radiation, although laser therapy and cryotherapy, a procedure in which the tumor is frozen with a special probe, may also be considered, due to the sensitive location of the tumor. If the tumor is caught early, the chances of total eradication of the malignancy are good. In rare cases, when the tumor has grown quite large, the eye may have to be removed. In a few instances, however, the tumor may actually start to shrink since, once it gets large enough, it chokes off its own supply of blood. This does not mean you should forgo treatment, however, since this form of spontaneous remission may not necessarily happen in your case.

DISCHARGE WITH REDNESS

Description and Possible Medical Problems

If you have a discharge from your eye that does not resemble normal watering and it's accompanied by redness and itching, you probably have a common condition known as conjunctivitis, also called pinkeye. In addition to the redness and discharge, your eye may feel as though there's grit in it. Although conjunctivitis is uncomfortable and the appearance of a reddened eye may make you want to stay inside until it clears up, pinkeye usually presents no threat to your permanent vision.

Conjunctivitis is easy to spot, but it's also easy to catch. Young children are extremely prone to conjunctivitis because of their still-developing immune systems and their tendency to share toys that have been contaminated by germs. But adults frequently get pinkeye as well.

Conjunctivitis can be caused by either a bacterial or a viral infection. When a bacterial infection is the culprit, both eyes are usually affected, and there will be a lot of discharge. The discharge will often form a crust while you sleep. A viral infection will cause less discharge, and only one eye tends to be affected.

Treatment

If you think you have conjunctivitis, you should see your doctor. If the infection is caused by bacteria, your doctor will prescribe an antibiotic ointment or eyedrops for you to apply to your eyes several times a day. Viral conjunctivitis will clear up without treatment, though your doctor may prescribe eyedrops that contain the antibiotic Neosporin or the corticosteroid prednisone to help soothe the inflamed eye. However, if you have glaucoma, your doctor will advise against these preparations because they can make the glaucoma worse. You should also refrain from wearing contact lenses until the infection is cleared up, which will take only a couple of days. If it lasts longer, you should see your ophthalmologist. During the period of infection, you should take precautions to avoid both contagion and reinfecting yourself. Wash your hands after you touch your eyes, and use a clean towel and washcloth each time. Don't use makeup, and stay out of swimming pools. It's also a good idea to make sure that other people keep their distance while your infection is active.

Tips and Precautions

To prevent future bouts with conjunctivitis, I always advise women to throw their eye makeup away after a few months of use. And you should *never* use mascara or eye shadow that belongs to someone else.

BODY SIGNAL ALERT

EYE, "CURTAIN" IN FRONT OF

Description and Possible Medical Problems

Behind the retina, at the back of your eye, lies a thin layer of blood vessels called the choroid. These blood vessels supply the entire eye with blood and oxygen, which help keep it functioning and healthy.

Sometimes the retina of one eye can suddenly tear away from the choroid, causing you to see a "curtain" or shadow in front of the affected eye. Your vision may also be blurred, and you may see flashing lights. You will, however, probably feel no pain. This condition is called retinal detachment, and you need to see your doctor immediately. Any delay in treatment could result in a permanent loss of vision.

Retinal detachment most often occurs when a hole or tear already exists in the retina. This may be caused either by trauma or as the vitreous humor, the gelatinous substance that makes up most of your eyeball, shrinks due to age; as the vitreous humor pulls away from the retina, it can take some of the retina with it, creating a gaping hole in the retina. The retina may then become detached from the choroid when the vitreous humor, which can seep in between the retina and the choroid, accumulates in the gap. This can cause pressure to build up, which can eventually force the retina to separate from the choroid.

Retinal detachment affects men more often than women, and unfortunately, if one of your parents had a detachment in the past, your chances of having the condition increase. Midlife adults also become more prone to retinal detachment with age due to the changes in the vitreous humor. Frequently, just before the retina detaches, you may see flashing lights and black floating shapes directly in your line of vision, not off to the side; if you blink, the lights and shapes will still be there. Only one eye at a time is affected, though retinal detachment may occur in the second eye after an initial detachment in the other one.

Treatment

A "curtain" will appear in front of your eye when the retina begins to tear away from the choroid. This is considered a medical emergency, and, once you see your doctor, he will usually perform surgery within a few hours of the initial detachment.

Most of the treatment for retinal detachment involves laser surgery, which will reattach the retina to the choroid. The procedure is painless and takes about two hours. You may be given either local or general anesthesia. If you catch the detachment early, your vision will be fully restored to its previous state. If a day or more elapses before you seek treatment, however, your vision may be permanently damaged.

Frequently, lasers are being used to repair the retinal tear or hole that usually precedes a retinal detachment. Your ophthalmologist will be able to detect any retinal problems before they worsen, which is why it is so important to have a regular vision checkup at least once a year over the age of 50.

EYE, DRYNESS

Description and Possible Medical Problems

A normal part of the aging process is that certain parts of the body begin to dry out. In some cases, such as oily skin, this is cause for celebration. The eye also begins to dry out somewhat with age, and, though it may not be a reason to celebrate, having dry eyes isn't a serious health problem. It's also relatively simple to treat.

It's common for problems with the tear ducts, which are also called the lacrimal glands, to flare up in midlife adults, though overproduction of tears is as common as underproduction.

When the tear ducts produce fewer tears, the eye can become red and irritated and may feel gritty at times. If you have a tendency toward dry eyes, you'll find that the condition will often occur in both eyes, not just one at a time. Men and women who have rheumatoid arthritis are also prone to dry eye syndrome. More women than men are affected, and chronic dry eye syndrome—also called keratoconjunctivitis sicca—usually makes its first appearance in midlife, usually about the age of 50, when the tear glands begin to produce fewer tears.

Sometimes people with dry eye syndrome find that their eyelid does not completely close during sleep. Again, this is nothing to worry about.

Treatment

If your eyes are frequently drier than you're used to, you should see your eye doctor. He may recommend that you use artificial tears to moisten your eyes. Artificial tears are a prescription medication that comes in either eyedrops or an ointment. You should use them as needed.

Tips and Precautions

Don't make the mistake that some people with dry eyes make of relying on over-the-counter solutions such as Visine that primarily reduce redness and irritation in the eye. The chronic use of any over-the-counter preparation isn't a good idea without your doctor's approval, and products such as Visine work by shrinking the tiny blood vessels in the eye. Using these products beyond the manufacturer's recommended length of time may not only cause you to develop a dependency on them but may permanently damage your eyesight. If your eyes are frequently dry and uncomfortable, see your eye doctor for a diagnosis; he'll prescribe the right kind of medication.

EYE, EXCESSIVE WATERING OF

Description and Possible Medical Problems

Though midlife adults commonly complain of having dry eyes, eyes that water excessively are also frequently seen. When one or both eyes won't stop watering, the problem can be caused by a number of conditions, most of which are easily treated.

Entropion is a condition in which the lower eyelid begins to droop and turns slightly inward because of the gradual loss of strength in the muscles that control the eye. When the lower lid sags, the eyelashes can irritate the eye, which may cause it to water excessively. Excessive tearing can also be caused by ectropion, a condition in which the lower eyelid turns outward. In this case, the tears that lubricate the inside of the lower lid are unable to drain into the tear duct. As a result, they'll run out of your eyes and down your cheek.

The nasolacrimal ducts of the eye serve to drain your tears from the eye into the nose. Sometimes these ducts can become blocked as a result of an infection, which again means that your tears have nowhere to go except down your face.

Some people's eyes tend to water more in cold weather. This is actually a sign that your eyes are healthy and reacting normally.

Treatment

Eyes that water excessively are an easy condition to treat. Both ectropion and entropion can be treated with a minor surgical procedure in which your doctor will tighten the muscles of the lids, which will prevent them from turning either outward or inward. When excessive watering is caused by a blocked tear duct, it can be opened manually or with surgery if the blockage is extensive. At the same time, it's important to treat any existing infection with medication to be sure that the blockage doesn't recur.

EYE PAIN IN BRIGHT LIGHT

Description and Possible Medical Problems

As we age, the eye takes longer to adjust to changes in light, due to changes in the retina and vitreous humor. But if your eyes actually hurt when they're exposed to bright light, aging is not the culprit; your mouth or sinuses are.

The sinuses, oral cavity, and eyes are located so close together that sometimes a problem in one area will spill over to one of the others. The ears and throat can also sometimes be responsible for the pain you feel in your eyes when they're exposed to light.

Treatment

If you have a toothache or other dental problem, or if your sinuses are acting up, it's possible that the pain you're feeling is responsible for making your eyes more sensitive to light. If you treat the toothache or sinus condition, the pain you feel in your eyes when you look at a bright light should go away.

If, however, this sensitivity to light remains after your toothache or sinus headache has cleared up, you should see your doctor in order to determine the true cause. Eye pain that's caused by exposure to light is also a symptom of uveitis, an inflammation of the part of the eye that includes the iris; conjunctivitis; and Graves' disease, a malfunction of the thyroid gland. Uveitis is usually treated with eyedrops containing prednisone. Graves' disease is treated by addressing the overactive thyroid; medication may include beta-blockers or even a dose of radioactive iodine to help diagnose and then treat the thyroid gland.

See also "Discharge with Redness" above and "Bulging, Both Eyes" above.

BODY SIGNAL ALERT

EYE PAIN WITH CYLINDRICAL FIELD OF VISION

See "Vision, Cylindrical" below.

BODY SIGNAL ALERT

EYE PAIN WITH TENDERNESS IN FOREHEAD AND TEMPLES, AND/OR SUDDEN BLINDNESS

Description and Possible Medical Problems

Sometimes, when you have a headache, you've probably noticed that your eyes hurt as well. Eye pain frequently accompanies a headache because the nerves that enable you to move your eyes become inflamed. Not only does this create a pain in your head, the pain will probably feel even worse every time you move your eyes to look at something. If you are prone to developing migraine headaches, you may have to stay in a darkened room due to the pain in your eyes.

If you have a headache with eye pain and don't have a history of migraines, rest assured that your headache will clear up within a day or two. However, if your headache is accompanied by eye pain and the artery that runs up the side of your neck and through your temple is swollen and painful, you may have temporal arteritis. Temporal arteritis is a disease in which the temporal arteries, which run from the heart to the brain, become inflamed. Because one of the temporal arteries is the ophthalmic artery, which supplies blood to the eyes, your eye pain may be accompanied by blurring, double vision, and even sudden blindness.

It's not known what causes temporal arteritis; however, like migraine, the condition tends to be hereditary. Temporal arteritis is most common in people over the age of 50 and affects women twice as often as men. Whites are also more prone to the disease than blacks are.

Treatment

If you think you have temporal arteritis, you should see your doctor immediately, especially if you have experienced sudden blindness. He will conduct a blood test that includes a test for the erythrocyte sedimentation rate, or ESR, which will check how quickly red blood cells settle in the bottom of a test tube. A high ESR is an indication of an inflamed artery, as in temporal arteritis. Your doctor may also perform a biopsy of the temporal artery in order to make a positive diagnosis.

If you do have temporal arteritis, you will need to treat it with a regimen of corticosteroid medication such as prednisone on a long-term basis, possibly for months. This will help reduce the swollen artery to its normal size. In order to prevent future problems, however, you will need to continue taking the medication for a year or more; regular blood tests that monitor the ESR in addition to your symptoms will help your doctor to guide your treatment.

BODY SIGNAL ALERT

EYE PAIN WITH REDNESS

Description and Possible Medical Problems

When you feel a pain in one or both eyes, it is usually one of several symptoms that accompany other eye problems. However, when it appears by itself and is accompanied by redness, it is usually due to an inflammation of one of the parts that make up the eyeball. Just as conjunctivitis, or pinkeye, is an inflammation of the conjunctiva (the membrane that lines the insides of the eyelids and part of the eyeball), other parts of the eye can also become inflamed. These include the iris, which is the colored part of your eye, and the sclera, a transparent film that serves as the outermost layer of the eye.

The choroid is located in the back of the eye, between the retina and the sclera. The choroid is the layer of the eye that contains the many blood vessels that nourish the eye, and, like the other parts of the eye, the choroid can become inflamed.

Iritis, or inflammation of the iris, is sometimes known as uveitis, since the iris is part of the uvea, a membrane that lies just underneath the sclera. The retina at the back of the eye can also become irritated.

Some of these conditions—such as scleritis—are more likely to appear in a person who has rheumatoid arthritis, while others may arise for no apparent reason. Because it will be difficult for you to detemine the cause of the pain yourself and the only symptom you'll have is generalized pain in your eye with perhaps some redness, it's important that you see your doctor.

Treatment

Diagnosis and treatment of the inflammation of a particular part of the eye will depend on a number of factors, ranging from how long you've had the pain to other diseases—such as rheumatoid arthritis—that may be present.

However, no matter what part of the eye is inflamed, your doctor will probably prescribe eyedrops or an ointment that contains a corticosteroid such as prednisone for you to use for a few days. This will help reduce the inflammation. Cold compresses can help reduce the redness. If you have choroiditis, the medication will be injected near your eye, since the choroid is at the back of the eye. Your doctor may recommend aspirin or a prescription painkiller if the pain is particularly severe. If you wear contact lenses, check with your physician to see if you can wear them during the infection; if he's like me, he'll turn thumbs down on the idea, since contacts usually aggravate the infection. Disregard your vanity and wear your glasses until the infection clears up totally.

The good news is that any inflammation of one or more parts of the eye will not permanently impair your vision, and it's easy to treat. Once you begin treatment, the inflammation should begin to clear up within a few days.

EYE, RED

Description and Possible Medical Problems

Have you ever found yourself in this situation: You're going about your normal day, happen to glance in the mirror, and suddenly notice a small patch of blood on the white of your eye. "What now?" you shriek.

Sure, you become alarmed, but rest assured that this spot of blood—known as an eye hemorrhage, or a subconjunctival hemorrhage—is relatively common and usually harmless.

The conjunctiva, the membrane that lines the inside of the eyelid and part of the eyeball, contains many tiny blood vessels. Frequently, a vessel on the conjunctiva on the eyeball will burst or leak, causing a small spot of blood to form on the white of the eye. Though a hemorrhage can happen spontaneously, sometimes it can be caused by a cough or sneeze.

Treatment

A subconjunctival hemorrhage is usually nothing to worry about; most disappear on their own within a few days. If, however, the spot is painful or reappears, you should see your doctor for a thorough examination. If the spot of blood on your eye hurts, it could be a sign of a blood disease or a trauma to the eye. Frequently, people who are taking an anticoagulant medication like Coumadin to treat recurrent or potential blood clots find they are more prone to subconjunctival hemorrhages than when they were not on the medication. If this is the case, your doctor will monitor your medication by taking periodic blood tests so that he can check for evidence of bleeding.

BODY SIGNAL ALERT

EYE, SENSATION OF FOREIGN BODY IN

Description and Possible Medical Problems

From time to time, we've all had the feeling that there's something stuck in our eye and we can't get it out. Usually, after we examine the eye carefully and try to make it water, the feeling goes away.

But sometimes it doesn't. If you feel as though there is something stuck in your eye but you can't see anything, you should see your eye doctor immediately, because your cornea, a clear film that covers the front of the eyeball, may have been damaged through either trauma or infection.

Because the cornea works in tandem with the retina to transmit images to the brain, any damage to the cornea may result in your vision being impaired, either temporarily or permanently.

Corneal tissue is so thin that it's not difficult to see how it can be damaged so easily. The cornea can be scratched by a grain of sand or by prolonged exposure to ultraviolet light. Even if the damage has been caused by a foreign body, once the offending particle has been removed, it may still feel as though there's something in your eye, and the cornea can become infected or ulcerated. You will also feel a sharp pain in the affected eye, and your vision will be diminished if the corneal damage has been caused by an infection or a physical trauma. Your eye may also become sore and red. With an infection, the cause is usually the herpes simplex virus, the virus that is also responsible for cold sores, and it will hurt. If a white spot appears on the surface of your eye, you probably have an ulcer on your cornea. An ulcer may be due to a physical injury but can also be caused by a fungal infection, which can be very serious but occurs only rarely.

Treatment

No matter what the cause, damage to the cornea can be healed within a few days with proper treatment. If the culprit is a scratch or injury by a foreign particle or a bacterial infection, your doctor may prescribe an antibiotic ointment such as Cortisporin or gentamicin ointment for you to use two or three times daily for a few days until the injury heals. When the herpes simplex virus is the cause, your physician may prescribe a special antiviral medication such as Zovirax to apply topically in either eyedrops or ointment.

If a corneal ulcer or infection is caused by a fungus, the ulcer is usually invisible to the eye, but it will be painful. If this happens, your doctor will recommend an antifungal medication, though a fungal infection can be stubborn and may reappear in the future.

Regardless of what caused the damage to your cornea, you should take care never to touch your eyes while they're healing, as foreign matter or a new bacterial, fungal, or viral strain can be introduced very easily, prolonging the corneal infection.

Tips and Precautions

Whenever you have an eye infection, you should be careful to follow this advice:

1. Never use eyedrops or ointments from a previous infection.

2. Wash your hands frequently, especially after you touch your eye.

3. Take a break from wearing contact lenses until your doctor tells you otherwise.

4. When you do have to touch the infected eye, don't touch the other one, as this can easily spread the infection.

EYELID, DROOPING

Description and Possible Medical Problems

If the upper eyelid of one of your eyes appears to droop a little lower than the other, and if it seems to have sagged more with age, you have a condition known as ptosis.

Ptosis occurs when the muscle responsible for raising the upper eyelid becomes weak over time or when the nerve that controls the muscle is damaged in some way. Ptosis is usually hereditary, and both diabetes and myasthenia gravis—a rare condition in which the nerves of the muscles weaken progressively over a period of time—can aggravate the condition. The degree of droopiness can also vary widely over the course of the day; it may hardly be noticeable in the morning, but by nightfall the eyelid may droop considerably.

Treatment

The good news is that, by itself, ptosis is not a serious problem unless the drooping lid begins to interfere with your vision, or if you believe it is aesthetically unattractive. If this is the case, you should opt for cosmetic surgery that will stop the lid from sagging by removing excess skin from the upper lid.

It's important for you to determine if the eyelid began to droop suddenly or if the deterioration was gradual, which is a normal sign of aging. If, however, your ptosis is caused by either diabetes or myasthenia gravis, a very rare neurological disease (see "Eyelids That Droop as the Day Progresses" below), you and your doctor need to first address and treat the disease. The drooping lid should return to its previous state after proper treatment of the disease.

EYELIDS, DROOPING LOWER

Description and Possible Medical Problems

As you know by now, although getting older generally means you don't have as much muscle tone as you once did, it usually is a gradual process and doesn't tend to affect the body in any harmful way. The muscles that control the eye, like the rest of the body, also gradually lose some of their strength with age. This includes the muscles that control the movement of the eyeballs and help the lenses to focus, as well as the muscles of both the upper and lower eyelids.

When the upper lid starts to lose its muscle tone, it will gradually begin to droop, but this does not usually happen until a person is in her 70s. When the lower lid loses muscle tone, it can begin to turn outward from the eye, a condition called ectropion. It may also sag inward, which can cause the lashes to rub against and irritate the eye. This condition is called entropion. While aging is usually a factor in the development of these conditions because of the naturally diminished muscle tone, they can also be caused by lupus erythematosus, a disease of the connective tissue (see "Rash on the Face" in Chapter 9 for more information about this disease).

Treatment

Because the eye is more exposed when the lower eyelid sags, it's more at risk for damage to the cornea. In addition, because the lower lid is slack, the tears that are normally held against the eye have nowhere to go and run out of the eye, which may make it seem as though the affected eye is watering excessively. A sagging eyelid is also more prone to infections.

Fortunately, a sagging lower eyelid is easy to treat. When ectropion or entropion is a by-product of the aging process, your doctor can perform a simple operation under local anesthesia that will return your eyelid to its normal appearance. If it is caused by lupus erythematosus, treating the disease (see "Rash on the Face" in Chapter 9) will help reverse the sagging. In either case, it's a good idea to see your doctor as soon as you notice that your lower eyelid is beginning to droop.

See also Eye, "Excessive Watering of" above.

EYELIDS THAT DROOP
AS THE DAY PROGRESSES

Description and Possible Medical Problems

It's natural for your eyes to droop a bit as you get older, but if your lids appear to be normal in the morning but then sag noticeably as the day goes on, you may have myasthenia gravis, a rare neurological disease. You may also have diplopia, or double vision. Myasthenia gravis gradually progresses to the rest of the body if left untreated.

Myasthenia gravis is a rare condition in which the body chemicals that control the neurotransmitters that transmit electrical impulses from the nerves to the muscles, particularly acetylcholine, fail to work properly. In effect, the nerves run out of gas. The cause of myasthenia gravis is not confirmed, but we think it's due to a defect in the immune system. The disease affects primarily the facial muscles, particularly the eyelids and the muscles that control swallowing and the movement of the vocal cords. In addition to eyelids that progressively droop as the day goes on, a person with myasthenia gravis may find that she also starts to blink incessantly and uncontrollably, which can result in fatigue.

Treatment

Myasthenia gravis is such a rare disease that there's a good chance your drooping eyelids are a normal sign of aging. However, if your eyelids continue to droop noticeably over the course of the day, you should see your doctor. Myasthenia gravis is thought to be caused by a reaction by the immune system. It is commonly treated with regular medical checkups to monitor your condition and the avoidance of certain medications such as antibiotics, beta-blockers, and psychotropic drugs, which can make the symptoms of myasthenia gravis worse.

But some medications, such as the decongestant ephedrine hydrochloride, and corticosteroids, are routinely prescribed to treat the disease. These medications can help bolster the immune system and ease the symptoms of myasthenia gravis. They can also prevent the breakdown of acetylcholine, allowing the nerves to continue to send messages to one another and the muscles.

EYELIDS, FLAT YELLOW GROWTHS UNDER

Description and Possible Medical Problems

If you wake up one day and find a flat yellow growth on the underside of an eyelid, the first thing you should do is call your doctor to have your cholesterol checked. This flat yellow growth, called a xanthelasma, is a cholesterol deposit that has gathered under the eyelid. Flat yellow growths can also occasionally occur in diabetics.

Treatment

Xanthelasimae are not in themselves a health problem; however, whether or not you're predisposed to high blood cholesterol and triglyceride levels, if these flat yellow growths appear under one or both of your eyelids, you should definitely monitor your cholesterol levels and start proper treatment with diet, exercise, and medication.

If you think the deposits are unsightly, your doctor can remove them on an outpatient basis. They may, however, grow back, especially if you do not treat your high cholesterol.

EYELID, LUMP IN

Description and Possible Medical Problems

"I have a sty in my eye." Most of us have experienced a sty, an infection that occurs at the root of an eyelash, at one time or another. It may feel as though a tiny pea or pebble is stuck in your eye, and, because it is an irritant, the entire eye may become red and sore. Some people develop another kind of lump on the eyelid, called a chalazion, which is similar to a sty except that the infection occurs near the edge of the eyelid in the skin of the lid next to the eye. A chalazion looks like a lump in your eyelid, and you may feel as though you have a foreign body in your eye. A chalazion forms when one of the glands that lubricates the edge of the eyelid, called a meibomian gland, becomes blocked. But, unlike a sty, a chalazion doesn't hurt.

Treatment

In most cases, you can take care of a sty or chalazion yourself. In fact, treating a sty yourself will speed up the healing process and relieve the pain. Simply apply a warm, damp washcloth to the area two or three times an hour. When the sty looks as though it's about to burst, you can either pull out the eyelash near the sty or let the sty burst by itself. Once all the pus has run out of the sty, wash the area with warm water. The area will heal totally in a day or two.

To treat a chalazion, you should gently rub the swelling toward the edge of the eyelid. This usually causes the meibomian gland to become unblocked and the pus to drain quickly. Again, make sure to wash the eyelid with warm water. As with a sty, the lid will quickly heal.

Unless the infection grows so large that it begins to interfere with your sight, you may decide to wait out a sty or chalazion. But once it becomes larger than a small pea, it can distort the appearance of the eye and become unattractive, so you'll probably want to treat it purely for aesthetic reasons.

If either of these self-help remedies doesn't work, you should see your eye doctor, who will probably lance the sty or chalazion to allow it to drain and then treat the site with a topical antibiotic such as Bactrim, applied two or three times daily for about a week.

EYELID, SWOLLEN

Description and Possible Medical Problems

If your eyelid is swollen but you haven't injured it and you have none of the other symptoms listed in this chapter—since swelling accompanies some of these symptoms—it's highly likely that you're having an allergic reaction or your eyelid has been bitten by an insect.

Treatment

In either case, a swollen eyelid is easy to treat and usually disappears quickly. If you're having an allergic reaction to a food or other substance, try to avoid the allergen if you know what it is, and treat the other traditional signs of allergy, such as a runny nose, with your regular allergy medication (see "Eyes, Itchy and Burning" above). The swelling should disappear within a day or two.

If you think the swelling has been caused by an insect bite, examine your eyelid to see if the stinger is still intact. If it's still there, you can apply a wet, warm washcloth for a few minutes and then gently try to pull the stinger out with a tweezers. Then place a cold washcloth on your eye to reduce the swelling.

If the stinger doesn't come out easily or the swelling doesn't go down after a couple of days, see your doctor.

EYELID, TWITCHING

Description and Possible Medical Problems

If you're like most people, occasionally you'll find your eyelid will twitch for a few seconds for no apparent reason. It's not unusual to be alarmed at the twitching, simply because you're not sure what is causing your eyelid to flutter. The good news is that most eyelid twitches are nothing to worry about, and they usually go away within a few minutes.

Treatment

A twitching eyelid is often caused by anxiety or fatigue. Most of the time, however, there is no obvious cause.

However, to stop the twitching, which can be annoying, you should try one or more of the following suggestions. Relax. Do some exercise. Listen to your favorite music, or else try to get some rest if you're over-tired.

If all else fails and your twitching eyelid becomes an annoyance, your doctor may decide to prescribe a small dose of Valium as a last resort to help you relax. This method, however, will bring only short-term results. To benefit in the long term, you need to reduce the amount of stress in your life.

In rare cases, a twitching eyelid can be a sign of a serious underlying disease such as multiple sclerosis or another neurological condition that affects the facial muscles. However, with these diseases, other, more severe symptoms are usually present that will help a doctor make a clear diagnosis.

EYES, ITCHY AND BURNING

Description and Possible Medical Problems

In the old days, it seemed as if people who are prone to allergies experienced flare-ups only in the summer, when ragweed is in full bloom. Today, however, it seems as if allergies occur all year round. The chemicals that we use both at home and at work are frequently the culprits, from pollutants, cosmetics, and detergents to the chemicals thrown off by copy machines. In fact, I have a friend who's also a doctor, and he's allergic to the formaldehyde in the carpets in his new home.

Whether you're allergic to animal hair, pollen, or floor cleaner, one of the universal symptoms of allergy is that your eyes become red and itchy, and boy, do they burn!

Though no one knows exactly why an allergy develops in a particular individual, if you have a particular allergy, there's a good chance one of your parents or siblings has it, too.

An allergy develops because the body is unable to process a particular substance—dust, food, or another substance—due to a void in the immune system. Actually, the way your eyes react to the offending substance is pretty remarkable. As if on cue, upon initial exposure to that substance, they begin to water and itch as if to literally push it out and away.

Treatment

If you are allergic to a particular substance, the first thing you should do is try to avoid the allergen. If it's inside the house, open the windows; if the allergen is outside, keep your windows closed.

There are many over-the-counter preparations you can use in a variety of formulas, from pills and capsules to nasal sprays and eyedrops. A diphenhydramine hydrochloride preparation, such as Benadryl, or a chlorpheniramine maleate preparation, such as Chlortrimeton, helps relieve the symptoms of allergy but causes drowsiness. If this is a problem, you should see your physician to find out about taking some of the new prescription allergy formulations that don't cause drowsiness, such as Claritin, Hismanal, or Seldane. However, the latter medications tend to be less effective in treating your symptoms than the former are, so it's your call.

In any case, if your allergy symptoms are particularly severe and include wheezing or shortness of breath, you should see your doctor because you may need to use a bronchodilator spray like Ventolin to help you breathe.

If you think you have hay fever but it's accompanied by a yellow nasal discharge and head pain, you may actually have sinusitis, a sinus infection. (See "Sinuses, Painful, with Fever" in Chapter 6 for more information about sinusitis.)

FLASHING LIGHTS

Description and Possible Medical Problems

Flashing lights are pretty when they're part of a Christmas or Fourth of July display, but when they regularly occur as part of the early stages of a migraine headache, they quickly lose their luster.

Migraines have the reputation of being able to totally disable a person, and for good reason. If you've ever experienced a migraine, also known as a vascular headache, you know that the pain in your head can be so intense that you're physically unable to do more than lie in bed in a darkened room and wait for the pain to subside.

Before a migraine hits fully, the flashing lights appear because the constricted arteries reduce the flow of blood to the part of the brain that controls your vision. In addition to the flashing lights, you may experience blind spots, vertigo, and nausea. These are all signs that a migraine is imminent.

We don't know exactly what causes a migraine headache. However, at a migraine's worst, the carotid and vertebral arteries in the brain, which supply it with blood, first narrow and then swell up, sometimes to twice their normal size. This decreases the amount of blood supplied to your brain. The combination of the swollen arteries and the reduced blood supply is the reason for the crushing pain that can totally incapacitate you. Most migraines last from a few hours to several days. After the pain subsides, you'll probably feel groggy and lethargic for a while.

For a full description of migraine headaches and their treatments, see "Headache with Sensitivity to Light, Nausea, and Vomiting" in Chapter 3.

FOCUSING, PROBLEMS IN

Description and Possible Medical Problems

If you have had trouble focusing your eyes lately, you should check to see if other symptoms are present. You should also ask yourself whether the focusing problem has come on suddenly or has appeared gradually. If your inability to focus appears all of a sudden, the problem is frequently just one of several symptoms—such as redness and irritation—that signal a temporary eye disorder such as conjunctivitis, the inflammation of another part of the eye, or a corneal ulcer.

Treatment

If you've only recently noticed that you find it difficult to focus easily, the problem is usually easy to fix. Maybe all you need is to have the strength of your glasses or contacts increased. Deterioration of vision is a given for most midlife adults, but the good news is that after the age of 65, usually no further vision loss takes place. In fact, some people have discovered that the shape of their eyes has changed in such a way that they don't have to wear glasses at all. If, however, your inability to focus has appeared suddenly and your eyes are red and painful, you probably have an eye infection, and you should see your eye doctor to clear it up. For treatment details, see "Discharge with Redness" above.

Rest assured that if you're having trouble focusing and it's not accompanied by any other eye problem, it's a normal sign of aging and is usually nothing to worry about.

GLARE

Description and Possible Medical Problems

If you're driving and there's a lot of glare through the windshield, not only is it uncomfortable, it's also dangerous because it hides part of what you need to see to stay safely on the road.

When glare occurs by itself without the influence of strong sunlight, it might be an early symptom of glaucoma or cataracts. Then again, it may only be a sign that your contact lenses need to be cleaned.

A certain amount of glare occurs naturally with age, since the lenses and vitreous humor change in size and scope, affecting how light is diffused across the retina.

Treatment

If you are experiencing a constant glare in your field of vision and your contacts—if you wear them—are relatively clean, you should see your doctor. Glaucoma and cataracts are serious threats to your vision, and early treatment is essential in order to restore as much of your vision as possible.

See also "Vision, Slow, Progressive Change in, Accompanied by General Cloudiness" below.

VISION, BLIND SPOT IN THE CENTER OF

Description and Possible Medical Problems

If you've recently developed a blind spot in the center of your field of vision and you've noticed that your vision is slowly worsening, it may be because the part of the retina called the macula is deteriorating, as it tends to do with age. The retina is a thin layer of tissue that covers the back of your eyeball and contains the rods and cones—microscopic structures within the eye—that help detect and process light images before sending them on to the brain via the optic nerve. The rods and cones are visible only when eye tissue is observed under a microscope; they cannot be seen by the naked eye. The macula processes the images that appear in your central field of vision. The choroid is another layer of tissue that lies behind the retina and contains the blood vessels that supply the eye with blood. When arteriosclerosis starts to harden the veins and arteries throughout the body, the vessels in the choroid are also affected, altering the macula and your central field of vision. Macular degeneration is usually slow and painless, and many people don't realize that anything is seriously wrong until they discover that even a magnifying glass won't help them see objects up close anymore; however, it is a condition that usually doesn't begin to show up until the 70s and 80s. Macular degeneration usually affects both eyes—sometimes both at the same time, sometimes one after the other—and many times a person who has had surgery to have her cataracts removed is more prone to developing macular degeneration.

The blood supply to the retina can also be reduced if the blood vessels in the choroid are leaking. When a reduced blood supply is the cause of macular degeneration, the condition is easier to treat.

Even though macular degeneration is the number one cause of legal blindness among Americans today, it's actually not the disability it was once considered to be. Because macular degeneration affects only the central field of vision, the vast majority of people who have the condition and are legally blind can still get around on their own because they can still see objects on the outer edges of their visual field.

Treatment

If you detect a blind spot in the center of your vision, it's important to see your eye doctor right away. First, he will run several tests to determine the degree to which your vision is affected. If your macular degeneration has not advanced significantly, your doctor may use laser therapy to repair the macula and reattach it to the retina. This will not eliminate the damage to your eye but will slow its progression. Laser therapy can also help to close the blood vessels that are leaking and therefore depriving the macula of blood.

Laser surgery can be performed on an outpatient basis in your ophthalmologist's office, and you can go home the same day. Your vision may be slightly impaired after the procedure, and you'll need to visit your ophthalmologist for close follow-up for about a month after surgery.

Even though laser surgery will help restore the central vision in many cases, it should not be considered a panacea, since the results are not always fully successful. When the macular degeneration cannot be treated with laser surgery, special prescription eyeglass lenses can help to restore some degree of central vision.

VISION, BLURRED

Description and Possible Medical Problems

We are all affected by blurred vision at one time or another. Fatigue, poor light, and alcohol can all make it difficult to focus clearly. And when you wear eyeglasses or contacts and it's time for a stronger prescription, your vision may be blurred more frequently.

If objects occasionally appear blurry to you and your eyesight is otherwise good, whether it's corrected by lenses or not, the condition is usually temporary and easy to treat. Blurriness is usually due to changes in the pupil, the part of the eye that is the first to react when our line of vision changes in some way.

The pupil is a black disk in the center of the colored part of the eye, which is called the iris. The pupil's function is to regulate the amount of light that enters the eye, and it is controlled by involuntary muscles that respond to stimuli. Around the age of 50, as is true of many other parts of your body, the pupil's reflexes start to decrease somewhat; it may take just a bit longer for the pupil to dilate or contract in response to the amount of light it can detect. This slowed reaction due to aging is a given, and there's nothing you can do to improve it. The pupil can also become wider or more narrow in response to certain medications, such as atropine, which is prescribed to calm an irritable or spastic bowel, pilocarpine, or cocaine, as well as when you're physically or mentally excited.

With many of the problems that occur in the eye, blurred vision is one of several symptoms including headache, dizziness, and bright flashes of light. However, if blurred vision appears by itself slowly over time with no other symptoms, the problem is usually easy to fix. The solution will probably lie in your glasses or contact lenses.

Treatment

The first thing to do if your vision is blurry is to check your glasses or contacts to see if they're dirty or smeared. Frequently, blurred vision is caused by a problem with your corrective lenses, whether they've been scratched or just need cleaning. If you've worn the same nondisposable pair of contact lenses for more than a year, the protein buildup on the lenses can be so extensive that even the recommended weekly enzyme cleaners won't remove it. Sometimes a slight tear in a contact lens can also cause blurred vision, so it's a good idea to check for this as well.

If you wear glasses, examine the lenses for scratches. Even scratch-resistant lenses can become marred.

After you clean your glasses or contact lenses thoroughly, your vision should be crystal clear. If, however, your vision is still blurry, see your eye doctor. All you may need is a stronger prescription.

BODY SIGNAL ALERT

VISION, CYLINDRICAL

Description and Possible Medical Problems

You know how it is when you look through a telescope—even though you are focusing on an image, you're still aware that you're looking through a tube.

But what if you have this sensation without looking through a telescope? If you notice that you are gradually losing your field of vision in one eye, you may have glaucoma, which is one of the most common eye problems today and one of the leading causes of blindness. In addition to your monocular field loss, other symptoms of glaucoma may include eye pain, blurred vision, and redness. Though glaucoma usually begins in one eye, it will eventually affect the vision in both eyes. As a result, both eyes will have to undergo treatment at the same time, even if only one eye shows symptoms of the disease.

Glaucoma is a condition in which the aqueous humor, the fluid that lubricates the outside of the eyeball, is unable to drain out of the eye normally. This usually occurs because of a blockage in the drainage channel that allows the fluid to drain out of the eye and into the veins that surround the eye.

When the drainage channel is blocked, the fluid drains away more slowly than usual or may become totally blocked. When this happens, the fluid builds up in the eye, creating pressure on the vitreous humor, the gel-like substance that makes up the internal part of the eyeball. This, in turn, presses on the vessels that provide the optic nerve with a steady flow of blood, slowing it down or stopping it completely. And when the blood flow ceases, the nerve begins to die, resulting in a gradual decline of vision.

Glaucoma usually begins to show up in people around the age of 40. There is also a genetic tendency to glaucoma; if a relative had the condition, you should be alert to changes in your eyesight and get medical attention promptly if you notice a one-eye field loss or develop a feeling of looking through a tube.

Treatment

If you think you might have glaucoma, it's important to act quickly, since once the blood flow to the optic nerve starts to slow down, your vision may be permanently affected. Prompt treatment will save much of the optic nerve and thus your vision. Your doctor will prescribe special eye drops and medication such as Betoptic and Pilocarpine, which will open the drainage channel and decrease the amount of aqueous humor your eye produces. This will allow the aqueous humor to drain as well as decrease the pressure on the vitreous humor, and your vision will return almost immediately. In order to prevent future problems caused by glaucoma, these medications will probably become part of your daily routine for the rest of your life. The good news is that your eyesight will probably stay the same.

In rare instances, medication will not be effective in reducing the pressure on the optic nerve. If this is the case, you will probably be advised to undergo a surgical procedure that will permanently improve the drainage from the eye. The operation will consist of making a small cut that will increase the size of the drainage channel. This is usually done with laser surgery or by inserting a small tube through which the fluid can drain. Either procedure will ensure that your vision is saved.

Tips and Precautions

Once you've been diagnosed with glaucoma, you'll need regular eye checkups at least once a year. This is especially true if you are over 60 or if you have diabetes or hypertension.

VISION, DISTORTED

Description and Possible Medical Problems

When you first wake up in the morning, it's not that uncommon for your vision to be distorted. The digital numbers on your clock may appear a bit wavy, or the cat may look thinner than she really is. Usually, blinking your eyes a few times or just sitting up to regain your equilibrium is enough to make your vision return to normal.

You can blame this funhouse mirror act on your retina and the gradual, yet harmless, deterioration it undergoes as our eyes age. Since the retina's function is to decode the light that enters the eye through the lens before sending it on to the final processor, the brain, when the retina becomes less flexible with age, the image your brain "sees" will be temporarily distorted in some manner. Some people will notice a slight difference in their vision; for others, the change will be quite dramatic.

Treatment

A certain amount of deterioration in the retina is natural and starts to become noticeable after the age of 60. As aging affects the retina, it becomes dull, and the amount of time it requires to process the light entering the retina increases.

Unfortunately, there's not much you can do to prevent deterioration of the retina. The good news is that a stronger eyeglass or contact lens prescription can frequently cure the distortion. You should, however, be alert to changes in your vision, because sometimes the distorted images you're seeing as the result of an aging retina can lead to more serious retinal problems, such as macular degeneration and retinal detachment.

See also "Vision, Blind Spot in the Center of" above and "Eye, 'Curtain' in Front of" above.

VISION, DOUBLE

Description and Possible Medical Problems

If you cross your eyes, you'll see two of whatever you're looking at. But if you begin to see double without purposely crossing your eyes, you should see your doctor, since this condition can be a symptom of diabetes, hypertension, or arteriosclerosis.

Double vision, also known as diplopia, occurs when one of your eyes crosses by itself or when the picture one of your eyes receives is not being processed properly by the brain. Ordinarily, the muscles of the eyes work together to coordinate two images into one picture. However, when one of the body's major operating systems goes awry—such as with diabetes or hypertension—it can affect how the ocular muscles operate. Sometimes a trauma to one of the nerves in the brain that controls the eye muscles—such as an aneurysm—can affect your eyesight.

When double vision is caused by an aneurysm, a condition in which the wall of an artery swells, the aneurysm can press on some of the nerves that affect sight. Arteriosclerosis can reduce or completely stop the flow of blood to the optic nerve, and diabetes frequently affects circulation to the retina.

Double vision tends to occur in diabetics who have had their disease for ten years or more. The altered metabolic processes that are a symptom of diabetes can sometimes deprive the retina of oxygen, with one result being double vision.

Treatment

Sometimes double vision disappears by itself in one to three months, no matter what the cause. But because double vision is often a symptom of a serious medical condition, you should see your physician so she can begin treatment if necessary.

Treatment for double vision depends on its cause. When an aneurysm is responsible, surgery is the primary treatment, and after the aneurysm is repaired you will need to be closely monitored by your doctor to make sure your blood pressure remains under control. Your doctor will probably recommend that you switch to a low-fat, low-salt diet so that your high blood pressure and/or arteriosclerosis doesn't worsen. Both conditions can aggravate an aneurysm and cause it to burst.

If diabetes is causing you to see double, the best thing you can do is to follow the program your physician has recommended to control your diabetes; in this case, your double vision should disappear in a week or two. Double vision caused by diabetes may disappear on its own a month or two after it first begins. Nevertheless, it's important to see your doctor to make sure you don't have an additional medical problem—such as high blood pressure or arteriosclerosis—that can make it worse. It's best to have your doctor monitor your health regularly.

VISION, FLOATING SPECKS AND FLASHES OF LIGHT IN

Description and Possible Medical Problems

A recently retired schoolteacher came to my office a few months ago for a routine visit. At 63, this woman has incredible energy and devotes most of her time to caring for an extensive backyard garden that she has been working on for years. "I feel absolutely terrific," she told me, "except for one very strange thing. Every once in a while, I think I've got fireflies in my eyes!"

As odd as that description may sound, her problem is actually quite common. If you're seeing specks of flashing light, ask yourself the following questions:

1. Do I see lines, particles, webs, and clusters of dots that move slowly across my field of vision?

2. Does this occur most frequently when I'm outside in the sunshine, when I'm looking at something against a plain background, or when I'm in an exceptionally well-lit room?

3. Do these floating specks seem to speed up when I move my eyes?

4. Do they come to a halt when I keep my eyes still?

5. Do I see flashing vertical lights (as opposed to steady glare)? Do I see lightning streaks in one eye at a time?

If you've answered yes to these questions, chances are you have the usually harmless disorder known as "floaters" and "flashes."

Treatment

Floaters and flashes are signs that the vitreous humor, the gelatin-like substance filling the space between the retina and the lens, is aging. In the early part of your life, the vitreous humor is clear, but the aging process makes it appear opaque in certain spots, which can cause vision problems. Many people begin to feel the effects of vitreous humor decay and shrinkage by the time 50 or 60 rolls around.

One form of vitreous humor degeneration causes tiny clumps to detach from the retina and float freely inside the eye's fluid. These microscopic specks cast shadows on the retina, and you see them as "floaters." Both nearsighted people and those who have had cataract surgery are especially vulnerable to floaters, but the problem seems to affect the over-50 population in general.

Floaters are certainly annoying but are usually nothing to worry about. The bad news is that there's really no cure for ordinary floaters, and they occasionally may get in the way of reading. The good news is that you can expect them to disappear over time.

However, if your floaters come in heavy showers accompanied by flashing lights, you may have a detached retina, and the shower of floaters may be a sign of retinal bleeding. If this is followed by fixed dark spots, you may already have retinal scarring. See your ophthalmologist immediately if you experience these symptoms. A detached retina can be repaired through laser surgery as long as you take care of the problem quickly.

Flashes originate because the vitreous humor starts out like Jell-O but becomes more liquified as the years pass. This change weakens the bond between the vitreous humor and the retina. In this weakened state, eye movements can tug at the vitreous humor, stimulating the retina automatically and causing you to see brief flashes of light. The flashes you see will be fleeting and probably confined to one eye. Be careful not to confuse this sensation with steady glare, a benchmark symptom of cataracts.

If you see flashes in both eyes that last for 10 to 20 minutes and are accompanied by pain, you're probably suffering from a migraine headache.

If the flashes are accompanied by a loss of vision or another change in your visual acuity, especially if your field of vision seems as though it is covered by a veil, make an appointment with your ophthalmologist immediately. These may be signs of a detached retina.

Tips and Precautions

Again, there's not much you can do to get rid of these little annoyances but wait them out. However, here's a helpful strategy: When one of those floaters appears, shoo it away by moving your eye around. Movement activates your eye's fluid, which may swirl the floater out of your line of vision.

VISION, GRADUAL DETERIORATION OF

Description and Possible Medical Problems

For most of us, a certain amount of deterioration in our vision is almost inevitable as we grow older. I find I can no longer work on models with small parts, as I have trouble focusing my eyes. I refuse to give in, however, which runs counter to the advice that my own ophthalmologist has given me. I will not wear reading glasses or bifocals, mostly for reasons of vanity. Instead, I wear contacts. The lens in one eye is for distance, while the other lens helps me to do close-up work.

I've found that what is almost universal among midlife adults and older is the gradual appearance of a kind of farsightedness called presbyopia, in which you will find it increasingly necessary to hold a book or newspaper farther away from you in order to see clearly. Whether you've traditionally been nearsighted or farsighted in the past doesn't matter. And if you've always been envious of a friend who's enjoyed 20/20 vision most of his life, relax, because there is such a thing as divine retribution—even people blessed with perfect vision are affected by presbyopia to some degree.

Presbyopia most often starts to appear in your mid-40s. You may find it also takes longer for your vision to adjust when you switch from looking at a faraway object to one that is up close—and vice versa. And the amount of time it takes for your eyes to adjust to the dark may also be longer. Sometimes presbyopia is accompanied by headache and eye-strain as you try to adjust to your altered sense of vision.

These symptoms are part of the normal aging process. As we get older, the structure of certain parts of our eye changes. The lenses become stiff, which makes it harder for them to adjust so that they can focus on objects that are close up.

Presbyopia, as well as nearsightedness (myopia) and farsightedness (hypermetropia), are vision problems that result when the rays of light that enter the eye are not bent or refracted properly. The light that reflects off an object enters the eye through the cornea, where it passes through the lens, which then bends the rays. If this refracted light hits the retina at its focal point, your eyes have 20/20 vision and the images are sharp and clear; no correction with eyeglasses or contact lenses is necessary. The image is then sent on to the brain via the optic nerve.

When a person is nearsighted, the focal point occurs behind the retina. In farsightedness, the focal point occurs in front of the retina. Glasses or contact lenses can correct either problem.

With presbyopia, the focal point is the same; it's the gradual hardening of the lens that causes the eye to work harder to focus on an object.

If you think you have presbyopia, try this simple test. Open the phone book to the white pages, and focus on a few telephone numbers. Slowly move the book away from you until you find that you don't have to strain to focus on the numbers. If you find you need to have your arms almost fully extended before the numbers come into focus, you probably have presbyopia.

Treatment

For people who have presbyopia, bifocals—glasses with two different strengths of lenses in them—are the most common solution. The top half of the lens will help you see more clearly at a distance, while the bottom half will improve your reading as well as your ability to focus on objects you need to see up close. Nowadays, new types of bifocals are available in which there is no "line" between the upper and lower halves, so that no one can tell that you're wearing bifocals.

However, as baby boomers can be as vain as I am when it comes to wearing glasses, there is hope in the form of contact lenses. Bausch & Lomb makes a special bifocal contact lens called Multifocal that is designed to be worn when you don't want to wear glasses.

Unfortunately, ophthalmologists recommend that you increase the strength of your prescription every three to four years after the age of 40, since the lens of your eye will continue to become stiffer, which will ultimately alter your vision. Fortunately, eyesight stops deteriorating at about the age of 65, making further prescription upgrades unnecessary.

VISION, SLOW, PROGRESSIVE CHANGE IN, ACCOMPANIED BY GENERAL CLOUDINESS

Description and Possible Medical Problems

Everyone's vision changes to some extent with age. However, if your vision continues to become blurry regardless of a change in your glasses or contacts prescription and is accompanied by a general cloudiness, you may have developed cataracts on the lenses of your eyes. Ask yourself the following questions:

1. Do I have poor night vision?

2. Do I find it hard to see in bright light?

3. Do I sometimes think my eyesight is actually improving because I am temporarily able to read without my glasses, a condition known as "second sight"?

If you have some or all of these symptoms, you should see your doctor as soon as possible, because they are a sign of cataracts. For most people, a cataract will start to form in one eye, but the condition will quickly spread to the other. Sometimes a cataract will also cause pain and inflammation of the eye.

It's not known precisely what causes cataracts. However, a chemical reaction is believed to be the first step in the process that begins to alter the composition of the lens. Some of the conditions that have been implicated in the later development of cataracts include a physical trauma or injury to the eye; a condition called iritis, which is an inflammation of the iris of the eye; and diabetes. If you've been taking corticosteroid medications for a long period of time or have spent a lot of time outdoors in bright sunlight or indoors on a tanning bed, you may also be more prone to developing cataracts due to the damaging effects ultraviolet rays have on the eyes and skin.

Though infants are sometimes born with cataracts, the vast majority of people who have the condition are age 50 and over. In fact, by age 60 most adults have cataracts to some degree, whether mild or severe.

If your doctor tells you that your deteriorating vision is due to cataracts, you shouldn't worry. In the past, a diagnosis of cataracts was virtually a guarantee of future blindness. But today, with more than half a million people undergoing cataract surgery in the United States each year, the operation is common and recovery with clear vision is almost assured.

Treatment

If you're one of those people who develop a mild case of cataracts and your vision remains relatively stable, your doctor may suggest that you do nothing for the time being. She may prescribe special eyedrops, which will enlarge the pupil and thus reduce the effect the cataract has on your vision, and take a wait-and-see approach. But if the cataracts develop and begin to hamper your eyesight, the only treatment is surgical removal.

Because cataract removal is such a common and relatively simple procedure, the surgery can be done under local or general anesthesia on an outpatient basis. During the operation, the lens of the affected eye is removed and a new, artificial lens is inserted in its place. The surgery takes about an hour, and the new lens may negate the need for glasses or contact lenses, since the surgeon can tailor a lens so that it will be the only corrective lens you'll need.

My mother had her cataracts removed several years ago, and after the surgery she had to wear an eye patch for about a week. The family arranged for my sister to stay with her during that time, because we were concerned that she might fall because of her temporary loss of vision. Three weeks later, she was back to driving her car without wearing glasses.

For some people, however, a lens implant is unwise because of the shape and structure of the eye. In this case, when the lens is removed and no artificial lens is inserted, you will become farsighted. However, this condition can be corrected with eyeglasses or contact lenses.

Cataract removal with or without lens implantation will improve most people's vision. Sometimes, however, the eyesight will remain poor. In this case the problem may lie with the retina, and your doctor will be able to treat this condition as well.

See also "Vision, Blind Spot in the Center of" above.

BODY SIGNAL ALERT

VISION, SUDDEN CHANGE OF IN ONE EYE

Description and Possible Medical Problems

Gradual changes in your eyesight may be a symptom of aging or an easily treated problem with the eye itself. Sometimes, however, your eyesight will suddenly worsen—for instance, you may not be able to see the entire left side of your field of vision while you're looking straight ahead. If this happens, you may have a headache or vertigo or may be slurring your speech or be unable to use an arm or leg—or both—on the same side of the body. This is usually an indication of a vascular injury to the brain, such as a stroke, and you should see your doctor immediately.

Several parts of the brain that enable you to see are located in different parts of the organ. One part of the brain, called the frontal eye field area, which is located just above the frontal lobe, controls your field of vision. A pair of cranial nerves that jut out from the brain stem helps to control eye movement. A small part of the brain called the primary visual area, which is located at the very back of the brain behind the occipital lobe, processes the pictures the optic nerve sends it. A trauma that affects any of these parts can cause you suddenly to lose your sight.

In some cases, however, a small stroke that causes an interruption of the blood flow to one eye can cause sudden blindness in that same eye. This is called amaurosis fugax, and it is most often caused by the narrowing of the carotid arteries. This condition appears frequently in people in their mid- to late 60s who are heavy smokers.

Treatment

Because there are many cerebral problems that may be responsible for a sudden loss of vision, you need to see your doctor right away. A slow-growing brain tumor could be putting pressure on one of the parts of the brain that influences your eyesight. A trauma or blow to the skull can also cause you to lose part or all of your vision in both eyes for a few days.

See also "Bulging, One Eye" above, "Vision, Sudden Loss of in One Eye" below, and "Visual Field, Sudden Loss on One Side of" below.

BODY SIGNAL ALERT

VISION, SUDDEN LOSS OF IN ONE EYE

Description and Possible Medical Problems

If you are suddenly unable to see in one of your eyes, see your doctor immediately. The most common cause of losing the sight in one eye is a disease or trauma to the carotid artery, one of the arteries that provides your brain with the blood supply it needs to function. Any interruption in this flow could temporarily or permanently affect one of the parts of the brain that controls eyesight. A carotid artery that has developed arteriosclerosis due to the plaque buildup that is a result of excess fat and cholesterol in the diet may also cut off some of the blood supply to the brain, resulting in a sudden loss of vision in one eye.

The carotid artery provides blood to the optic nerve, iris, and retina. When the blood flow to these is reduced, temporary blindness can occur. In this case, you may experience the sensation of a curtain being drawn across the eye and then suddenly opened.

Sometimes men and women who have carotid disease and blindness in one eye will experience fatigue and numbness in the arm and/or leg on the side of the body that's opposite the affected eye. Some people also find that they experience temporary blindness in one eye when they bend over or stand up quickly or when they look at a bright light.

Given this, you should ask yourself the following two questions so that you'll be well prepared with answers for your doctor:

1. When I cover one eye, is the vision in the other eye normal?

2. Have I lost part of my vision, such as the left-hand side of the field of vision in both eyes?

Treatment

Carotid disease is a progressive disease. People who experience monocular blindness—or an inability to see out of one eye—due to carotid arteriosclerosis have already experienced some degree of arterial blockage in their arteries.

If your doctor suspects that carotid artery disease is causing your one-eyed vision loss, he will probably order an ultrasound examination of your head and neck, both to measure the degree of blockage and to determine the amount of blood that is reaching the brain. An angiogram, in which a harmless dye is injected into your arteries in order to get a clear picture of your blockage, may be done if the results of the sonogram are unclear or if your doctor believes the arteriosclerosis is severe.

Depending on the severity of the buildup on the walls of your carotid artery, your doctor will choose one of several treatment options. If the disease is still in its early stages, a daily dose of aspirin is usually all that's needed. Aspirin has been found to have anticoagulant properties, which will help keep your blood thin and prevent it from forming clots. If the blockage is more severe, your doctor may prescribe either warfarin or heparin. Warfarin is an anticoagulant, but is more powerful than aspirin. Heparin is also an anticoagulant but is usually prescribed when arteriosclerosis is more pronounced.

Your doctor may suggest you undergo an endarterectomy, or the surgical removal of plaque from the walls of an artery, if he thinks a stroke seems imminent because of blockage and/or the presence of blood clots in your carotid artery. Though an endarterectomy presents a risk because the blood flow to the brain through the carotid artery is stopped during the operation, once you undergo the procedure, it is unlikely that plaque will develop on the walls of the artery again.

There are two carotid arteries, and sometimes both are clogged. The worst one would have the endarterectomy first, and the second one would be untouched now, and be performed at a later date.

BODY SIGNAL ALERT

VISUAL FIELD, PARTIAL LOSS OF

Description and Possible Medical Problems

It's not unusual to suddenly lose part or all of your vision for a few seconds as a result of a physical injury—for instance, when you see stars during the impact of a car accident. Your sight will usually be fully restored within a few days.

But what happens when you suddenly become unable to see within a small area or visual field or can see only some of the objects located within that area?

Partial loss of a visual field is commonly known as a scotoma, and it affects people in a variety of ways. A scotoma may result in total blindness to all objects within the affected field, or the affected person may be able to pick out certain large objects but not smaller ones. Sometimes the scotoma will be visible as flashes of light that occur only within a partial visual field; this is called a scintillating scotoma.

A number of health problems can cause a scotoma. Certain eye diseases, such as glaucoma, the inflammation of the optic nerve called optic neuritis, and a retinal disorder called macular degeneration, can cause a scotoma. A scintillating scotoma frequently occurs in people who suffer from migraine headaches. Prompt treatment is necessary in order to prevent permanent damage to your vision.

Treatment

To treat a scotoma, your doctor will first have to address the underlying condition that is causing the partial loss of a visual field. Scotomas that are caused by glaucoma or macular degeneration lessen or disappear when these conditions are treated. A scintillating scotoma will disappear when a migraine subsides. However, with optic neuritis, the vision loss will last until the inflammation of the optic nerve subsides, which can take up to three weeks or more. Since optic neuritis can sometimes be painful, your doctor may recommend that you remain still and quiet and try to restrict your eye movement to hasten your recovery. Optic neuritis can also be an early symptom of multiple sclerosis, so your doctor will want to monitor your health closely to check the progress of the disease.

BODY SIGNAL ALERT

VISUAL FIELD, SUDDEN LOSS ON ONE SIDE OF

Description and Possible Medical Problems

If you suddenly lose all or part of your ability to see on one side of your entire field of vision, and if your eyesight decreases markedly over the course of only a couple of hours, you must see your doctor immediately because this is a sign of a stroke.

A stroke, also known as a cerebrovascular accident, occurs when the flow of blood to the brain is interrupted, even for as little as a minute. A stroke can be due to several different types of blockage. In one type of stroke, called a cerebral thrombosis, the arteries that supply blood to the brain have become lined with plaque (this is known as arteriosclerosis). A blood clot may form where the plaque lines the artery and eventually block the flow of blood to the brain. In a cerebral embolism, a blood clot or a small piece of plaque or arterial wall from another part of the body breaks off and travels through the arteries until it lodges in an artery, creating a blockage. Another type of stroke is a cerebral hemorrhage, in which the affected artery starts to leak or ruptures and blood flows into the brain. The accumulation of blood can then create pressure on the parts of the brain in which it masses and clots, cutting off the flow of blood and oxygen to the brain. If your loss of vision is accompanied by a severe headache, you have probably had a cerebral hemorrhage.

The loss of vision symptoms for all three types of stroke are similar, except that a cerebral hemorrhage usually causes more damage and is more often fatal than the other two are.

Stroke is most common in men and women over 60, but men are more prone to stroke and die more frequently from it. About one third of all strokes are fatal, while another third leave the person with permanent damage. Nevertheless, one third of all stroke victims suffer no permanent damage at all. If you fall into this last category, you may have had a transient ischemia attack, or TIA, which is a mild form of stroke in which the blockage and impaired vision last less than 24 hours. With a cerebral thrombosis or cerebral embolism, the symptoms tend to be permanent.

If you have had a TIA, you should begin treatment for arteriosclerosis immediately, since a TIA is an indication that you will probably have another stroke—perhaps a more serious one the next time around.

Treatment

If you have experienced a sudden loss of vision due to a stroke, your doctor will administer a series of tests in order to make a positive diagnosis. These may include an electrocardiogram, X rays, and possibly a CAT scan to determine which parts of the brain have been injured. To reduce the risk of a TIA or stroke recurring, your doctor will prescribe medication that will help control your high blood pressure, a daily dose of aspirin, which serves as an anticoagulant and discourages future clots from forming, and a low-salt and low-fat diet, which will also help lower your blood pressure.

Your vision will probably return to normal after a TIA; with a cerebral thrombosis or embolism, the damage may be permanent.

In some cases, surgery to remove arterial plaque may be necessary.

See also "Vision, Sudden Loss of in One Eye" above.

Chapter 6

EARS AND NOSE

BODY SIGNAL ALERT

Call your doctor or ear, nose, and throat specialist immediately if you experience any of the following symptoms:

SYMPTOM	POSSIBLE MEDICAL CONDITION
You have a rash or group of pimples along your ear	*Ramsay Hunt syndrome*
You have a sudden loss of hearing that's also accompanied by pain, dizziness and/or buzzing in your ears with fever	*Ear infection*
You have a sudden loss of hearing in one ear and feel dizzy	*Acoustic neuroma*
You are bleeding steadily from the nose	*Hypertension, injury, medication*

HOW THE EARS AND NOSE AGE

The human ear is sensitive to an amazing range of sounds. From a ticking watch—which clocks in at a safe 20 decibels—to a dangerous 140-decibel shotgun blast, not much escapes the healthy ear.

But as we age the years of lawn mowers and loud music take their toll. Men and women are usually in their 40s and 50s when they first become aware that their hearing is not what it used to be. Typically, they first notice a loss when they can no longer hear some of the higher frequencies, such as a whistle or the notes of a flute. Gradual hearing loss is the result of slow damage to the nerves of the inner ear, which sends sounds to the brain and helps you maintain your sense of balance. It can also occur because the bones of the middle ear become less flexible; the middle ear is responsible for conducting sound to the inner ear. The eardrum can also thicken with age, which can interfere with the quality of your hearing.

Fortunately, most ear conditions are easily treated. Modern technology has provided us with small, unobtrusive hearing aids, a tremendous advance from the clunky appliances of just a few years ago. With these advances, preventing further hearing loss is easy.

As we age the nose also changes, though it's usually one of the parts we're least concerned with. Over the years the nose loses cartilage, which may cause the tip of the nose to fall, but gravity's cumulative effects can also play a part. Though for most people the thinning cartilage brings only slight physical changes, in some the fall is so pronounced that the nose narrows and lengthens considerably. This can result in nasal obstruction, which makes it difficult to breathe. This loss of cartilage is a major reason why older people may snore more or breathe through their mouths when they sleep.

The mucus membranes in the nose also become thinner with age. Often the nose produces less mucus, which makes the nose feel drier. In addition, the sense of smell decreases with age, since the olfactory nerves become less effective after the age of 60.

DECREASED SENSE OF SMELL

Description and Possible Medical Problems

Mrs. C., a regular patient, visited me for a checkup and complained that food just didn't taste right to her anymore.

When I pressed her for details, she became visibly upset. "Oh, I don't know," she said. "Ever since I turned 60, it's as if all my senses have deteriorated. It just takes more of everything for me to smell anything lately."

She described how, in particular, food tasted bland and even the flowers in her garden didn't smell as sweet as they had the year before. Though, as a rule, women tend to retain their senses in later years better than men do, the sense of smell starts to fade when a person reaches his 50s and 60s. Since the sense of smell is closely connected with the ability to taste, sometimes the first sign that there's a problem will arise when foods don't taste the way they usually do. And sometimes certain diseases can hasten the loss.

If your loss of smell is sudden, it's probably not due to aging. Illness or allergies—whether they're seasonal or year round—can affect your sense of smell. So can the medication you're taking for it. In fact, taking any kind of prescription or over-the-counter medication can result in a decreased sense of smell.

To discover if your reduced sense of smell is due to regular aging or an illness, allergy, or medication, ask yourself the following questions:

- Can I pinpoint exactly when my sense of smell or taste began to decline? Or was it more gradual?

- Have I started to take a new medication recently?

- Have I recently recovered from a lengthy respiratory illness?

- Have I had major dental work done recently?

- Do I tend to lose my sense of smell at the same time every year?

Treatment

Though many people start to notice a decline in their ability to smell as early as their 40s, the loss usually doesn't become pronounced until they reach their 60s. In fact, there are many elderly men and women who can't smell at all.

Severe colds, the flu, and infections of the upper respiratory tract can completely take away your ability to smell. In this instance, as well as when medication is causing the decreased sense of smell, you just have to be patient. When you're better and/or have discontinued the medication, you'll be able to smell again. And if you've recently had major dental work done, your ability to smell will return after you've completely healed.

Occasionally, nasal polyps will result in a loss of smell. If you have trouble breathing due to these obstructions, see your doctor, who will probably recommend surgical removal of the polyps.

If you lose your sense of smell suddenly, it's important to keep in mind that the condition is probably reversible. If your loss is more gradual, aging is the culprit.

DIFFICULTY BREATHING

Description and Possible Medical Problems

Everyone occasionally suffers from a stuffed-up nose and the inability to breathe during a cold. This usually passes when you begin to feel better.

A certain amount of change in the structure of your nose as you get older can cause you to feel stuffed up. You can tell if your clogged nose is due to aging if you slightly raise the tip of your nose with your finger and find it's easier to breathe. Usually, however, the changing structure of the nose doesn't begin to interfere with clear breathing until the age of 60 and up.

However, when you find that it's difficult to breathe and you don't have a cold or flu, something else is causing it, probably a cold or a respiratory infection.

Treatment

A large number of adults are chronic users of nasal decongestants. If you're one of them, you probably first used an over-the-counter spray to clear up a stuffy nose from a cold, and then discovered that once your cold was over you couldn't breathe easily without them.

Some people quit their nasal spray habit gradually, while others feel that cold turkey is the only way to go. Whatever you choose, you should be prepared for discomfort and more stuffiness than you're used to for anywhere from a few days to several weeks. And the next time you have a cold with a stuffy nose, be sure to use nasal sprays sparingly, as directed on the package. Then, when your cold is over, stop using them.

See also "Decreased Sense of Smell" above, "Sinuses, Painful, with Fever" below, and "Wheezing" in Chapter 11.

EAR, CLOGGED FEELING IN

Description and Possible Medical Problems

You know how you feel when you're on a plane and coming in for a landing or driving down a mountain: your ears suddenly feel clogged. Usually, a good swallow or two will take care of it.

But what if this doesn't help? A clogged sensation in your ear is frequently caused by an accumulation of earwax and has a simple solution. In most cases, you can even take care of it yourself.

Treatment

First, check to see if your ear is filled with earwax, or cerumen. Take a windup clock and see if you hear the ticking at the same volume in both ears. Another trick is to hum. If you can hear the humming louder on one side, that's the side with the accumulation of wax. If you do find that one ear is filled with earwax, fill an eyedropper with mineral oil and place a few drops in the ear daily for a few days until the wax plug softens. Then flush out the wax with warm water in a plastic syringe.

There's always the possibility that a bug has crawled into your ear or that a plug of cotton from an ear swab has dislodged and became stuck in your ear canal. Gently flushing the ear with mineral oil followed by water will probably do the trick for either problem. If you have no luck, contact your physician immediately and have her dislodge the offender. Don't poke around yourself; you may puncture the eardrum.

TIP FOR FREQUENT FLYERS

There is a new device available that eliminates the painful earaches that are due to pressure changes on ascent or descent. They are called "Earplanes" and look like a small set of earplugs. They can be purchased in drugstores and airports.

Special Mention for the Elderly

In the elderly, earwax can actually accumulate for years through inattention. The cerumen can become hard as a rock in some cases. This requires medical attention to remove the wax and avoid aggravating the chronic infection that usually accompanies a large accumulation of hardened earwax.

See also "Loss of Hearing, Sudden" below.

EAR, ITCHY

Description and Possible Medical Problems

As you age, your skin becomes thinner because of the breakdown of collagen. Even though you may spend time worrying about the effects aging is having on the skin on your face, aging also affects the skin on your ears.

If your ears have been itchy lately, it could be due to one or more of a number of conditions, such as excess earwax or allergies. Ask yourself the following questions to help you find an answer for your itchy ear.

1. Have I recently switched to a new soap or shampoo?

2. Does my skin get noticeably drier in the winter?

3. Do I bathe more frequently in the summer?

Treatment

If your ear itches, it's probably easy to cure.

Aging skin is more sensitive to the chemicals used in soaps, shampoos, and other cosmetics. It's not unusual for a midlife adult suddenly to develop an allergy to a substance that previously caused no problem. Or, if you've recently started using a new soap or hair spray, it may contain an ingredient that is causing your skin to itch.

One at a time, go through a process of elimination to determine which product is causing the problem. It may be more than one. Switch to hypoallergenic products if you get no relief.

Excess earwax can also cause an itchy ear. Also, your skin naturally becomes drier in the winter—even the skin on your ears. You might just need to dab some moisturizer on your ears at the same time as you apply it to your face. Bathing less often can also help, since water is a drying agent.

Though the skin diseases eczema and psoriasis occur mostly on the scalp, knees, and elbows, they can also appear on the ears.

EAR, PAIN IN

Description and Possible Medical Problems

Frequently, men and women who were serious runners in their 20s and 30s turn to swimming in their 40s and 50s because they discover that their bones and joints can't take the constant pounding anymore.

Unfortunately, avid swimmers frequently contract occasional ear infections of the ear canal and outer ear known as otitis externa, or swimmer's ear. Swimmer's ear is commonly caused by water that becomes trapped in the ear canal or by poking and probing in the ear with a foreign instrument. Since the ear feels as though it's filled with water, many people with otitis externa try to alleviate their symptoms by sticking hairpins, cotton swabs, or other objects into the canal. This usually just makes the condition worse and may permanently damage your hearing.

An itchy ear and/or flaky skin are also signs of otitis externa. You may also have a constant earache, sharp ear pain when you move your head, and secretions from the ear. Changes in pressure can also cause pain in your ears if you have otitis externa. Children often contract numerous ear infections throughout childhood without their hearing being affected. Midlife adults, on the other hand, can suffer partial or total hearing loss if otitis externa is left untreated. The infection can also spread, damaging bones and nerves and eventually causing paralysis. Fortunately, it's easy to treat.

Treatment

If you suspect you have otitis externa, it's important to get treatment for it right away. Applying a heating pad and taking aspirin or acetaminophen will help ease the pain before you can get to your doctor. Your physician will clean the canal and remove excess water with suction or a special cotton swab before prescribing an oral or topical antibiotic medication or eardrops.

A painful ear that's caused by a change in pressure is easy to fix. If swallowing a few times doesn't do the trick, head for a lower altitude or just wait awhile. If your ears don't unclog after a change in pressure, it may be an indication of an underlying problem and you should see your doctor.

Tips and Precautions

To prevent recurring infections, which are common among swimmers, try not to get any water into the infected ear while it is healing. Once the infection disappears, it's a good idea to wear earplugs whenever you swim, and also to remove all water from your ears when you're finished.

See also "Ear, Itchy" above and "Ear, Clogged Feeling in" above.

BODY SIGNAL ALERT

EAR, PIMPLES OR RASH ALONG

Description and Possible Medical Problems

If you develop a painful rash along your ear—commonly known as shingles—then it's safe to say that you had chicken pox as a kid.

Ramsay Hunt syndrome, a form of shingles that commonly appears along your ear, is a form of the herpes zoster virus, the same virus that causes chicken pox in children.

What causes the chicken pox virus suddenly to appear after years of latency? It's sometimes difficult to pinpoint the culprit, but too much emotional and/or physical stress can often trigger the immune system to become depressed, which may "wake up" a latent virus. And people who have weakened immune systems are prone to repeated bouts with the virus—and attacks of shingles.

To find out if the rash on your ear means you are having your second bout with chicken pox, ask yourself the following questions:

1. Do I have a painful rash or pimples on my outer ear?

2. Did I have chicken pox as a child?

3. Have I lost my sense of taste?

4. Am I sometimes unable to move one side of my face for short periods of time?

Treatment

As with any viral infection, the most severe period is the initial flare-up. When your physician determines that your rash is Ramsay Hunt syndrome, he will treat it with corticosteroidal preparations in either oral or topical form. But because the virus hides in the nerves of the spine for many years, it may cause permanent nerve damage when it surfaces after being dormant for decades. Though this is rare, you should see a neurologist at the first sign of a flare-up.

Special Mention for the Elderly

When an elderly person is affected with Ramsay Hunt syndrome, an extremely painful condition called postherpetic neuralgia can sometimes occur. Men and women 60 years and older are prone to postherpetic neuralgia because of their naturally lower immune systems. Postherpetic neuralgia is signified by facial paralysis, constant headache, and severe pain where the rash initially occurred.

Medications such as Zovirax and pain medications will help lessen the outbreak. If pain persists, a medication such as Zostrix can be very helpful in alleviating it.

See also "Pimples, Painful, on One Side of the Face" in Chapter 9.

EARS, BUZZING AND HISSING SOUNDS IN

Description and Possible Medical Problems

If hitting the buzzer on your alarm clock each morning does nothing to relieve the constant ringing or buzzing in your ears, you probably have tinnitus. And you have probably lost some of your hearing as a result of the aging ear.

Tinnitus is a ringing in the head. It is usually caused when the arteries in the ear—like elsewhere in the body—begin to narrow; as a result, the ear "hears" the blood rushing through the ear. And sometimes a person with tinnitus can hear his own heartbeat. Regardless of the particular sound, however, tinnitus tends to get worse at night, when there is a lack of sounds to drown it out. And some people may feel they need to seek psychological treatment, because the constant sound can begin to drive them crazy.

Treatment

It's sometimes difficult to pinpoint the sudden onset of tinnitus, since the cause can be due to an infection or obstruction, or to an underlying disease such as anemia or arteriosclerosis. If you have tinnitus, it's important for you to see a doctor to rule out the possibility of a serious disease.

To diagnose tinnitus, your physician will go through an elimination process. Sometimes the culprit is as simple as removing an accumulation of earwax, which is the first thing she will check for. Next, she will test your hearing with a tuning fork to see if you have a problem hearing it. She will also do a neurological exam to check your coordination and balance, and if she finds that you have lost some degree of control over your balance in addition to having a significant hearing loss, you will be referred to a hearing specialist.

It might be a good idea to eliminate caffeine, alcohol, and cigarettes, since these can frequently aggravate tinnitus. People with constant tinnitus find that playing the radio at night helps drown out the ringing enough so they can fall asleep. Others have found that a sound machine that emulates water can help mask the ringing, as can a fan or air conditioner. Or, if you live in the city, just open the window. Often, a standard hearing aid will help ease the ringing of tinnitus because it decreases the internal buzzing and amplifies external noise.

EXTERNAL EAR, LESION ON

Description and Possible Medical Problems

When you were a kid spending your summers on the beach, remember how the tops of your Uncle Herman's ears always turned beet red? He was a good candidate for contracting basal or squamous cell carcinoma on this part of his ears later in life.

The increase in cases of skin cancer in the last decade has been alarming. The parts of the body that are frequently exposed to sun are those that are most susceptible to developing carcinoma. As with most cancers, both squamous and basal cell carcinoma can spread to other parts of the body if not caught early, so it's a good idea to pay attention to any changes in a mole or mark.

The American Cancer Society recommends that people follow the

"ABCD rule" and see their physician immediately if they see any changes that look suspicious. The ABCD rule is as follows:

• *Asymmetry:* The shape of the mole or mark is irregular.

• *Border:* The edges of the mole or mark are ragged and uneven.

• *Color:* The mole or mark is not uniform in shape and may be blotchy in appearance.

• *Diameter:* The size of the mole or mark is increasing and/or is larger in diameter than a pencil eraser.

Squamous cell lesions or tumors are usually painless, but they can spread very quickly if unchecked. They tend to appear as a reddish nodule on top of the skin surface or as a flat scaly lesion. Basal cell tumors resemble a small pearl-colored bump.

Though basal cell carcinoma is the most common type of malignant skin cancer, the ear is more susceptible to squamous cell carcinoma. Interestingly, squamous cell tumors on the outer ear occur more frequently in men, whereas in women they are found closer to the ear canal. You should also be aware that squamous cell tumors are more likely to spread to the ear canal in people with a history of chronic ear infections. And basal cell tumors can occur especially in people who have a history of otitis media, an ear infection. If you have had either of these conditions regularly throughout your life, be sure your doctor regularly checks your ears for these lesions.

A nodule on the external ear, however, is not always cancerous. Another cause of lesions on the ear is rheumatoid arthritis. Rheumatoid nodules can sometimes become sore and infected, though most of the time they are not painful.

In addition, people who have gout, which is a disease caused by an excess of uric acid accumulating in the body, sometimes have an ear affliction called gouty tophi, in which the uric acid accumulates and forms lumps in various places in the body, including the cartilage of the ear. Like rheumatoid nodules, gouty tophi can be painful.

Treatment

Treatment for both kinds of tumors requires a biopsy to determine the diagnosis. Squamous cell tumors are often treated with a type of surgery called Mohs' technique, a type of surgery that's ideal for cases where it's difficult to tell the exact size and depth of the tumor—like on the ear. Basal cell tumors are also treated with Mohs' technique, though other surgical methods, such as cryosurgery and radiation, are often used. The surgery can be performed in an outpatient surgical unit; you can usually go home the same day. If the lesion is small, a local anesthetic will be used; general anesthesia will be used if the lesion is larger, and you will probably need to stay overnight at the hospital for observation. Your doctor will recommend that you take Tylenol for the pain, and you'll feel better in a few days.

If the lesion is caused by gout, your doctor will prescribe a medication such as Allopurinol, which will help reduce the amount of uric acid in your blood stream. If you have rheumatoid arthritis, your doctor will recommend you use a nonsteroidal anti-inflammatory medication such as aspirin or Naprosyn to reduce the pain and inflammation.

Tips and Precautions

Though more than 95% of basal and squamous cell cancers are eliminated if caught early, if you've had cancer once, unfortunately you're predisposed to having it coming back. To prevent a recurrence, always apply sunscreen liberally. And take a lesson from your Uncle Herman— wear a hat whenever you're out in the sun.

Don't Blame Rock 'n Roll

If you have noticed that your hearing has gradually declined since you entered your 40s, you may have written it off to too many loud rock concerts that you attended in your teens and 20s.

Guess again. The most common cause of hearing loss in midlife adults is occupational hazards. In other words, if your job regularly exposes you to loud noises above 85 decibels, you run the risk of damaging your hearing. Normal conversation usually runs around 60 decibels, while a loud rock concert can easily exceed 100. Some workplace noises that can definitely cause permanent damage are a jackhammer or jet engine at close range, or the constant drone of loud factory machinery.

If you work in a quiet office, however, you're not totally off the hook; your leisure time activities can also cause significant hearing loss. Motorcycles and even lawn mowers can emit noise that enters the high-risk levels of 85 decibels and above.

> The best thing to do if you're exposed to loud noises that can cause injury to the ear at work or play is to wear ear protection. The most effective kind resembles stereo headphones, while others choose the more unobtrusive earplugs.

LOSS OF HEARING, GRADUAL

Description and Possible Medical Problems

Since hearing loss due to aging occurs very gradually, many adults in their 40s and 50s are caught off guard when they notice that they are unable to hear as well as they used to. They don't realize that their ability to hear actually began to deteriorate more than a decade earlier.

The last time you went to a concert, it may have sounded as though some of the higher notes were missing from your favorite songs. This is presbycusis, a hearing loss that can be caused by damage either to some of the thousands of tiny hairs that line the inner ear or to the nerves of the cochlea, the cavity of the inner ear. Men are affected by presbycusis more than women are, and they also tend to suffer from more severe hearing loss.

If one or both of your parents suffered from poor hearing for most of their adult lives, and if you feel that your own hearing is deteriorating, you probably have otosclerosis. In otosclerosis, the bones of the middle ear grow abnormally, which puts pressure on the stirrup, or stapes bones, blocking entrance to the inner ear.

Presbycusis and otosclerosis are two common causes of hearing loss from midlife on. The major difference between them is that presbycusis is caused by damage to the inner ear and starts when a person is in his or her mid-40s. Otosclerosis affects the middle ear and is usually detected as a slight hearing loss in young adults that gradually deteriorates with age.

Prolonged exposure to loud noise, as well as high blood pressure and heart disease, are primarily responsible for the one third of men and women over 50 who suffer from a mild to substantial hearing loss.

If you've noticed that your hearing has seemed to diminish in recent years, ask yourself the following questions:

1. Do I have some hearing loss in both ears?

2. Do one or both of my parents need to wear a hearing aid?

3. Do my ears occasionally ring or buzz?

4. Do I frequently misunderstand what someone is saying?

5. Did I suffer from a sudden hearing loss when I was younger?

Treatment

Presbycusis is a slowly progressive disease that cannot be reversed by surgery or other means. However, the technical advances of hearing aids in recent years—as well as their increased comfort—are a definite boon to men and women with mild or severe hearing loss.

With otosclerosis, the good news is that since this form of hearing loss is conductive, involving a bone obstruction, most of your hearing loss can usually be restored through surgery.

BODY SIGNAL ALERT

LOSS OF HEARING ON ONE SIDE WITH DIZZINESS

Description and Possible Medical Problems

Any type of hearing loss will frighten most anyone, but when you also feel as though like the room is spinning, it's time to call your doctor. You may be suffering from acoustic neuroma, a condition in which a non-cancerous tumor grows between the inner ear and the brain. Because the tumor is benign and grows slowly, some physicians suggest you don't need to act on it right away. However, as the tumor grows, it may put pressure on your nervous system and the brain.

If you should lose part of your hearing in only one ear, ask yourself the following questions so you can communicate the answers to your doctor:

1. How long have I been unable to hear in one ear?

2. Do I hear a constant ringing or buzzing?

3. Have I felt dizzy lately?

Treatment

Acoustic neuronoma is diagnosed with a CAT scan of the brain. Because it's important to prevent the benign tumor from growing and putting pressure on a number of vital brain structures, surgery is the only treatment. Fortunately, removal of the tumor is performed with microsurgical techniques that have been proven quite effective and don't cause any severe complications.

LOSS OF HEARING, SUDDEN

Description and Possible Medical Problems

Small children are no strangers to the pain of ear infections, which can cause the ear to feel very full, but adults in midlife years and older can get them, too, though they tend to occur less often. Ear infections are sometimes accompanied by pain and fever.

If you suddenly lose some of your ability to hear and also have a fever and an earache, and/or you feel nauseous, you probably have an ear infection known as otitis media. You may also feel dizzy and be aware of a faint buzzing in your ears.

There are four kinds of otitis media, which range from mild to severe. In serous otitis media, fluid is present in the middle ear, while in otitis media with effusion, fluid also collects in the middle ear but is accompanied by an infection. Secretory otitis media alters the cells that line the middle ear so that the trapped fluid thickens and oozes from the ear. In acute purulent otitis media, pus accumulates in the middle ear, making it the most dangerous type of ear infection since the pus can build up enough pressure to burst the eardrum.

Treatment

Since it's difficult to know which of the four types of otitis media you have, it's important to see your physician whenever you have an ear infection. She will probably prescribe a decongestant such as Seldane, Claritin, or Hismanal for you to take for two weeks or longer, which will help to unclog the middle ear. She may also prescribe an antibiotic such as penicillin or Keflex when an infection is present. An untreated infection can lead to a chronic ear infection, which, in some cases, can lead to permanent hearing loss.

See also "Ear, Clogged Feeling in" above.

LOSS OF HEARING WITH BUZZING

Description and Possible Medical Problems

Sometimes when a midlife adult complains of hearing loss or a low, constant buzzing and his physician comes up empty-handed, the diagnosis is simpler than either one may have thought.

It's ironic, but sometimes a drug that is used to treat an ear infection can actually contribute to hearing loss. Several kinds of drugs are notorious for inducing a temporary hearing loss that's usually accompanied by buzzing.

To determine if your hearing loss is due to medication, go through the following checklist:

1. Do I take a lot of aspirin?

2. Has my doctor recently prescribed an antibiotic to treat another illness?

3. Do I frequently take diuretics to control my weight?

If you answered yes to any of these questions and you've recently had a noticeable loss of hearing, it's possible that the medications—both over the counter and prescription—are responsible.

Treatment

Though three classes of drugs—diuretics, antibiotics, and aspirin—are among the most commonly used and prescribed, they can be extremely toxic to the ear, or ototoxic. The inner ear is affected since these drugs can damage the tiny hairs and other parts of the inner ear. The ensuing hearing loss, especially in the elderly, may be irreversible. And patients who already have substantial hearing loss shouldn't be prescribed these ototoxic drugs at all.

Fortunately, less toxic formulations of these drugs are available, so if you've had any problems with your hearing in the past, be sure to alert your doctor before he prescribes these medications.

Special Mention for the Elderly

Elderly people with chronic health problems frequently visit several different doctors, who may not always be aware of the medications their colleagues are prescribing. Even though one may prescribe a low-toxicity antibiotic, if another doctor prescribes a similar medication for a separate condition, the combination might be enough to permanently damage an adult's hearing.

Make sure that each doctor you or an elderly family member sees knows about all the medications that are being taken.

NOSE, BROKEN

Description and Possible Medical Problems

Though most midlife adults don't have to worry about having their nose broken unless they box or play football, a broken nose can be more common in the elderly than in prizefighters, since the cartilage can weaken and become extremely thin and brittle with age. Frequent falls also make people 65 and over more susceptible to breaking or fracturing their noses.

Treatment

If you think you've broken or fractured your nose, see your doctor. If you attempt to let it heal by itself, the cartilage may fuse incorrectly, which may lead to breathing problems later on because of an obstruction.

Your doctor will treat your fracture by first setting the cartilage into place and then inserting a special packing material into your nose to support the cartilage as it heals. The packing will stay in place for about a week or so and won't interfere with your breathing.

NOSE, RUNNY

Description and Possible Medical Problems

Frequently, a cold that starts out with a stuffy nose will end with a runny nose, also called rhinorrhea. It's the body's way of ridding itself of the cold germs and viruses that are on their last legs as you begin to feel better.

Treatment

There's not much you can do for a runny nose except wait it out. Some people use antihistamines, which cause mucus to thicken, but the downside of using these preparations is that your cold may stick around longer than it would otherwise. Thickened mucus helps to keep germs and viruses in the body longer, and just when you're feeling better, a virus or germ can get its second wind and attack again.

And the older you get, the longer a cold tends to stick around. So it's a good idea to avoid using antihistamines for a runny nose and drink lots of fluids, which will hasten the end of your runny nose.

See also "Sinuses, Painful, with Fever" below.

NOSE, STUFFY

Description and Possible Medical Problems

You may think your stuffy nose is due to a cold—after all, you've never been allergic to anything—but think again. Adult-onset allergies are more common than most people think, especially with the increasing numbers of people who suffer from environmental allergies, in which rugs, furniture, and even hair spray can trigger an allergic reaction.

If your stuffy nose is due to an allergy and not to a cold or flu, you'll probably answer yes to these questions:

1. Has my clogged or runny nose lasted far longer than a cold usually does?

2. Do my symptoms seem to appear and disappear without warning?

Treatment

Allergies can occur at any time of the year, although spring, when pollen is at its most abundant, and fall, when ragweed is in bloom, are the seasons when allergies and the accompanying nasal discomfort become most severe. At other times of the year, allergies to household mold and dust can cause a reaction.

When it's impossible to avoid the offending allergic substances, you can treat your stuffy nose with over-the-counter antihistamines or decongestants. Look for antihistamines that don't make you sleepy, and don't overdo it with the decongestants, especially the sprays—it's easy to become hooked on them.

See also "Difficulty Breathing" above.

BODY SIGNAL ALERT

NOSEBLEED

Description and Possible Medical Problems

Though a nosebleed usually arrives without warning and is alarming, it's usually not a serious condition, and it disappears as quickly as it came.

In midlife adults and older, nosebleeds can occur for no apparent reason, or they may be due to a blow to the nose or even breathing dry air. This type of nosebleed starts and stops suddenly. The blood vessels on the front of the septum—the cartilage that divides the nose—are thin and fragile, and it doesn't take much for them to break. However, there are some instances in older adults where a nosebleed can indicate a serious condition that warrants immediate medical attention, and that's why it's a Body Signal Alert.

More serious nosebleeds usually originate further back in the nose and may be caused by a number of factors, from an excess of anticoagulant medication such as aspirin to the rupture of an artery, or even as a symptom of a worsening case of hypertension.

If your nosebleed recurs several times over the course of the day, or if the bleeding is constant, you should see your doctor right away.

Treatment

To stop a mild nosebleed, don't lean your head back or lie down. Instead, sit up straight and pinch your nose so that you're applying pressure to the septum. Apply ice; the bleeding should subside within a few minutes.

As far as a recurring or constant nosebleed is concerned, do not attempt to treat this more serious type by yourself. Your doctor will first apply gauze soaked with anesthetic to the septum to shrink inflammation and stop the bleeding. If this is not successful, your doctor may choose to cauterize the site of the bleeding or to surgically place a temporary nasal balloon against the septum. This will help control the bleeding.

SINUSES, PAINFUL, WITH FEVER

Description and Possible Medical Problems

You've probably seen the television commercials that tout the latest over-the-counter medication for sinus infections and headaches. The woman on the tube pops a capsule, and in the next scene she's smiling.

Sinus infections are common occurrences in many midlife and older adults, but people frequently confuse sinusitis—an infection of the sinuses—with an allergic reaction or migraine headache.

Sinusitis is often caused by a cold, when the mucus membranes near the nose become so swollen that the passages to the sinuses close. Since the sinuses are unable to drain, pressure builds up in them, which can become extremely painful, especially if the sinus openings remain closed for a period of time. Frequently, a tooth infection or abscess will spread to the sinuses. Unfortunately, sinusitis can sometimes persist for weeks.

Sinusitis can be caused by either a bacterial or viral infection. A viral infection causes the nasal secretions—also called postnasal drip—to be clear and watery, while the mucus accompanying a bacterial infection will be thick and sticky, with a greenish tinge.

You probably have sinusitis if you answer yes to the following questions:

1. Do parts of my face behind and under my eyes feel painful to the touch?

2. Do I have a fever and/or chills?

3. Do I find it difficult to breathe through the nose?

4. Do my sinuses become painful when I bend over or walk up and down stairs?

Treatment

If you have viral sinusitis, the best course of action is patience, drinking fluids, and taking an over-the-counter or prescription painkiller such as Tylenol with codeine to relieve the pain. Bacterial sinusitis requires at least a two-week course of antibiotics—penicillin or one of the new types such as ciprofloxacin—prescribed by your doctor. For either viral or bacterial sinusitis, decongestants can help open the sinus passages so they can drain.

Acute sinusitis is usually the by-product of a cold or flu. Chronic sinusitis, which can persist for months, comes when a series of acute infections is left untreated. Nasal corticosteroid sprays such as Nasacort have gained wide use in treating sinusitis. Sometimes surgery is necessary to widen the sinus passages and improve drainage.

Tips and Precautions

If you have had acute or chronic sinusitis in the past, there are a few things you can do to reduce the chances of recurrent infections.

If you smoke, stop. Cigarette smoke can irritate the lining of the sinuses and nasal membranes, causing the opening between them to swell and narrow. Also, if you have allergies, follow the treatments recommended by your doctor to lessen your chances of swelling. Also take precautions around people who have colds, to lessen your risk of becoming infected.

Treatment

Allergies can occur at any time of the year, although spring, when pollen is at its most abundant, and fall are the most common times. Dust and pets can cause allergic symptoms all year round. Allergies can even be caused by noxious fumes given off by new carpets and some household chemicals.

Chapter 7

MOUTH, TEETH, AND GUMS

===== **BODY SIGNAL ALERT** =====

Call your doctor immediately if you experience any of the following symptoms:

SYMPTOM	POSSIBLE MEDICAL CONDITION
You have a bleeding sore in your mouth that does not heal	*Oral cancer*
Your dentures don't fit comfortably	*Aging, bone degeneration*
You have severe bad breath that does not respond to improved oral hygiene	*Lung disease*
You have loss of tongue movement	*Tumor*
You suddenly lose your sense of taste or your mouth becomes dry	*Stone in salivary duct, side effect of medication, possible stroke or lung tumor*
You have numbness around your mouth	*Stroke*
You have extremely swollen and red gums	*Gum disease, medication, leukemia*

HOW THE MOUTH AGES

Thanks to water fluoridation and a conscientious dental campaign by the American Dental Association, many children today will go through life cavity free. The rest of us weren't so lucky. Although Americans as a whole practice better oral hygiene today, years of neglect and regular childhood visits to the dentist for another round of cavities to be filled mean that your teeth are still at risk because fillings can crumble unnoticed, leaving the tooth open to further decay and eventual loss.

In normal aging, the muscles that control the mouth gradually lose their strength when people reach their late 60s and early 70s, which can result in problems with chewing. When you lose some muscle tone, you may find that it's difficult to close your mouth fully.

The bone mass of the jaw also becomes more porous with age, in addition to a decrease in exercise and less calcium in the diet. This can lead to loosening of the teeth, but it's never too late to increase your intake of calcium as well as start to walk a mile or two each day, which will help reverse the loss of bone. It's also possible foods you once thought were overly spicy seem almost bland due to a decrease in your sense of taste. Aging reduces the number of taste buds on the tongue, as well as the sensitivity of the ones that remain. Although your taste buds may at last be able to handle Tabasco sauce, your stomach may tend to rebel more than before as it becomes more sensitive.

Undoubtedly, the loss of taste sensation combined with a loss of teeth will probably affect your diet. The good news is that, for many people, a loss of taste means that you may finally lose some of those unwanted pounds. But you should be careful not to lose too much weight, since a significant weight loss can result in a lowered immune system.

Fortunately, oral health can be improved with regular attention and professional treatment and becomes acute only later in life if you have neglected your teeth and gums. It's easy to improve your oral health by visiting your dentist annually, or more often if you want to play it safe.

BODY SIGNAL ALERT

BAD BREATH

Description and Possible Medical Problems

The majority of Americans believe that to have anything less than clean, minty breath 24 hours a day is something akin to sacrilege.

Of course, sweet-smelling breath is a real asset in life, but frequently, eliminating bad breath isn't just a matter of brushing your teeth and gargling with mouthwash. After all, mints, toothpaste, and mouthwash will only partially mask bad breath that doesn't respond to improved oral hygiene. Sometimes gingivitis, or gum disease, or a serious health problem such as lung, kidney, or liver disease or any mouth or throat infection is responsible for persistent halitosis. Most of the time, however, the problem can be solved easily with a simple change in diet.

Treatment

The first thing to check—and the easiest symptom to treat—is your oral hygiene habits. If you're not brushing and flossing properly—or cleaning your dentures thoroughly each day—you should immediately start to pay closer attention to your dental routine. Advanced cases of gingivitis or gum disease (see "Gum Pain, Bleeding, Red, Swollen Gums, Receding Gum Line" below) can also cause persistent bad breath.

If you improve your dental hygiene program but you still have bad breath, you should give yourself a nutritional checkup, since, as you age, your digestive system can slow down considerably. And if you eat a lot of processed and refined foods—which take longer to digest than unrefined foods do—the food can stay in your stomach longer and ferment, producing a noxious gas. Low-calorie diets are notorious for causing bad breath, as ketones, a by-product of digestion, are produced by the digestion of excess protein and expelled through your mouth as a foul-smelling gas. If improving your diet doesn't work, you may have a problem in your gastrointestinal tract, which is often responsible for releasing foul-smelling gas through the mouth.

Lung disease and its primary cause—cigarette smoking—can also cause bad breath that doesn't go away with brushing and flossing. Other serious diseases, such as kidney or liver failure or diabetes, can also cause the breath to smell foul, as can any infection that occurs in your mouth or throat. If your bad breath has appeared suddenly and doesn't respond to your own treatment, see your doctor to rule out these diseases as the cause. Over-the-counter cold remedies and antihistamines such as Benadryl and prescription medications, especially antidepressants such as Elavil and others that cause your mouth to become dry, can bring on bad breath since adequate saliva production helps to keep your breath fresh. Ask your doctor about switching to another medication.

BODY SIGNAL ALERT

DENTURES THAT DON'T FIT PROPERLY

Description and Possible Medical Problems

Because the structure of your mouth and jawbone changes as you age, if you wear a partial or full denture, you should expect the fit of the denture to change as well. In fact, because of the loss of teeth, the jawbone, which supports the dental appliance, will shrink even more quickly than if your own teeth were intact.

Your lower jawbone is especially at risk if you wear a full or partial lower denture, since the base plate of the denture places an abnormal amount of stress on the natural gums and underlying bone. This can cause the jaw to deteriorate even more. As the bone changes, you'll probably find that you have to change the dentures to fit better. Fortunately, new technology is making possible dentures that fit better and adjust to changes in pressure. They're also better able to absorb the shock of chewing and biting down, thus redirecting some of the stress away from the gums.

Treatment

The most important thing to do to prevent damage to your gums and your remaining teeth if you wear dentures is to go for regular dental checkups so your dentist can detect any tiny changes that occur in the fit of the dentures and make appropriate adjustments. It's important to see your dentist immediately upon noticing any change in the way your dentures fit. And, as your bone structure changes over the years, your dentist will occasionally need to make a new denture for you.

The abrasion of the denture against your bone and the resulting irritation may occasionally result in an infection of the soft tissue of the gum. If this occurs, your dentist will prescribe an oral solution of antifungal medication such as nystatin suspension or Mycelex troches, lozenges that you'll slowly dissolve in your mouth. Both should be taken three to five times a day for a week or two to totally clear up the infection.

Tips and Precautions

Some people sleep with their dentures in, but this can aggravate and speed up the deterioration of gum and bone tissue. Your gums need a break from the pressure the dentures place on them. That's why it's important to clean them thoroughly each night and to store them in a glass of water each night to prevent them from warping.

BODY SIGNAL ALERT

GUM PAIN, BLEEDING, RED, SWOLLEN GUMS, RECEDING GUM LINE

Description and Possible Medical Problems

You can be sure that one thing most adults have in common by midlife is some form of periodontal disease or gum recession. Periodontal disease is the major cause of tooth loss in adults 40 and older. Gum disease is caused by plaque, a colorless film of bacteria that forms on the tooth. Plaque damages the tooth by eating away at the enamel and the underlying structure of the tooth. It affects the gums by building up at the gum line and aggravating the tissue, making them hurt and bleed easily. When this occurs, you have gingivitis. If the plaque is not removed regularly with brushing and flossing, gingivitis will progress into periodontitis, in which the plaque hardens into calculus, forming pockets between the tooth and gum. Bacteria can then accumulate in the pocket and cause an infection. The infection may spread to the underlying bone, which can loosen the teeth even more.

To find out what type of periodontal disease you have, ask yourself the following questions:

1. Do my gums bleed when I brush my teeth?

2. Are my gums frequently swollen and red?

3. Have my gums receded visibly?

4. Do I have bad breath that doesn't respond to regular brushing and a change in diet?

5. Is one or more of my teeth loose?

If you answered yes to the first two questions, you have gingivitis. If you answered yes to all five, you have periodontitis. If your gums have become swollen and visibly enlarged, you should see your dentist immediately.

Possible Medical Problems and Treatment

Poor oral hygiene is to blame for most cases of periodontal disease, though diabetics and people with bruxism, a condition in which people grind their teeth, are especially prone to gingivitis and periodontitis. Enlarged, red gums can also occur as a reaction to the drug Dilantin, which is used to control epileptic seizures, or as a first sign of systemic leukemia, though this is rare.

To treat gingivitis, it's important to change your hygiene habits to prevent the disease from progressing further. Your dentist or hygienist will show you how to brush and floss properly and may recommend the use of a plaque-disclosing solution such as Viadent or Plax so you can see if you're effectively removing plaque from your teeth.

If you're in the advanced stages of periodontitis, you may need surgery to prevent further loss of teeth and bone. In one type of periodontal surgery, a periodontist cuts the gum in order to remove the underlying calculus. Any infections must be treated before the gum is pulled up to cover the root of the tooth. Two other types of surgery are a gingivectomy, in which the loose gum is cut away, and a gingivoplasty, in which the loose gum is cut away and the remaining tissue is reshaped around the teeth.

Fortunately, it's possible to stop and even reverse the progression of both gingivitis and periodontitis if you improve your oral hygiene habits and have your dentist treat them, then follow up with regular visits.

Tips and Precautions

Numerous tartar control toothpastes, special toothbrushes, and other over-the-counter products designed to fight plaque have proliferated in recent years. All this is in response to the spotlight that dentists and toothpaste manufacturers have thrown onto the problem of plaque. However, it's important not to rely exclusively on these products as replacements for flossing and dental checkups. Although special tartar control toothpastes can help prevent the plaque from progressing into calculus on the tooth surface, they do not affect the formation of plaque and calculus where periodontal disease starts: below the gum line and between the teeth. Regular use of these products should be only one part of a good dental hygiene program.

LIPS, CRACKED

Description and Possible Medical Problems

Everyone has experienced dry, cracked lips at one time or another, usually during the dryness of winter or the heat of summer. They may feel chapped, raw, and painful.

Sometimes, however, cracked lips may be caused by a vitamin B deficiency. You'll be able to tell if this is the case if your lips do not heal despite the use of medicated lip balms, ointments, and other salves.

Treatment

When your cracked lips are due to a vitamin B deficiency, increasing your intake of foods rich in vitamin B—whole grains, dairy products, poultry, and fish—should help soothe them. A B-complex supplement that contains 100% of all of the B vitamins will also help heal them. Check the chart below for a complete list of foods containing the family of B vitamins.

See also "Mouth, Cracks in the Corners of" below.

Because the B vitamin family is so important to good health, here's a list of foods that are rich in them:

B vitamin	Foods rich in this B vitamin
Vitamin B1 (thiamine)	Whole grains, legumes, enriched flour, meat (especially pork), brewer's yeast
Vitamin B2 (riboflavin)	Milk, eggs, grains, lean animal protein, fish, poultry, dark green vegetables (such as broccoli, spinach, and asparagus)
Vitamin B6 (pyrodoxine)	Beef, pork, veal, poultry, fish, nuts, bananas, bran, yeast, lima beans, soybeans

Vitamin B12   Foods of animal origin—the highest levels are
(cobalamin)   found in organ meats such as liver, while lesser
                amounts are found in fish (especially sardines,
                salmon, tuna, and shellfish), egg yolks, and dairy
                products

MOUTH, CRACKS IN THE CORNERS OF

Description and Possible Medical Problems

Do you have cracks in the corners of your mouth that never quite seem
to heal? You apply Vaseline, lip balm, and maybe even an over-the-
counter bacitracin ointment, but nothing seems to help.

This annoying problem is called angular cheilitis, or perlèche, and is
caused by any one of a number of underlying conditions. The most common cause is dentures that no longer fit properly. When this happens,
your bite is naturally altered, and the dentures may rub against the
insides of your mouth, causing irritation and sores in the corners of your
mouth that never totally disappear.

Another less common cause of angular cheilitis is a vitamin B deficiency. Do you eat a lot of refined foods made with white flour and
other processed grains? If you have cracks in the corners of your mouth
and you don't wear dentures and your bite hasn't changed recently, you
may need to eat more foods that are rich in vitamin B (see page 149), as
well as taking a vitamin B supplement.

Treatment

Cracks in the corners of your mouth are relatively simple to treat; all
you have to do is address the underlying cause.

If you believe that poorly fitting dentures are the cause of your cheilitis, you should visit your dentist, who will make the necessary adjustments in your dental appliance. After wearing the newly adjusted denture
for a few days, the cracks in the corners of your mouth should disappear.

If you don't wear dentures, and you know that your diet is low in vitamin B, you can start to cure the cracks in the corners of your mouth by
eating whole-grain breads and cereals instead of refined ones. It's also a
good idea to take a B-complex vitamin supplement, which will quickly
help clear up the cracks.

MOUTH, DRY

Description and Background

After a routine exam, a 55-year-old patient cleared her throat as she was getting ready to leave. "Doctor," she said, "one more thing."

I motioned to her to sit down. She did, seeming almost embarrassed to bring up what was bothering her.

"My mouth has seemed rather dry lately," she said. "I find that it's harder for me to eat, especially foods like toast and crackers." She added that she had begun to drink water with her meals to help her swallow, which she had never done before.

Dry mouth, or xerostomia, may be due to illness, a change in medication, or a problem with the salivary glands. A stone in the salivary duct can also cause your mouth to become dry. In this case, you'll definitely know the cause because, in most cases, a salivary duct stone causes a section of the temple or upper neck to swell up. You may also feel a sharp pain in your mouth. A stone is formed by certain chemicals in the duct which then harden and block the duct.

Though doctors once believed that a decrease in saliva production was a natural sign of aging, they now dismiss it. More often, it is something else that affects the salivary glands, although sometimes a patient will complain of the sensation of a dry mouth, or xerostomia, when salivary output is normal.

Though most people might think that having a dry mouth is just an inconvenience, it can lead to other health problems, including an increase in tooth decay.

If you've recently developed dry mouth, or if it's plagued you on and off for years, it's important to determine the cause, since it can also be a symptom of some serious diseases.

Treatment

If you've recently started to take a newly prescribed medication, it may be the culprit. Antihistamines such as Benadryl, over-the-counter painkillers such as Motrin or Tylenol, and medications used to treat depression, like Elavil, are other drugs that can cause your mouth to suddenly turn dry. Some medications such as over-the-counter diet pills, diuretics like Diyzide, and any antispasmodic such as Levsin can also cause dry mouth. If this is the case, the dryness will disappear once the medication is stopped or switched. If you are undergoing radiation or chemotherapy, these treatments can also alter the salivary glands: the former by damaging them, the latter by altering the saliva's makeup.

If you can't change your medication or if your dry mouth persists, you can help alleviate the symptoms by drinking liquids while you eat as well as by sipping water frequently during the day. Some people have found that chewing gum or sucking on mints helps. Others have found some relief by using artificial saliva drops, such as Salagen tablets, which are available over-the-counter.

If you have a stone in the salivary duct, your physician will either remove it with surgery or attempt to push it out with his fingers and treat the pain and residual swelling.

If none of these treatment methods works, your doctor might prescribe the medication pilocarpine for you to take, 5 milligrams three times a day; this medication will stimulate your salivary glands.

Tips and Precautions

Many people experience dry mouth when they're under stress. Simple anxiety and stage fright can also cause your mouth to become dry. If you consistently wake up with a dry mouth, it's probably due to sleeping with your mouth open; the best thing to do is to keep a glass of water on your nightstand so you can take a sip when you wake up.

MOUTH, EXCESSIVE SALIVA IN

Description and Possible Medical Problems

The production of sufficient saliva is important to proper digestion. Besides producing enzymes that help to break down food so the body can use it, saliva helps to prevent tooth decay and also makes swallowing easy. Though a decrease in saliva production is more common in adults, an increase—known as sialorrhea—does occasionally occur.

Treatment

Dry mouth, or xerostomia, is often a side effect of a particular medication. However, an increase in the output of saliva can also result from taking a new drug. Bethanechol chloride, which you may be taking if you have a urinary retention problem, and neostigmine, a medication that alleviates the symptoms of myasthenia gravis, a neurological disease that results in a loss of muscular control, can also cause your glands to produce more saliva than usual.

Sialorrhea is virtually always reversible when your doctor switches your medication. If your doctor does not want to change your medication, I recommend that you take the antihistamine Benadryl in pill or capsule form twice daily. Seldane is another antihistamine that will also help to dry your mouth, but it doesn't cause drowsiness like Benadryl does; I suggest you take Seldane once or twice a day. It's also important to know that increased salivation can be a sign of the progression of Parkinson's disease, a result of the muscles of the throat becoming lax and hard to control (see "Face Resembles a Mask, Drooling, Change in Voice, Difficulty Walking, Trembling Hands" in Chapter 3 for more information on Parkinson's disease).

MOUTH, METALLIC TASTE IN

Description and Possible Medical Problems

If you've ever been able to receive radio waves through the fillings or orthodonture in your mouth, you probably found that the broadcast is usually accompanied by a metallic taste in your mouth.

Whether or not you fall into this category, if a metallic, slightly bitter taste stays around for a period of time, something besides the radio is causing your symptoms. Indeed, changes in the sensation of taste are usually caused by a recent or progressive change in your physical health. A metallic taste disorder may be due to a vitamin deficiency—most often the B vitamins or the mineral zinc—or to a cold or flu, during which the pus resulting from an upper respiratory infection can taste bitter. A benign or malignant tumor on the tongue can also cause a metallic taste.

Certain medications such as antihypertensives and any antibiotic can also cause a metallic taste. In some cases, the altered taste will disappear after your body adjusts to the medication; in others, it will remain as long as you're taking the medication.

If the metallic taste in your mouth doesn't go away on its own, it's a good idea to see your doctor.

Treatment

Your doctor will diagnose the cause of the metallic taste in your mouth by analyzing any changes in your diet and looking for the presence of a chronic respiratory infection. He will also examine your tongue for signs of a tumor. I had one patient who had a metallic taste that was caused by a tumor of the lung lining; the metallic taste preceded the cancer diagnosis by several months.

See also "Mouth, Dry" above.

BODY SIGNAL ALERT

MOUTH, NUMBNESS OF

Description and Possible Medical Problems

If you've ever had novocaine at the dentist's office, then you know what a numb mouth feels like.

Some people who are chronic worriers bite their lips a lot, which can result in a lack of sensation in the lips. But if you discover that the area around your mouth is numb, it might be a sign of a lack of blood flow to the brain. This could be a signal of impending stroke.

Frequently, when a stroke has occurred, your mouth will feel numb either around the lips or on one side of them. Most people who have had a stroke also have a numb arm and/or leg—if both, they'll be on the same side of the body—and difficulty with their speech and/or vision.

Sometimes numbness around the mouth caused by poor circulation to the brain can also be accompanied by a sudden loss of consciousness.

Treatment

Many times, treatment will include aspirin, but only after a vascular flow study of the vessels of the neck that lead to the brain, along with, possibly, an angiogram and a CAT scan or MRI (see Chapter 11, "Chest, Heart, Lungs, and Circulation," for a further description of these medical tests). A low-salt, low-fat diet is prescribed, along with prescription medication that will lower blood pressure.

MOUTH SORES, COMMON

Description and Possible Medical Problems

We've all had canker sores at one time or another. These small, white sores that form inside your mouth can appear for no reason, and they're usually painful.

Canker sores—also known as aphthous stomatitis—are usually no more than a nuisance, however, and they normally last for only a week or two. Sometimes they'll appear when you first start to get a cold, although physical or emotional stress can also cause them to surface.

However, a small, painful mouth sore might also be a cold sore, caused by the herpes simplex virus. A cold sore first appears as a blister, which frequently crusts over a couple of days after it first appears. It usually takes about a week from the initial onset until the cold sore completely disappears. Like a canker sore, a cold sore tends to reappear because even though the sore may disappear, the virus remains dormant in your body, ready to strike when you're stressed.

A cold sore usually appears around the outside of your lips, while a canker sore tends to appear on the inside of your lip or cheek and sometimes on your tongue, which may make it difficult to eat and talk properly.

Treatment

It's not clear exactly what causes canker sores, though it's thought that they may be hereditary or reactions to changes in the immune system. Some sores are caused by dental nicks or cuts by a dentist's tool. These canker sores tend to recur over time.

Since canker sores tend to appear and disappear within a matter of days, many people simply grin and bear the discomfort. If they bother you or are painful, there are a number of over-the-counter preparations like Orajel and Zilactin medicated gel that you can use as needed to lessen your discomfort.

If a canker sore should linger for more than two weeks, you should contact your doctor, who will prescribe an antibiotic to treat the underlying infection.

There's not much you can do to prevent cold sores from recurring, though some physicians believe that taking 500 milligrams of the amino acid lysine every day will help prevent future attacks. They also believe that eating foods high in lysine, such as meat, milk, fish, beans, eggs, and brewer's yeast, will keep cold sores from coming back. At the same time, avoiding foods that are high in the amino acid arginine—such as chocolate, cereal grains, gelatin, nuts, seeds, and raisins—may also help to cut down on the incidence of cold sores.

Once a cold sore is on the verge of appearing—you'll know because the spot where it previously appeared will start to hurt and tingle—it's a good idea to apply a topical solution of acyclovir, a prescription antiviral drug that may prevent the sore from becoming full blown.

During the attack, it's important to wash your hands frequently to avoid spreading the virus to other parts of your body.

BODY SIGNAL ALERT

MOUTH SORES THAT WON'T HEAL

Description and Possible Medical Problems

We all get common but minor oral irritations such as canker sores, abrasions, and cold sores. They're an annoyance, and we have to avoid certain foods for a few days, but usually they disappear on their own within a week to 10 days. These sores are usually painful.

But what if the sore doesn't disappear? Or it takes on another form, such as a small whitish bump or lesion anywhere in the mouth? The sore may be cancerous, and early detection and treatment are essential. Oral cancer is one of the most common kinds of cancer. People who smoke and drink alcohol are more prone to oral cancer than those who don't. Children and young adults are rarely affected, but once you reach midlife, cases of oral cancer can increase significantly.

Treatment

If the sore in your mouth doesn't heal within three weeks after it first appeared, see your doctor immediately. Sadly, many people with oral cancer who aren't treated right away do not survive because oral cancer can spread quickly to the nearby lymph nodes and then rapidly to other areas of the body through the lymphatic system. If oral cancer is caught early, however, your doctor will be able to cure you totally.

Tips and Precautions

Most dentists today routinely check for oral cancer. If you're like most people, you probably put off dental visits past the recommended period of time.

Just as many women regularly check their breasts for tumors or cancerous growths, men and women should get into the habit of examining their mouths for cancer as well. Once a month, you should check for any new lumps or growths on the top, side, and underside of the tongue, as well as on the roof and floor of your mouth and the inside of your cheeks. Also press on your tongue to check for new growths there.

BODY SIGNAL ALERT

TASTE, LOSS OF SENSE OF

Description and Possible Medical Problems

If you've been reaching for the salt shaker more often lately because food doesn't seem to taste as good as it used to, you need to determine whether the change has been gradual or sudden.

A gradual loss of taste is probably due to the fact that you don't have as many taste buds as you once did—and those that remain gradually lose their effectiveness. However, a noticeable loss of taste doesn't usually occur until a person reaches the 70s or 80s, if at all. A vitamin deficiency—of zinc and/or vitamin B_{12}—can also cause a gradual loss of taste. And habitual cigarette smoking is one of the most common causes of taste loss.

A sudden loss of taste is usually caused by a specific medical condition; it may be a sign of stroke, infection, or a tumor in the lung.

Treatment

There's not much you can do if you find you're gradually losing your sense of taste. Quitting smoking or taking zinc and/or vitamin B_{12} can help you to determine if these are responsible for your loss of taste. Taking a multivitamin with 100% of the RDA of all recommended vitamins and minerals each day will provide you with sufficient dosages of both zinc and vitamin B_{12}.

However, if you suddenly lose your sense of taste, you should check for recent changes in your lifestyle or health. For instance, antihistamines are frequently responsible for reduced taste sensation, which is frequently accompanied by a dry mouth. And because taste is so closely related to smell, if you have a cold or an upper respiratory infection, you'll probably lose some if not all of your sense of taste. Psychotropic medications that alter your consciousness—such as marijuana and cocaine—are another cause.

However, if none of these is the cause, you should check with your physician as soon as possible to determine what the cause is. Your doctor may give you a taste test to determine the kinds of tastes you can detect—sweet, salty, sour, and bitter—that is akin to a scratch-and-sniff test. He will place sugar, lemon, bitters, and salt on your tongue in order to determine what specific tastes you can detect.

After a thorough examination, if your physician determines that your taste loss is temporary, you should concentrate on selecting foods that give you at least some sensation of taste. Tangy, sweet, or spicy foods, along with foods that are crunchy or have some texture, will help alleviate the annoyance of not being able to taste your food. If, however, your doctor suspects that your loss of taste is due to an underlying illness, such as a stroke, he will probably order more tests to make a positive diagnosis and then begin treatment for the illness itself.

TEETH, PAIN IN

Description and Possible Medical Problems

If you feel a sharp pain in a tooth, chances are you have a cavity.

If you've gotten to this point in life and have never had a cavity, you should get a medal. Though there are many young people who haven't had to go under a dentist's drill due to recent advances in dental treatment and widespread water fluoridation, most midlife adults have had plenty of experience with the dentist's drill. Though many got their cavity quota out of the way in childhood, cavities in midlife can lead to infection, root canal, or loss of a tooth.

Though sometimes a cavity will not be discovered until a dental exam, the more advanced stages of decay will cause a sharp pain in the tooth when eating, drinking, and/or breathing.

If you're susceptible to adult-onset cavities, you'll answer yes to the following questions:

1. Do I brush and floss only when it's convenient?

2. Do I eat a lot of sugary, sticky foods?

3. Did I have frequent cavities as a child?

4. Do I visit my dentist less often than every six months?

5. Do I feel pain when eating or drinking a hot, cold, or sweet food or liquid?

Treatment

Cavities form when the bacteria that are naturally found in the mouth combine with the sugars in food to form plaque, a sticky substance that can eat away at tooth enamel and the exposed tooth roots of adults who have gum disease. Midlife adults who have even a minor case of gingivitis are especially prone to cavities on the tooth root because there's no enamel on the exposed surface. And when a cavity forms on the root, it can hasten an advanced case of gum disease. Saliva does help to wash away excess bacteria. But since saliva production decreases with age, you'll need to pay close attention to your dental hygiene.

Your dentist will treat a cavity by first removing the decay and then placing a filling in the tooth. Fillings are made of gold, a porcelain cement that blends in with your natural tooth color, or silver amalgam, which is a combination of silver, mercury, and copper.

If the decay is extensive and threatens the tooth, your dentist may suggest a root canal, which removes the deep decay and the tooth nerves but allows the tooth to remain.

Your dentist will also map out a detailed home care plan designed to prevent future cavities.

Tips and Precautions

The many different brands of fluoride treatment on the market today can go a long way toward protecting your teeth from decay. Your dentist or hygienist may prescribe a special gel or paste for you. You may find that some are painful to your sensitive teeth, so it's a good idea to experiment until you find the kind that works best for you.

TONGUE, BLACK, HAIRY

Description and Possible Medical Problems

When you were a kid, your imagination may have run away with you at night when you thought you saw a black, hairy monster under the bed, and you called for Mom and Dad to come take a look.

Now that you're an adult, the sudden appearance of a black, hairy tongue is just as disturbing as it was when you were a kid. Your imagination may also take over just as it did in childhood, as you ponder the possible causes and come close to driving yourself to the emergency room.

Relax. Have you been taking penicillin or other antibiotics to treat a bacterial infection? If your tongue turns black or brownish in color, it's probably in response to a lengthy course of antibiotic treatment. The papillae, or tiny, hairlike protrusions on the tongue, can turn dark due to a proliferation of bacterial growth on the tongue. In addition to the color change, you may have bad breath, due to the foul odor of the excess bacteria.

If you're a cigarette or pipe smoker, regular use of tobacco products can also cause a black, hairy tongue.

Treatment

A black, hairy tongue is harmless. Once you stop taking antibiotics, your tongue should return to normal.

If you still have a few days or weeks to go on your antibiotic therapy, however, you can improve your oral hygiene in the meantime by brushing and/or scraping your tongue at least once a day or as often as you need to.

And if you smoke and you believe this is the cause of your black, hairy tongue, my best advice is simply to stop.

TONGUE, BURNING

Description and Possible Medical Problems

Because the tissues of the mouth and tongue change with age, becoming thin and less elastic, they tend to become more sensitive to extremes in temperature. A burning feeling in the mouth and on the tongue is one result of these changes.

In addition to the changes that come with age, a vitamin B deficiency is frequently to blame for a burning tongue. Studies show that a lack of iron might also be a contributing factor to a burning tongue. Some women who have gone through menopause and don't take estrogen replacement therapy complain that their tongue feels as though it's "on fire." Studies have shown that a decrease in estrogen levels is linked with the appearance of a burning tongue.

But a burning tongue can occur in anyone at any age, and spicy foods as well as foods with a high acid content can make it worse. This is a related condition called glossodynia.

Treatment

To alleviate the symptoms of a burning tongue, it's a good idea to start taking a multivitamin supplement such as Z-Bec that contains 100% of all of the B vitamins to see if this helps. One tablet or capsule each day is the recommended dosage. For postmenopausal women, beginning a program of estrogen replacement therapy may help ease a burning tongue.

However, if these methods don't work, some temporary treatments are available. You can buy benzocaine in several over-the-counter preparations to apply to your tongue when the burning becomes severe. Anbesol in gel or liquid form applied three to four times a day can also offer relief. Some people also find that increasing their consumption of dairy products helps to soothe the burning, at least temporarily.

TONGUE, ENLARGED

Description and Possible Medical Problems

When you accidentally bite your tongue, it may swell up for a few hours before it returns to its normal size. It may leave behind a sore that might last a day or two.

But when your tongue becomes enlarged and stays that way without biting it, this could indicate that you have a vitamin B deficiency or pernicious anemia, which occurs because of a deficiency in vitamin B_{12}.

Treatment

It's been said that the eyes are the mirror of the soul. Many physicians believe that the tongue is the window of your physical health, since changes in the tongue frequently show up when there's something amiss in another part of the body.

A vitamin deficiency is among the first medical conditions to show up on the tongue. Since most people don't get enough B vitamins in their diets due to their consumption of processed, refined foods, which contain a fraction of the B vitamins of their unrefined, whole-grain counterparts, the body can quickly become depleted. A deficiency of B vitamins—niacin, thiamine, and riboflavin are several—can result since these vitamins are not stored in the body like vitamins A and D.

Pernicious anemia is another cause of an enlarged tongue, which is primarily caused by a deficiency in cobalamin, or vitamin B_{12}, another nutrient that is difficult to get enough of without supplementation. If you are deficient in vitamin B_{12}, your doctor may decide to give you an injection of 1000 micrograms of vitamin B_{12} once a month or more often.

Improving your diet by eating whole-grain breads and cereals and eating more lean red meat will help curb these deficiencies (see page 149 for a listing of foods rich in B vitamins). Taking a multivitamin supplement that provides 100% of the RDA for all the B vitamins will help return an enlarged tongue to normal size.

BODY SIGNAL ALERT

TONGUE, LOSS OF MOVEMENT OF

Description and Possible Medical Problems

If you find you are unable to move your tongue around easily, you may have a tumor. If the tumor is benign, you may not have noticed it as it's grown, since a benign tumor can take years to develop. Some people may even dismiss the growth as a normal sign of aging.

A benign tumor usually starts out as an almost imperceptible lesion that is lighter in color than the tongue. It tends to grow slowly over the course of several years. Though it may occasionally bleed, it won't hurt.

A benign tumor can turn into a malignancy, however, so your physician will want to examine it regularly.

If the growth has appeared suddenly, it's likely the tumor is malignant, and it can quickly spread to other parts of the mouth and body. Like a benign tumor on the tongue, a malignant tumor is not painful, and in its early stages it resembles a benign tumor. However, it grows quickly and can become ulcerous and bleed frequently. A malignant tumor can also stiffen the tongue to the point where it is almost impossible to eat and talk. The cause of a malignant tumor on the tongue is usually a long history of pipe, cigar, or cigarette smoking.

Treatment

While a benign tumor of the tongue is certainly a nuisance, it's easy to treat and doesn't pose a threat to your health.

A benign tumor can be removed with laser surgery. If a tumor of the tongue is caught early, it can be successfully removed. A malignant tumor will be treated like any other cancer, with surgery, medication, and/or radiation. As with any other cancer, the earlier it is detected, the better your chances are of beating it.

If the removal of the tumor hampers your ability to talk in some way, you will need to work with a speech pathologist to improve your speech. Your sense of taste may be affected, depending on the area in which the tumor appeared, and so may your ability to swallow.

However, even though a portion of the tongue will have to be removed along with the tumor, with therapy most people are able to function as they did before the surgery.

TONGUE, SORE PATCHES ON

Description and Possible Medical Problems

Does your tongue resemble a topographic map? Have some parts of its surface smoothed out, leaving bright red and sometimes painful craters behind? You may have geographic tongue, a disorder in which some of the papillae, which form the rough surface of the tongue, wear away over time.

A healthy tongue is covered with hairlike tissue called papillae. Each papilla is surrounded by taste buds, which help detect flavors.

Sometimes, the papillae will become deformed and may disappear in spots for a time. The patches can become sore and turn dark red. Alcohol, tobacco, and spicy foods can make the condition worse; they might even be the cause of it.

Geographic tongue may appear and disappear for no apparent reason. Glossitis is a related condition in which the papillae disappear completely and the entire tongue is sore and red. The exact cause of geographic tongue is not known, though it is not considered to be a serious problem. Glossitis usually results from—guess what?—a deficiency in vitamin B.

Treatment

There is no known cure for geographic tongue or glossitis. Spicy foods, cigarette smoking, and alcohol can aggravate geographic tongue and increase the pain; avoiding them may help prevent a recurrence. An antiseptic mouthwash will help soothe the pain; some physicians prescribe the use of a special medication such as viscous lidocaine to coat the tongue and ease the pain. The recommended dosage is application of a thin coating three or four times daily.

Glossitis is frequently caused by a B vitamin deficiency. A regular program of supplementation may help, as well as increasing your intake of foods that are high in vitamin B (see page 149 for a list of foods that are rich in vitamin B).

TONGUE, VEINS ON

Description and Possible Medical Problems

As we age, we become more aware of the minute changes in our bodies, from that slight ache in the knee that now comes after a brisk walk, to the gray hairs that seem to multiply with great regularity.

You'll probably notice veins on the surface of your tongue that weren't there before. And, if you look closely, you may also see that the veins in the floor of your mouth and underneath your tongue seem more pronounced.

Treatment

The good news is that this increased varicosity is a part of normal aging and not a sign of illness. It means you're healthy, so there's nothing to treat or worry about. If, however, the veins begin to bleed, you should see your doctor to rule out an underlying cause such as a tooth trauma or a blood-clotting disorder, especially if you are taking an anticoagulant medication such as Coumadin.

Another sign of aging that shows up on the tongue is a greater tendency toward injury from trauma; for instance, if you bite your tongue, it may take longer to heal. In addition, the surface of your tongue may become thinner and smoother. All of these conditions will go away by themselves and are nothing to worry about.

TONGUE, WHITISH AND THICK

Description and Possible Medical Problems

Everyone's tongue feels coated at one time or another, especially after a few drinks, but a whitish, thick tongue is an indication of oral candidiasis, commonly known as oral thrush.

Oral thrush is caused by the same fungus that causes vaginal yeast infections in women. *Candida albicans* is a fungus that exists in your body in relatively small numbers. It can rapidly multiply to create oral thrush.

Treatment

Frequently, oral thrush strikes when your immune system has been disturbed in some way. This might be due to illness, to certain medications that can affect your immunity, such as antibiotics or corticosteroids, or to chemotherapy. If not treated, the infection can spread to the roof of your mouth as well as to the tonsils and esophagus. If you think you have oral thrush, see your doctor, who will recommend an antifungal prescription medication such as Mycelex tablets, which slowly dissolve in your mouth, or a nystatin mouth rinse, both of which should be used three to four times a day. Unlike a vaginal yeast infection, oral thrush is not caused by an underlying yeast infection, so home remedies such as drinking cranberry juice and eating yogurt are not effective.

Chapter 8

NECK AND THROAT

BODY SIGNAL ALERT

Call your doctor or ear, nose, and throat specialist immediately if you experience any of the following symptoms:

SYMPTOM	POSSIBLE MEDICAL CONDITION
You start to wheeze and feel your throat close up	*Allergic reaction*
Your neck spasms painfully or "locks up"	*Reaction to Medication*
You have what you think are swollen glands in your neck or throat that persist for longer than three weeks	*Hodgkin's disease or non-Hodgkin's lymphoma*
You are sick and have a sore throat that is painful and makes it difficult to breathe or swallow	*Strep throat, viral infection*
Your voice suddenly changes	*Polyps on vocal cords*

HOW THE NECK AND THROAT AGE

The muscle tone of the neck and throat can gradually become lax over the years, but these changes don't happen to everyone. For those who do experience a weakening of the muscles inside the throat, the voice may change in timbre as the space between the muscles responsible for the vibration of the vocal cords and the resonance of your voice narrows. This really isn't terrible; you may finally get that deep, husky voice you've always wanted. While most people experience no discomfort, sometimes the weakening of these muscles can bring on a scratchy throat that is difficult to alleviate. The lining of the throat may also become drier, especially when speaking, so it may be necessary to drink more water throughout the day, which is never a bad thing. The good news is that the swallowing mechanism was designed to last a lifetime and rarely causes any problems.

The most common concern about the way the neck muscles age is primarily a cosmetic one, since the skin and outside muscles of the neck gradually weaken and lose their tone. This typical aging of the neck is one of the telltale signs of growing older and is the reason why the field of cosmetic surgery has grown by leaps and bounds. Cosmetic surgery of the neck can help to reestablish the sharp angles of youth.

Unfortunately, the effects aging has on the throat and neck are largely irreversible; although they're frequently touted as effective, neck exercises do little to tone the muscles of the neck. And if your throat muscles are weakening, talking more won't help tone them up. A lifelong regimen of regular cardiovascular exercise and good eating habits is still the best cosmetic defense to help keep every part of your body looking and feeling young.

CHIN, SWOLLEN AREA UNDER OR AT JAW OR TEMPLE

Description and Possible Medical Problems

When you feel a swollen area under both sides of your jaw, you probably know you have swollen glands. You also know they're no fun. Because swollen glands are caused by an infection, patience, antibiotics, and more patience are all necessary for treatment. So it helps if you view your prescribed rest period as a well-deserved break from the usual grind and use it as an excuse to catch up on the soaps or that stack of paperback novels you never got around to last summer.

If, however, you think you have swollen glands but only one side of your face is affected, you probably don't have swollen glands at all. Instead, you may actually have a problem with your salivary gland. The enlargement may also appear in front of your ear or directly under your chin. Regardless of the location, the swelling will probably not be painful. There are three salivary glands: the submandibular gland, which is located under the front of your tongue; the sublingual gland, located behind the submandibular gland; and the parotid gland, which runs from your jawbone to your temple.

If only one side of your face or the area directly under your chin is swollen, the swelling is probably caused by a small stone in one of the salivary ducts. Other telltale signs of this condition include a dry mouth or if the swelling grows when you're eating. In fact, some patients who have an enlarged salivary gland caused by a stone have told me they can actually feel the gland swell up when they begin to eat.

Though they are extremely uncommon, tumors of the salivary glands can develop, most often in either the parotid or the submandibular gland, and on only one side of the face. Unlike a swelling that is caused by a stone in the salivary duct, a tumor grows slowly over the course of several years; it rarely becomes malignant. Women between the ages of 40 and 70 are most likely to develop a tumor of the salivary gland. However, if you ignore it and don't seek medical attention, it can eventually become malignant and spread to the rest of your body.

Enlarged salivary glands that appear on both sides of the face frequently occur in people who have a long history of alcohol abuse. The salivary glands on both sides of the face can also swell up in people who suffer from bulimia, as their constant, forceful vomiting causes these glands to overreact and swell up.

Treatment

If you think you have an enlarged salivary gland, sucking on a lemon may cause the stone to pop out. If this doesn't work, call your doctor. He may want to try to push the stone out of the gland manually, which will reduce the swelling and solve your problem.

If, however, the swelling doesn't go away, you should see your doctor. If he determines that you have a tumor, he'll recommend that it be surgically removed. But most likely, the enlargement is due to a "stone."

COUGHING

See Chapter 11, "Chest: Heart, Lungs, and Circulation."

GLANDS, SWOLLEN, THAT LAST LONGER THAN THREE WEEKS

Description and Possible Medical Problems

You probably didn't notice it when it started to grow, or else you ignored it completely. After all, it was just a little lump or bump on the side of your neck. Nothing to worry about, right? It didn't hurt; you may actually have thought it was a pimple.

But that small bump on the side of your neck didn't go away. In fact, it continued to grow—either rubbery or hard in texture—but still very slowly. "Something to do with aging," you told the first person who noticed. "Nothing to worry about."

The fact is that a slowly developing growth on the side of your neck is something to worry about, since it might mean you have lymphoma, or cancer of the lymph nodes.

There are two kinds of lymphomas: Hodgkin's disease and non-Hodgkin's lymphoma. The symptoms of both are generally the same; their causes, however, differ. Hodgkin's disease is caused by a malignant cell in the lymphatic system called a macrophage, while non-Hodgkin's lymphoma is caused by a malignant white blood cell that multiplies and spreads.

With both Hodgkin's disease and non-Hodgkin's lymphoma, the cancer can spread through the lymphatic system from the lymph nodes into the chest, to the spleen, and down to the lymph nodes in the abdomen. The initial bump grows slowly over a period of three or more weeks, and the glands are usually not painful. The bump may also seem as if it is unable to move, as though it's permanently attached to your neck or jaw. Other symptoms of Hodgkin's disease and non-Hodgkin's lymphoma include night sweats, fever, general malaise, and weight loss.

Treatment

Your doctor will run a series of tests and perform a biopsy to make a diagnosis. With proper and prompt treatment, I have many patients with lymphoma who have lived well into their 80s and 90s.

Radiation therapy is the primary form of treatment for Hodgkin's disease; chemotherapy may also be used. In some cases of Hodgkin's disease, bone marrow is removed after the initial radiation treatment to allow for higher doses of medication and chemotherapy. The marrow is then replaced after the treatment.

Unfortunately, non-Hodgkin's lymphoma is more difficult to treat and cure. Both chemotherapy and radiation are used to treat non-Hodgkin's disease, though usually only in the beginning and middle stages of the cancer. Non-Hodgkin's lymphoma is an incurable disease, though the survival rate can be as high as 75% for 10 years if it's caught and treated early.

Today, if Hodgkin's disease is caught early, it can be cured. There are even many professional athletes who have returned to successful careers after treatment for Hodgkin's disease. I have seen many young patients with lymphoma who, when treated early and aggressively, have thrived and gone on to live long, healthy lives. One good example is the hockey player Mario Lemieux.

Non-Hodgkin's lymphoma is more serious and frequently involves a prolonged course of chemotherapy and radiation treatments. Like Hodgkin's disease, non-Hodgkin's lymphoma must be treated early and aggressively for the best results. Non-Hodgkin's lymphoma is more common in people over 50, such as Jackie Kennedy Onassis.

HOARSENESS

Description and Possible Medical Problems

We all get hoarse from time to time. Sometimes it's due to over-enthusiastic cheering at a sporting event; at others it's due to talking too much. Hoarseness can also result from a cold, perhaps accompanied by a sore throat. Whatever the cause, hoarseness occurs when the larynx—which contains the vocal cords—becomes irritated and inflamed, a condition that is known as laryngitis.

Whenever I hear hoarseness in a patient's voice, I'll immediately suspect he or she is a smoker. I always ask, "How many cigarettes do you smoke?" It always amazes my patients that I know they smoke. In turn, I'm surprised that they're not aware of their smoker's voice. From then on, at every checkup I'll know to look for the possibility of polyps—

abnormal growths that are common in smokers—on their larynxes.

For people who do not smoke but are frequently hoarse nonetheless, the cause is usually raising the voice or talking loudly. Like smokers, people who talk loudly or who frequently shout or scream are prone to developing polyps on the larynx.

While some folks may joke that the periodic bouts of laryngitis some people have finally allow others to get a word in edgewise, the fact is that persistent hoarseness and/or laryngitis may in fact be an indication of a more serious disease, such as polyps or a tumor on the larynx or in the lung.

Treatment

Usually, the best way to treat hoarseness is to rest your voice, learn to talk at a normal volume, and let the raspiness run its course. Drinking warm beverages, such as hot tea with honey, is also quite soothing. And if you smoke, stop. If the hoarseness is accompanied by a cold or flu, you should treat your other symptoms as well as limit your conversation.

If you become hoarse only after certain instances—like after a late night out—and your voice returns to normal after a few days, you have nothing to worry about. However, if you have chronic laryngitis or your hoarseness lasts more than a week, or if your voice changes, you should see your doctor immediately to rule out the possibility of polyps or a more serious problem. He or she may refer you to an ear, nose, and throat specialist, who will use a laryngoscope to check your vocal cords for polyps or other growths. A laryngoscope is a thin, small, flexible tube that your doctor will insert through your nostril so that she can look down into your throat. The procedure lasts only a few minutes and requires a local anesthetic.

Tips and Precautions

Many people gargle with salt water or an antiseptic mouthwash when they become hoarse. Although you're probably just doing what your mother told you to do when you were a kid, you may actually be doing more harm than good. First, you should keep the use of your vocal cords—including both speaking and gargling—to a minimum in order to give the larynx a chance to rest and heal. Second, salt water and antiseptic may irritate the infection of a cold more, delaying a return to your normal voice.

LYMPH NODES, PAINFUL, BEHIND EAR, WITH FEVER AND LETHARGY

Description and Possible Medical Problems

Chains of lymph nodes run along the side of the neck from the ear to the shoulder. Lymph nodes feel like small peas under the skin. If they're swollen, they may also be painful to the touch, and you may also have flulike symptoms, such as nasal congestion, fatigue, and overall aches and pains. Feel along the line with your fingertips; it is important to know if you have one or more swollen lymph nodes.

If you have swollen, painful glands behind the ear and jawbone accompanied by a high fever and lethargy, you probably have a viral infection. Just a few years ago, if this happened to you, it wouldn't raise any eyebrows. You'd stay in bed for a few days, be patient, take aspirin, and drink lots of liquid if it was viral, and in a week or so you'd be back to normal. If it has a bacterial origin, then antibiotics would be added.

Today, however, the story is different. If you have what seems to be the flu along with swollen lymph nodes and it doesn't go away after about a week, you may have chronic fatigue syndrome, which is believed to be caused by the Epstein-Barr virus. However, though many people automatically jump to the conclusion that they have chronic fatigue syndrome, the condition is actually quite rare.

Chronic fatigue syndrome is actually a variation of infectious mononucleosis. Back in high school, mono, or "kissing disease," was a badge to be worn proudly. Adults who get chronic fatigue syndrome face the possibility that they will have to deal with it for the rest of their lives.

Other symptoms of both mononucleosis and chronic fatigue syndrome include a sore throat, low-grade fever, headache, and, of course, fatigue. The difference between the two diseases is that mononucleosis generally clears up within a few weeks; chronic fatigue syndrome can go on for years.

Treatment

If you think you have mononucleosis or chronic fatigue syndrome, see your doctor, who will do a physical exam that includes a throat culture. If you have mononucleosis, she will advise you to rest and drink plenty of fluids; antibiotics are not effective with mononucleosis since it is a viral infection. I also tell my patients to use analgesics sparingly, as they can further depress your immune system and exacerbate liver and blood problems.

The treatment for chronic fatigue syndrome, which some physicians refer to as chronic infectious mononucleosis, is similar, except that this course of treatment may not help. In order for your doctor to positively diagnose chronic fatigue syndrome, she will first rule out other diseases. You have to show that you've been fatigued and had the other symptoms of mononucleosis for at least six months before you can be diagnosed with chronic fatigue syndrome.

A definitive diagnosis for chronic fatigue syndrome is still tricky, however. While some people who have symptoms of chronic fatigue syndrome have not been exposed to the Epstein-Barr virus, there are many people who show antibodies to the virus but who don't have any symptoms. If you feel you do have chronic fatigue syndrome, the best thing to do is to work with your doctor to try different remedies that may help alleviate your symptoms. Sometimes multivitamins, good eating habits, and moderate exercise can make you feel better. But you should be aware of the many alternative therapists out there who make their living by supposedly providing cures for chronic fatigue syndrome. These include intravenous vitamin therapies, herbal preparations, and megadoses of vitamins.

LYMPH NODES, PAINFUL, ON BOTH SIDES OF NECK UNDER JAW AND BEHIND EAR

Description and Possible Medical Problems

Whenever both sides of the neck swell up, most people automatically think of swollen glands. However, you may actually have a condition in which nodules have formed on your lymph glands. The symptoms of both conditions are virtually the same—fever, a stuffy nose, body aches—with one important distinction: swollen glands are soft and palpable; lymph nodules are small, hard, and painful.

Sometimes, in the presence of a viral or bacterial infection, small, hard masses will form in the glands on both sides of the neck behind the earlobe. These nodules are similar in scope to the painful glands that occur with viral infections such as mononucleosis or chronic fatigue syndrome, though they can also be a symptom of a bacterial infection.

Treatment

If the nodules are caused by a viral infection, there's not much you can do but wait until the infection clears up on its own in about a week or two. Take aspirin or acetaminophen to soothe the pain of the nodules as well as the other symptoms.

For a bacterial infection, your doctor will prescribe an antibiotic that will clear up the infection and the ensuing symptoms. Be sure you finish all the medication prescribed, or the nodules and the infection may return before they're completely cleared up. Nodules on the lymph nodes that are caused by a bacterial infection are often painful and are difficult to differentiate from a viral infection. If they occur along the hairline, a hair gland is probably infected. The best treatment for a bacterial infection is warm, moist towels applied over the hair gland for about five minutes at a time, three or four times a day.

NECK, ENLARGED

Description and Possible Medical Problems

Have you ever seen a serious weight lifter with neck muscles that seem to bulge in all directions? It almost looks as though he has no neck, when in fact he's built up his neck muscles to the point where they've reached their peak size.

The neck muscles are extremely difficult to develop, so if you notice that your neck seems a bit enlarged, it's not because you've been pumping a few weights at the health club. Your enlarged neck is probably due to a goiter, which is a swelling in the thyroid gland, or to a growth that appears on the gland. The goiter usually appears on the side of your neck, halfway between your collarbone and the tip of your earlobe.

The thyroid gland is responsible for how our bodies metabolize food. In midlife adults, production of the thyroid hormone thyroxine frequently changes because of menopause or simple aging: the gland produces either too much (hyperthyroidism) or too little (hypothyroidism). However, a goiter can also appear when the thyroxine level is just right because of a lack of iodine. This is a condition known as euthyroidism, where there is a goiter but normal or euthyroid function of the gland which can be determined by a blood test.

A century ago, goiter was a relatively common health problem that was usually caused by a lack of iodine in the diet. As a result, iodized salt was introduced, and today goiter is most often caused by an iodine deficiency. Whatever the cause, goiter is painless most of the time.

Treatment

The treatment for goiter depends on its cause, which your doctor will determine after a blood test and possibly a consultation with an endocrinologist. In the case of hypo- or hyperthyroidism, in which the thyroid gland produces too little or too much thyroxine, your doctor will first do a physical examination and check your medical history. She will specifically check for any body tremors, nervousness, an intolerance to heat, or a weight gain or loss, all of which are signs of a thyroid condition. She will also place your fingers on your neck and ask you to swallow, which will help her check for a goiter or nodule on your thyroid. Your doctor will also conduct a blood test and perform a scan of your thyroid with a radioactive substance, which will help her to check both the activity and the structure of your thyroid.

If you have hypothyroidism, in which the thyroid doesn't produce enough of the hormone, treatment with replacement thyroxine medication usually eases the problem.

If the enlargement is due to a growth on the gland, surgery is usually recommended. In a few cases, the growth may turn out to be cancerous, so if it does not disappear after a week, you should see your doctor immediately. If surgery is required, the growth will be removed and you will feel better in several weeks.

See also Chapter 18, "When Your Whole Body Feels Lousy."

LUMP OR MASS?

To tell the difference between a lump or mass and a swelling in your neck, keep the following in mind. When I refer to a lump or mass, I'm describing a distinct area that you can definitely distinguish from other surrounding tissues with your fingers. In other words, it stands out. Also, it may or may not be painful.

A swelling in your neck is not as easily distinguished from other tissues in your neck. It tends to be painful, and the boundaries of the swollen area are not as distinct. Also, swelling tends to appear over a larger area and may cover the entire side of your neck.

NECK, ENLARGED MASS ON ONE SIDE OF

Description and Possible Medical Problems

When any part of the neck swells up—on either the side or the front—the thyroid gland is usually responsible.

If you see and feel a lump or mass on one side of your neck but are still able to eat and drink as usual, you'll probably be tempted to ignore it since it's not painful.

However, it's a good idea to see your doctor because you may have a condition known as thyroid nodules, which can be either a type of cyst or a benign growth known as an adenoma. A small percentage of thyroid nodules do turn out to be malignant tumors, which is why you should see your doctor so she can rule it out.

Treatment

If your doctor determines that your thyroid nodules are cysts, you probably don't have to do anything, unless you want them removed for cosmetic reasons. If, however, the mass turns out to be an adenoma, he may recommend that your thyroid gland be altered, either with medication or with radiation treatment. If you have a hyperactive thyroid, he may prescribe Inderal or another beta-blocker to slow down your rapid heartbeat. If you have hyperthyroidism, he may want you to take propylthiouracil, or PTU, which is a medication that is taken in conjunction with the beta-blocker to reduce the amount of hormone your thyroid is producing.

If he thinks the thyroid nodules may be malignant, he will perform a blood test and a thyroid scan to determine if they are cancerous or not. If they are, all or part of the gland will be surgically removed. After surgery, your doctor will conduct a blood test to determine if you will need lifelong thyroid replacement medication, such as Synthroid, to regulate the amount of thyroid in your body. He may also prescribe a series of radioactive iodine doses to ensure that all of the malignant growth is gone. You will also need to visit your doctor regularly so that he can monitor the functioning of the gland.

NECK PAIN UPON MOVEMENT

Description and Possible Medical Problems

Whether you call it a charley horse, a cramp, or a pulled muscle, if you get a pain in your neck that doesn't disappear after a few days, you'll quickly discover that your entire life will be affected, especially if the pain makes it difficult to turn your head. Everything becomes difficult: driving, cooking, sleeping, even bathing.

As it turns out, the term "pulled muscle" is an accurate description of the condition. When a muscle becomes stretched beyond its normal capacity, the muscle fibers lengthen and become strained and may actually tear. Afterwards, you may feel a dull pain in your neck that may take a week or more to disappear completely.

Frequently, a pulled muscle in the neck—which is also called torticollis—is the result of a quick, sharp motion. The pain usually shows up later, so you may be unaware of the cause. Other causes can be holding your neck in an awkward position while you drive or sleeping on an unfamiliar pillow. Recently, however, I have also been seeing torticollis appear in weekend athletes who overdo their exercise routines.

Treatment

To treat a pulled muscle in your neck, you should first try to massage the area gently with your fingers, kneading the sore muscle and stretching your neck at the same time.

In addition, try taking an over-the-counter pain medication such as Advil four times a day, as well as applying a moist heating pad three times daily to relieve your discomfort.

If these methods don't bring relief after a few days, see your doctor. He may prescribe a muscle relaxant such as Valium to ease the pain or a stronger nonsteroidal medication such as Naprosyn, Lodine, or Toradol.

And if these don't help, your doctor will suggest that you see a physical therapist several times a week for additional treatment, which may include hot packs or electrical stimulation. But it's rare that a pulled neck muscle will bring you to this point, since torticollis usually lasts only about a week.

Tips and Precautions

To prevent a pulled neck muscle in the future, try stretching more before you exercise. It's also a good idea to spread your exercise out over the whole week and not just restrict it to Saturday and Sunday. This will also help to cut down on your overall injury rate.

You might also try eliminating your pillow at night. Especially if you have been unable to trace the cause of the muscle pull, this may be a simple—and the only—solution.

NECK, PULSATION ON THE SIDE OF

Description and Possible Medical Problems

For people who are tuned in to every minute change in their bodies, anything that even remotely appears to involve either their heart or their circulatory system immediately sends up red flags.

One of these changes may be that the artery in the side of your neck is pulsating more vigorously than it did just a few years ago. Because any change in the circulatory system may indicate the presence of coronary disease or an impending heart attack, your first impulse may be to call your doctor immediately.

There's no need to worry. An increase in pulsation is a sign that you're in good health and that your arteries are functioning normally. In addition, any activity that causes your heart to beat faster—such as exercise or nervous excitement—will naturally cause the artery in your neck to pulse faster, too. So relax.

Treatment

If an artery on the side of your neck seems to be pulsating more vigorously lately, it means that you're healthy and you don't have to do a thing.

NECK, RED PATCHES ON

Description and Possible Medical Problems

As you get older, the sensitivity of your skin increases. For instance, you may find that you're able to stay out in the sun for only half the time you could 5 or 10 years ago before you start to burn.

This increase in your skin's sensitivity also extends to exposure to chemicals, cosmetics, and certain types of plants. If you notice that red patches suddenly appear on your neck, it's likely that your skin is reacting to a substance to which it is highly allergic. This reaction is a condition called contact dermatitis. Poison ivy is one form of contact dermatitis; so is a rash that forms when you try a new cosmetic.

Within a day or two after you're exposed to the new allergen, red patches will start to appear in the affected area, and they'll probably be itchy. In some people, blisters will also form a few days later. The entire episode, from the initial exposure to the allergen to when the rash clears up, usually lasts about a week or two.

A person can also have an allergic reaction due to anxiety or other emotional stresses in her life.

Treatment

Calamine lotion and hydrocortisone creams are the most commonly used over-the-counter preparations for contact dermatitis. If blisters start to form, you might want to cover them with gauze to prevent infection. And certainly you should stay away from whatever caused the red patches in the first place.

If the contact dermatitis does not clear up after two weeks or if the rash becomes severe, see your doctor, who may advise the use of corticosteroids or other prescription medication to treat the condition.

If you think your rash is caused by anxiety and flare-ups start to become regular events, your physician might suggest biofeedback or another relaxation technique to help you learn how to control your stress. In my practice, I see many adults whose necks turn beet red when I examine them. All they have to do, I tell them, is relax.

Tips and Precautions

For some people, their sensitivity is so acute that even calamine lotion causes an allergic reaction. If this describes you, try applying a mixture of baking soda or Epsom salts and water to the rash. Mix the two together to make a paste, and then spread it over the affected area. If the contact dermatitis doesn't improve after a week or two, see your doctor.

BODY SIGNAL ALERT

NECK SPASM WITH LOCKED MUSCLES

Description and Possible Medical Problems

If you've ever had writer's cramp or have been awakened in the middle of the night by painful leg cramps, you're familiar with the pain caused by involuntary muscle spasms. Relief comes when you knead the cramp or change the position of the affected area.

But sometimes a pain in the neck can turn into a spasm that doesn't go away no matter what you do. Torticollis spasmodic is a condition where the head becomes locked into one position and you're unable to move it. It may or may not "unlock" on its own and without warning. However, you should seek medical help immediately.

Torticollis spasmodic can be caused by a number of health problems, including hyperthyroidism, a congenital muscle imbalance, or a defect of the spine. In some cases, the spasm may appear from time to time before disappearing on its own after a few hours or days, while in others the torticollis spasmodic can get progressively worse.

The most dramatic kind of torticollis spasmodic is when the neck muscles lock up as a reaction to the class of drugs known as phenothiazines, which are used to treat psychiatric problems, or to Compazine, which is commonly used to treat nausea.

Treatment

If your neck muscles suddenly lock up and make it impossible to move your head, you should call your doctor immediately. In fact, if you've been taking phenothiazines and feel even a slight spasm in your neck, you should head for the emergency room. Whether the cause is medication or a health disorder such as hyperthyroidism, an injection of antihistamine will usually relieve the spasm and "unlock" the neck muscles.

However, this form of treatment should be provided only by your physician, since over-the-counter antihistamines in the form of pills usually won't work. Once treatment is successful, it's important that you avoid any medication that contains phenothiazines for the rest of your life.

NECK WITH RED "NECKLACE"

Description and Possible Medical Problems

In addition to poisonous plants and certain chemicals, there are many people who are allergic to nickel, which is found in many pieces of jewelry. When you wear a necklace that is nickel-plated and the metal touches the skin of your neck, contact dermatitis can occur, resulting in reddened skin and severe itching. Poison ivy and certain types of soap can also cause contact dermatitis.

Treatment

See "Neck, Red Patches on" above.

SWALLOWING, DIFFICULTY IN

Description and Possible Medical Problems

Everyone has found it difficult to swallow during a particularly emotional time, whether it's your child taking her first steps or graduating from high school. At those moments, you'd probably find yourself unable to swallow even your favorite food. An ordinary sore throat can also make swallowing hard.

However, if you're having difficulty swallowing and the sensation doesn't go away, it's a sign of a serious medical problem, since the act of swallowing is so essential to human health.

If you have difficulty swallowing because of a severe sore throat that hasn't gone away after a week or so, you may be experiencing the beginning of a serious illness that will be diagnosed by the symptoms that accompany the inability to swallow easily. For instance, symptoms such

as weakness in the face, arms, and/or legs along with difficulty swallowing is sometimes the first sign that a person has suffered a stroke.
Though disorders and diseases of the esophagus are rare, certain
esophageal problems such as heartburn or a hernia are all too common
and can make it difficult to swallow normally.

Hyperparathyroidism is a rare condition in which the parathyroid—
four small glands in the neck that release parathyroid hormone, which
regulates bone growth—produces an excess amount of the hormone.
Hyperparathyroidism usually starts when a small growth appears on the
parathyroid gland. This growth can then press against your windpipe,
making it difficult to swallow. Though hyperparathyroidism usually presents no symptoms, a blood test can show an elevated serum calcium
level, which is a sign of the condition.

If you have difficulty swallowing, ask yourself the following questions:

1. Do I have trouble swallowing liquids, solids, or both?

2. If I do have trouble swallowing solids, is meat one of the most
difficult?

3. Do I have heartburn?

4. Am I regurgitating pieces of undigested food?

5. Do I have a sore throat or a fever with swollen glands?

6. If an elderly relative complains of difficulty swallowing, has he or
she recently started to take a new medication or changed a medication?

Treatment

If you find that it's difficult for you to swallow easily, you should call
your doctor. She will conduct a physical exam and run some tests to
help her determine what is making it difficult for you to swallow. She
may do a blood test, as well as an upper GI series to see if a condition
affecting the esophagus is the cause of your swallowing difficulties.

If a sore throat is making it difficult for you to swallow, your doctor
will examine your throat to check if an infection is the cause. She may
also take a throat culture to see if you have strep throat. If you do, treatment may include antibiotic therapy for a week or more with penicillin
or erythromycin. For a common sore throat, over-the-counter lozenges

work well and Tylenol will help relieve the pain. It will also help if you eat mostly soft foods that are easy to swallow.

If heartburn is the primary cause, your doctor may simply recommend that you take antacids and raise the head of your bed at night. If you have hyperparathyroidism, she will probably recommend that the parathyroid gland be surgically removed

Special Mention for the Elderly

In the elderly, swallowing problems are a very serious matter and must be treated right away.

If you have a parent or other relative who has had a stroke or currently has severe Alzheimer's disease, swallowing can become an activity fraught with tension and apprehension because of the difficulty in coordinating the muscular and neurological movements that are necessary when swallowing. Such a person may even lose the desire to eat because it just becomes too difficult.

If swallowing becomes difficult, older people can choke on their food, or food can go down the windpipe instead of the esophagus. Since they lack the strength necessary to cough up even a small piece of food, the food particle may stay in the windpipe for a time. When this happens, a form of pneumonia called aspiration pneumonia can result.

If swallowing is difficult for an elderly parent or relative, her physician might recommend a nasogastric tube to help with feeding. The tube is inserted into the nose through the esophagus and directly into the stomach. Although family members may find this suggestion disturbing and quite unpleasant, it really does help the patient. These tubes are uncomfortable, however, and can eventually cause the skin in the nose to break down, so this feeding method should be used for no more than three months.

If a more permanent method is needed, the nasogastric tube can be removed and a small tube known as a gastric tube, or GT, can be placed directly into the stomach by a gastroenterologist. This is called a PEG procedure. The tube is then hooked up to an automatic feeding pump.

Again, although even the thought of this procedure depresses most family members, I've seen patients whose health and spirits pick up rapidly because the GT provides balanced nutrition after many years of being malnourished. In fact, many patients who have a GT placed soon regain their appetite, begin to eat regular meals again, and ultimately have the tube removed.

Before a gastric tube is prescribed, however, the physician will probably call on a team of other specialists, such as a nutritionist, speech pathologist, and/or an ear, nose, and throat doctor, to see if anything can be done to keep the patient eating real food for a while longer.

See also Chapter 13, "Abdomen and Digestive System."

BODY SIGNAL ALERT

SWALLOWING, DIFFICULTY IN, AS THE DAY GOES ON OR FOOD IS CHEWED

Description and Possible Medical Problems

Some people occasionally have trouble swallowing food or water. Usually it's due to nervousness or anxiety, and it tends to clear up as soon as they calm down a bit. Others, however, may find that one minute they have difficulty swallowing and the next this problem either improves or worsens.

If you're experiencing these symptoms, you may have a rare condition known as myasthenia gravis. Though it is an uncommon disease, many people are aware of it because of its striking, often fickle characteristics. Besides trouble swallowing and chewing, other symptoms of myasthenia gravis include muscle weakness, most often in the face and neck and later in the rest of the body. Your entire body might also become progressively weaker as you chew.

Women are affected more often than men by this disorder, which is caused by an immune system imbalance that affects the nervous system. In effect, the body actually experiences a series of electrical short circuits, which cause it to be fine one minute but weak the next. The thymus, a gland in the chest that helps regulate the immune system, is responsible for the development of myasthenia gravis in approximately 20% of the people who have the condition. In the other 80%, the cause is unknown.

Treatment

Myasthenia gravis cannot be cured, but the disease can be regulated with rest, improved diet, and medication, such as Tensilon or the corticosteroid prednisone, which may help stimulate your immune system. If your doctor determines that your myasthenia gravis is due to a malfunctioning thymus gland, he may recommend an operation to surgically remove the gland; after the procedure, your health will remain stable. Keep in mind, however, that myasthenia gravis is a rare disease. In fact, I have seen only three cases of the disease in all my years of practice.

SWALLOWING, DIFFICULTY IN, WITH A SENSATION OF A LUMP IN THE THROAT

Description and Possible Medical Problems

Often, one of the first physical signs that appears when a person is highly emotional is the sensation of a lump in the throat. Is there or is there not a lump? Or does your throat tighten up as a result of the hormones that naturally flow when your body is stressed in some way?

That is the question.

Globus hystericus is the clinical term for a "lump" in the throat. No lump actually exists; instead, it's the perception of a lump that you feel. You may also find that it's difficult to swallow. Globus hystericus can worsen in certain instances, usually during a heightened emotional state. Interestingly enough, a case of globus hystericus does not make it harder for a person to swallow, and for many people the condition actually disappears when they eat.

When the lump recurs frequently, however, or it doesn't fade away or is accompanied by occasional spasms, you should consult your doctor.

Treatment

If you occasionally feel as though there's a lump in your throat when you become emotional, do nothing. However, studies have shown that a constant feeling of a lump in the throat is a common symptom of depression, obsessive-compulsive disorder, or another emotional problem. When the underlying psychological issue is treated, the lump should disappear.

THROAT CLOSES SUDDENLY, WITH WHEEZING AND DIFFICULTY SWALLOWING

Description and Possible Medical Problems

We've all heard a sad story about a child who was allergic to peanuts or bee venom who unwittingly ate a cookie with peanut oil in it at a birthday party or was stung by a bee and died an hour later of anaphylaxis. Though children's allergies are at once more severe and more common than adults' because of the sensitivity of children's still-developing immune systems, adults can also experience allergic reactions severe enough to require a run to the emergency room.

Whether or not you're prone to allergies, if you suddenly begin to have trouble swallowing and breathing and you feel your throat closing up, get to a doctor or the emergency room immediately. These symptoms are signs of a severe allergic reaction that could become very serious if you don't seek medical attention right away.

Treatment

During an acute allergy attack, you'll need to see your physician immediately. She will give you an injection of epinephrine as well as oral antihistamines to relieve your symptoms. She may also decide to give you cortisone. After your symptoms subside somewhat and you're able to breathe and swallow freely again, your doctor will instruct you about the substances you should avoid and how to keep them to a minimum. If, for instance, you're allergic to dust, an air purifier can help remove dust from the air. It may also help to remove pieces of upholstered furniture, which tend to harbor dust. Some people are also increasingly sensitive to fumes in carpets and dry-cleaned clothes, as well as processed wood that produces toxic fumes.

If you know you are allergic to one or more common substances, it's imperative that you wear an ID bracelet or dog tag or carry a card that identifies the substances you are allergic to in case of future allergic attacks.

See also "Wheezing" in Chapter 11.

BODY SIGNAL ALERT

THROAT, SORE

Description and Possible Medical Problems

In the last several decades, an entire industry has evolved around the common problem of sore throats.

As with hoarseness, a sore throat usually arises because of a temporary condition—such as a cold or allergy or overstressing the throat and larynx by yelling and screaming—but it's important to run through a process of elimination to make sure it's not a sign of a more serious illness.

Ask yourself the following questions to help determine the cause of your sore throat:

1. Has the pollution in my area worsened recently, or have I been spending more time in an urban area?

2. Have I recently been diagnosed with a hiatal hernia?

3. Do I suffer from frequent sinus infections?

4. Is my mouth frequently dry?

5. Does my throat feel sore all day or just in the morning?

6. Do I have a fever as well as a sore throat?

Next, look into a mirror and open your mouth using a spoon to hold your tongue down. Now take a flashlight and look at your throat.

1. Is it fire engine red?

2. Are there white patches that appear to be filled with pus?

There are many causes of sore throat. If you've recently moved to an area where the pollution in the air is denser or are spending more time outside during the middle of the day, when pollution is usually at its worst, you may find yourself with a chronic sore throat. A hiatal hernia—a bulge in the lower esophagus that causes the stomach to press into the chest cavity—frequently causes stomach acids to back up into the esophagus, and you feel a burning in the back of your throat. Even if you don't have a hiatal hernia, if you eat and drink late at night and lie completely horizontal when sleeping, the digestive juices can back up into your esophagus, resulting in a morning-only sore throat.

Sinus infections can also cause a recurrent sore throat. If your sore throat is caused by a dry mouth, it may be that you tend to breathe through your mouth. People who snore often have this problem. And if your throat is very red and sore and you also have a temperature, you might have strep throat. However, if your red, sore throat also has white patches of pus, it's probably not strep but a viral infection. In a young adult, this infection is usually mononucleosis; in an older adult, it's a simple viral infection.

Treatment

Because there are so many reasons why your throat may be sore, the treatment will depend on the cause. If you think pollution is causing your sore throat, your only remedy is to stay inside more and to venture outside only in the early morning and on days when the air pollution index is low.

If you have a sinus infection, antihistamines can help alleviate a sore throat by stopping the postnasal drip. If your mouth is dry because of the sinus infection, sipping water frequently during the day will help keep your throat moist and more comfortable.

If I think a patient has strep throat, I'll take a throat culture. It's important to seek treatment for strep throat right away, since it can lead to scarlet fever or rheumatic fever if left untreated. If the culture comes back positive, I'll treat it with penicillin or erythromycin for a 10-day period. Although strep throat occurs more frequently in children than adults, you should know that if you have strep throat, you can easily pass it to your children.

Contrary to popular belief, however, antibiotics are not the panacea many people think they are. If your sore throat is caused by a bacterial infection, I will prescribe antibiotics only after I take a recent health history, do a physical exam, and conduct a few lab tests, including a throat culture and blood tests. Even with the antibiotics, you'll still have to rest, drink lots of liquids, and complete the entire course of medication. Otherwise the infection can return in a form even more severe than the first time around.

If you have a sore throat that's making it difficult for you to swallow, I'll look for a swelling behind the throat, or a tonsillar abscess, which is typically caused by a bacterial infection. If this is left untreated, the throat may actually begin to close up. If this occurs, the airway may become blocked, creating a life-or-death situation, which is why it's important to see your doctor in the early stages of a sore throat.

See also "Mouth, Dry" in Chapter 7.

THROAT, TICKLE IN

Description and Possible Medical Problems

We all get a tickle in the throat from time to time. It may be caused by a particle of dust, a hair, even a minute carpet fiber. In the winter, dry air can also be responsible for a tickle in the throat.

Sometimes, however, when a tickle in the throat doesn't go away, another culprit may be at work. If you have sinus problems, the post-nasal drip that frequently accompanies them can create a tickle in your throat. Sleeping with your mouth open can also dry out your throat. And a tickle in the throat can sometimes be a by-product of the aging process. As the muscles of the throat gradually lose their tone, touch one another, and even slightly fold in on themselves in places, you may experience the sensation of a chronic tickle in the throat. And as we grow older, the body's tissues tend to dry out gradually. Since this is true of throat tissue as well, dryness can cause the tickle.

Treatment

The good news is that a tickle in your throat is easy to treat. If it is caused by dry air or a dry throat or by the aging process, taking frequent sips of water, sucking on hard candy, or chewing gum can help lubricate the throat and cut down on the tickle.

You can also try turning down the heat in the wintertime and humidifying the air with a wet towel draped over your radiator or a humidifier, especially at night.

VOICE, CHANGES IN

Description and Possible Medical Problems

Teenage boys spend a lot of their time trying to control their cracking voices. And some men in their 70s and older discover that their voices start to change as well, becoming higher in pitch with a tremble that wasn't there before.

This vocal change late in life is caused by the gradual weakening of the vocal cords. As a result, they allow more air to escape as you speak, resulting in a higher voice.

When an adult in midlife undergoes a change of voice, the cause is usually more serious, such as polyps or a tumor on the larynx. Cigarette smoking is the number one cause of voice changes in the midlife adult due to cancer of the larynx or lung. More men than women develop tumors of the larynx and lung; since cigarette smoking causes the majority of cases of cancer of the larynx, and for many years more men smoked than women, men have an unfair "advantage."

Polyps and papillomae—a cluster of polyps—are two kinds of laryngeal tumors. Whether benign or malignant, any such tumor should be removed immediately and checked by your doctor.

In the elderly, neurological diseases such as Parkinson's will also cause the voice to change. And the aging process tends to make the voice seem softer. In addition, a change in dentures or the loss of a tooth can cause the voice to change.

A very serious cause of voice change is lung cancer, especially when it spreads to the vocal cords.

Treatment

I always take a voice change seriously, since it can indicate the presence of a more serious health problem. When a patient tells me that his voice has changed, I do a complete checkup, including blood tests, a chest X ray, and a visual examination of the throat. If I see polyps on the vocal cords, I'll refer the patient to an ear, nose, and throat specialist, who will do a biopsy to see if the polyps are benign or malignant. In most cases, regardless of the results of the biopsy, the specialist will recommend that the polyps be removed with laser surgery. Though little medical follow-up is necessary, the patient may want to see a speech pathologist, who will teach him how to talk in normal tones so that the polyps don't return. If the polyps are malignant, I'll then refer the patient to an oncologist for further treatment, which may include chemotherapy and radiation therapy.

In any case, if your voice suddenly changes and doesn't return to normal after a week, you should see your doctor immediately.

Chapter 9

SKIN

═══ **BODY SIGNAL ALERT** ═══

Call your doctor if you experience any of the following symptoms:

SYMPTOM	POSSIBLE MEDICAL CONDITION
You have a changed lesion on your skin that is scaly and hard	*Squamous cell carcinoma*
You have a new lesion on your skin that is brown with an irregular border	*Malignant melanoma*
You have a new lesion on your skin that is raised and pearly in color	*Basal cell carcinoma*
You have pimples on one side of your face that are painful	*Shingles*
Your skin has taken on a yellow tone	*Jaundice, other liver disease*
You have a rash over your entire body	*Reaction to medication*

HOW THE SKIN AGES

The skin is the body's largest organ, consisting of more than two square yards. Though the skin serves as the major outlet for many of the vital parts of the body—from sweat glands to nerve endings to blood vessels—it is the substance collagen that is responsible for the signs of aging that appear on the skin.

The epidermis is the top layer of your skin. It consists of cells that are eventually sloughed off from your skin. These cells contain keratin, a protein, and melanin, which colors your skin.

Beneath the epidermis is the dermis, which contains strong fibers of collagen along with elastic fibers called elastin. Together, they work to provide a strong, firm base.

As we age, however, the dermis starts to thin and the collagen and elastin become stiffer, which creates wrinkles as well as a paler skin tone. Years of gravity and possible obesity take their toll as well, resulting in a change in facial contours, a double chin, and sagging eyelids. Older skin also becomes drier, as the skin's oil glands no longer produce as much oil.

DRY, SCALY PATCHES THAT ITCH

Description and Possible Medical Problems

Dermatitis is an umbrella term for skin that is irritated and inflamed. If you have dry patches on your face and body that are scaly and itchy, you have eczema, a type of dermatitis. There are many other kinds of dermatitis, some caused by internal reactions, some by external reactions to, for example, a chemical or an allergen.

Though most people with dermatitis have a genetic sensitivity, eczema is a skin condition that is caused by an external reaction. There are also many types of eczema, from a condition called housewife's hands, a reaction to detergents and cleaning solutions, to seborrheic eczema, which occurs on the face.

Treatment

If your dry, itchy patches have appeared suddenly, you should see your doctor for treatment. He may prescribe a corticosteroid preparation to apply to the affected area. This medication will reduce the dryness and inflammation.

If your dry skin has appeared or worsened only since you began taking a new kind of medication, your doctor will switch you to another medication that is equally effective but does not have the side effects.

There's always the possibility that you have developed an allergy to a substance that previously gave you no trouble; this substance might be a new cosmetic or moisturizer. If you think this might be the case, try eliminating, one by one, any new cosmetics you have bought that may come into even brief contact with the areas of your skin that are affected. You might, for example, be using a new hand cream, and if you frequently touch your face, your skin may be irritated.

If this process of elimination doesn't help, see your doctor. You may be having a new allergic reaction to a certain food.

HEAT RASH

See "Rash Under Breast" in Chapter 12.

BODY SIGNAL ALERT

LESION, BROWN, WITH IRREGULAR BORDER

Description and Possible Medical Problems

We have all noticed minute changes in our skin, whether a new mole that has suddenly appeared or a scar that appears to be invisible—until we get a sunburn or a tan.

If you notice that a small patch of skin on your face or body has turned dark brown and has an irregular border, you may have malignant melanoma, which is the most dangerous type of skin cancer to have.

Basal cell carcinoma (see "Lesion, Raised and Pearl-colored" below) and squamous cell carcinoma (see "Lesion, Scaly and Hard" below), the other types of skin cancer, are easy to treat because they don't spread, or metastasize, to other parts of the body. Malignant melanoma, however, can quickly spread throughout the lymphatic system.

Melanoma develops as a lesion on the skin or inside moles or other skin growths; it starts in the cells that provide pigment to the skin. While some benign tumors later become malignant, malignant melanoma starts out as cancerous cells and does not develop from a previously benign growth.

As with basal and squamous cell carcinomas, malignant melanoma tends to occur in people who have had a significant amount of exposure to the sun, such as sailors, farmers, and construction workers.

Treatment

The moment you notice any change in a mole or in a dark brown, irregularly shaped patch of skin on your face or body, see your doctor. It's important to treat malignant melanoma before it has a chance to spread, because it does metastasize so rapidly.

Your doctor will take a biopsy of your skin to determine if the growth is benign or malignant. If it is malignant, she will remove the tumor under local anesthesia, usually on an outpatient basis. If the growth has appeared near a lymph gland in your neck, your doctor will probably remove the gland as well, to guard against further spread. If your doctor believes the melanoma has spread into the muscle or bone, he may also order chemotherapy or radiation treatment.

QUESTIONS TO ASK IF YOU HAVE A RASH OR SKIN LESION

If you have a skin lesion, whether it's a raised area of the skin that may or may not change in color, or if it comes in the form of a rash, ask yourself the following questions and then tell your doctor the answers. They will help determine your diagnosis and subsequent treatment.

1.   How long have I had the lesion? Did it appear in the last 24 to 48 hours, or have I had it for several months?

2.   If the lesion is in the form of a rash, does it itch? Is it red and flaky? Is there a break in the skin?

3.   Is the rash located in an area that has been exposed to a potential irritant? Have I changed soaps or detergents lately?

4.   Have I changed a medication or tried a new food lately?

5.   Is the rash localized to one side of the body, or does it appear on both sides?

6.   Is the lesion bleeding?

7.   Is the lesion flat or raised?

8.   Does cold temperature bring about the rash?

9.   Has my skin changed color?

10.   If I have a pimple or mole, has it grown or changed in some way?

11.   Do I have more rashes in summertime?

LESION, DARK AND ROUGH-TEXTURED

Description and Possible Medical Problems

It's a medical fact that fair-skinned people are more prone to skin cancer than those with darker skins are. An early sign of skin cancer in a light-skinned person is the appearance of a darkened lesion that feels like sandpaper. Since only sun-exposed areas of the skin have these lesions, called actinic keratoses, or solar keratoses, the face is especially vulnerable.

Though an actinic keratosis is a benign skin growth, it can turn into a malignant squamous cell carcinoma.

Treatment

Because doctors consider an actinic keratosis to be a premalignant tumor, your doctor will probably recommend that it be removed either surgically or with cryotherapy, in which the lesion is frozen off.

Another treatment is with a topical cream called 5-fluorouracil, or 5-FU, a medication that chemically removes the lesion over the course of two to four weeks. If your doctor treats you with 5-FU, the lesion will feel as though it's burning. The pain can be alleviated with the simultaneous use of a corticosteroid cream.

After the initial burning sensation, the lesion will begin to ulcerate before it begins to heal. At this point, the daily application of 5-FU should be discontinued.

Your doctor will also recommend that, to avoid future growths of actinic keratosis, you stay out of the sun as much as possible and use a sunscreen with an SPF of 15 or higher whenever you do go outside.

LESION, RAISED AND PEARL-COLORED

Description and Possible Medical Problems

If you notice a raised lesion on your face with a luminescent color, like a pearl, chances are you have one of the most common forms of skin cancer, basal cell carcinoma.

Basal cell carcinoma affects men and women who burn easily in the sun and who have had a significant amount of sun exposure over the course of their lives. Some doctors believe that heredity can increase your risk of contracting this malignant form of cancer.

But the news is actually very good. The fact is that basal cell carcinoma rarely spreads to other parts of the body, and it's one of the easiest kinds of cancer to treat.

Treatment

Though basal cell carcinoma rarely spreads to other parts of the body, your doctor will want to remove the tumor when biopsy shows a positive diagnosis. He will remove it surgically, with radiation, or by freezing it with cryosurgery.

After treatment has been successful and all traces of the tumor have been removed, your doctor will recommend that you stay out of the sun unless you regularly and liberally apply a sunscreen with an SPF of 15 or higher.

LESION, SCALY AND HARD

Description and Possible Medical Problems

As you've read elsewhere in this chapter, if you spent your youth and early adult years baking or working in the sun, you're more apt to get skin cancer than a person who has stayed in the shade.

If you begin to notice that the part of your skin that's been exposed to the sun begins to look scaly and feels as though it's hardened, you may have squamous cell carcinoma, a form of skin cancer.

Squamous cell carcinoma frequently appears on the lips, hands, or ears; people 50 and over are most likely to have squamous cell carcinoma.

In addition to the hardened scaliness, you may also notice that a small growth has appeared below the rough skin. This growth may resemble a wart or an ulcer, but if it doesn't clear up completely, you'll know it's squamous cell cancer.

Treatment

If you notice a growth that may be a squamous cell carcinoma, see your doctor right away. Squamous cell carcinoma can eventually spread to other parts of the body, making it harder to treat.

Your physician will probably take a biopsy of the tumor in order to determine proper treatment, which will probably include surgical removal of the tumor. Treatments in addition to surgery may include chemotherapy, cryotherapy, and radiation (see pp. 196-197 for more information). When a squamous cell tumor is detected and treated early, the survival rate is close to 100%. After treatment, you will need to see your doctor regularly to guard against other growths.

LIVER OR AGE SPOTS

Description and Possible Medical Problems

You may think of your grandmother when you hear the term "liver spots," and you may be alarmed when you begin to see these flat, reddish-brown patches on the backs of your hands and other parts of your body that have been exposed to the sun. Don't worry . . . it happens to the best of us!

Liver or age spots, also known as senile lentigines, begin to appear after the age of 50 and are a normal sign of aging.

Treatment

Some people decide to treat their liver spots by bleaching them or by using cover-up creams to hide them. Others choose to have them removed with cryotherapy, in which the spot is frozen with liquid nitrogen, then removed.

Many people choose to leave liver spots alone, because they don't grow larger or darker with time. After all, they do serve as a badge of all the experiences you've had in your life.

MOLES, CHANGES IN

Description and Possible Medical Problems

It seems as though almost everyone has a few moles on the body. Most of the time, a mole is nothing more than a cosmetic issue. Some people will have a mole removed, but in recent years celebrities like Madonna and Cindy Crawford have made moles appear sexy.

If you have a small, raised mole, possibly with a hair growing from it, you can usually leave it alone. However, if you notice that the mole has changed in any way, you should see your doctor, since any change could be a sign of melanoma.

Here are some of the ways in which a mole can change:

1. A change in pigmentation around the base of the mole

2. A change in the consistency, surface, or color of the mole

3. A sudden increase in the size of a mole

4. Loss of hair from a mole

5. Any amount of bleeding from a mole

Treatment

If you have a mole that has changed in appearance, you should see your doctor or dermatologist, who will consider your history and carefully examine the mole. If she determines that the change in the mole is a sign of melanoma, it will need to be removed with surgery or cryotherapy. This will not only remove the cancer but also stop its spread. You may also need chemotherapy along with an extensive medical follow-up.

PIMPLES

Description and Possible Medical Problems

I bet you thought you left acne and the occasional pimple behind in your 20s.

Guess again. Though acne flare-ups in adults do not occur to the degree they do in teenagers, midlife and older adults can indeed get pimples on their faces—and elsewhere on the body.

A pimple forms when an oil gland that surrounds a hair follicle becomes plugged by sebum, the oil produced by the gland. The male hormone androgen, which is produced by both men and women, plays a role in sebum production because an increase in the amount of andro-gen in the body means an increase in sebum.

There are several reasons why pimples may suddenly make an appearance in an adult. Androgen levels, for one, can be affected by medications such as birth control pills. But acne can also be aggravated by the use of certain cosmetics, especially heavy moisturizing creams, which can block the oil glands and produce a buildup of sebum or encourage an allergic reaction that produces pimples. Creams can also aggravate preexisting acne. Heredity can also play a role.

Treatment

If your acne has recently appeared only after you began using a new cos-metic, you should discontinue its use and see if it clears up. If a new medication is the culprit, ask your doctor which medication you should switch to.

There are a number of other steps you can try to treat it yourself. Benzoyl peroxide is an over-the-counter medication that causes your skin to peel. When this happens, the skin around the pimples begins to flake and the plugs in the oil glands fall out.

Some midlife women find that their acne flare-ups coincide with the onset of their menstrual periods. If this is the case, you can help reduce the incidence of pimples by keeping your skin clean enough so that it is slightly dry—again, to encourage the skin to peel and reduce the number of pimples. You don't have to worry that keeping your skin dry will cause it to wrinkle; if your skin is producing enough oil to make pimples, it has enough oil to keep it moist. But don't let it become too dry; the oil gland will overreact and produce even more oil, and therefore more pimples.

If your acne is severe, see a dermatologist. She may prescribe the antibiotic tetracycline, which can clear up the acne and prevent scarring.

Look at the bright side: having pimples may make you feel like a kid again, except this time you don't have to ask your parents what time you have to be home!

Tips and Precautions

Though you probably remember hearing as a teenager that your acne was caused by chocolate, greasy foods, oversleeping, or even masturbating, none of these things is true.

PIMPLES AND RED SKIN ON FOREHEAD AND NOSE

Description and Possible Medical Problems

Though acne isn't as common in adults as it is in teenagers, the fact is that there is a form of acne that only people over 40 can get, called rosacea. Rosacea is a type of acne that results in red skin with pimples; it usually appears on the nose, which may result in a thickened appearance to the nose. You may have only a few pimples or many that are concentrated in a small area.

Treatment

To treat rosacea, your doctor will prescribe a treatment that's similar to what she would recommend for a teenager with acne. This may be one of a variety of skin creams such as Metrogel. As with severe cases of acne in teenagers, if you have rosacea, the best person to diagnose and treat it is your doctor or dermatologist.

BODY SIGNAL ALERT

PIMPLES, PAINFUL, ON ONE SIDE OF YOUR FACE

Description and Possible Medical Problems

If you had chicken pox as a kid, chances are very good that the cluster of painful pimples that appears on one side of your face is shingles. Before the pimples arrive, you'll feel a sharp pain in the area where the pimples will appear, along with a burning sensation. The rash usually lasts about a week, but the pain may stick around for months after the pimples disappear. If the rash occurs near your eyes, you may find you have temporary or permanent problems with your vision.

Shingles, which can also appear on the side of your body just below your chest, is caused by the herpes zoster virus, the same virus that causes chicken pox in children. Shingles appear when the dormant virus is reactivated, which happens most often in adults over the age of 50.

It's believed that the virus spends its latent years in the ends of nerves that originate in the spine. It's not known exactly why it becomes active again—and not every adult who had chicken pox as a kid will get shingles. However, the virus's genesis in the nerves accounts for the sharp, localized pain that characterizes shingles.

Treatment

Once you have an attack of shingles and the rash has appeared, there's nothing you can do to lessen its severity. You can, however, treat the pain and inflammation of the rash with aspirin and calamine lotion. Cold compresses that have been soaked in a 5% solution of aluminum acetate—also called Burow's solution—can also help soothe the skin more than calamine lotion, especially if the rash is severe.

Some physicians prescribe the corticosteroid medication prednisone to help relieve pain and swelling, but, again, it will not reduce the amount of time you'll have to put up with the rash.

If the rash occurs near the eyes, there is a danger that it may cause a severe eye infection. If you develop conjunctivitis, also called pinkeye, along with the rash, you should see your ophthalmologist.

BODY SIGNAL ALERT

RASH

Description and Possible Medical Problems

The first thing you must know about skin rashes is that they cannot be diagnosed over the telephone; they need to be examined by a physician.

I've found that the way a patient describes the rash is almost never the way it appears, at least to my diagnostic eyes.

The causes of rashes run the gamut from a reaction to a new medication that you've just begun to take, such as penicillin, to a low blood platelet count (if a rash is bleeding). The latter is a condition that looks like a red rash or skin irritation when it first appears but can quickly start to ooze or bleed. The cause may be a viral or bacterial infection that causes a skin infection called cellulitis, or it may be recent exposure to a toxic chemical you've never handled before. And people who are highly emotional sometimes break out in rashes periodically. All of these conditions require medical attention, which is why it's so important to see your doctor for proper treatment when you first notice the rash.

First, however, ask yourself the following questions, since your answers will help your physician to determine the diagnosis and the proper treatment for your rash:

1. Have I recently been exposed to a chemical or a new medication?

2. Does the rash itch?

3. Is the rash flat, diffused, or pinpointed, confined to a certain area?

4. Where did the rash first appear?

5. Is it localized, or does the rash appear all over my body?

6. Do I have a fever and/or chills?

7. Have I recently been exposed to a person who has a rash?

8. Has my skin recently been broken due to a trauma or a bite?

Treatment

If the rash is generalized and appears over a large area of your body, a new medication is usually the culprit. Your doctor will recommend that you stop using the medication; he'll suggest an alternative. He'll also advise you to apply calamine lotion or over-the-counter Benadryl three or four times a day to soothe the itching. If the rash appears as a small area of bloodlike pimples on your lower legs and ankles, it may be due to a low platelet count, and the treatment will include drug therapy to increase the count, along with dietary iron supplementation. If the rash appears under the breast or in the groin, you probably have a fungal infection that is often seen in diabetics and obese people. Treatment will be in the form of an antifungal ointment such as Lotrimin three times a day.

If the rash appears as a redness around an area of skin that has recently been traumatized or broken, the cause is usually an infection, and treatment will consist of an antibiotic such as Keflex or Cipro taken by mouth. If the rash is particularly severe, you may need to be hospitalized in order to receive the antibiotic intravenously.

If the rash occurs on one side of your body, starting on your back and continuing around to the front of your torso, and the appearance of the rash is preceded by tingling and pain, you probably have shingles or the herpes zoster virus. Treatment will consist of a medication called Zovirax that can be taken orally or spread on in a cream to speed recovery. A viral rash or one that's caused by a drug reaction may be flat and might itch (see also "Pimples, Painful, on One Side of the Face" above).

If the rash occurs on your face and itches and is accompanied by pain and fever, and if you never had chicken pox when you were a kid, you should see your doctor right away. Chicken pox can be severe when it occurs in an adult, and a medication such as Zovirax will be used to treat it.

If the rash appears on your hands and feet and in your mouth, and you also have malaise and a fever, you probably have a common summertime virus called a coxsackievirus. This virus lasts about a week, and there is no known treatment for it.

Finally, if the rash occurs in a series of small clusters or as a large sore on your genitalia, possibly accompanied by a discharge of pus from the urethra, you may have herpes or gonorrhea, which will need to be treated with medication.

Again, since all these conditions require a doctor's attention, the moment you notice a rash starting to form, you should contact your physician for advice on what to do.

RASH ON THE FACE

Description and Possible Medical Problems

From time to time, we all get one of these common conditions: skin rashes, pain in the joints, and a feeling of fatigue. Usually, however, these conditions appear by themselves.

When they appear simultaneously, it's probably not a coincidence, but a disease called lupus erythematosus. Lupus has long been considered to be somewhat of a mystery due to its various symptoms, which may change in severity from one day to the next. This occurs because lupus is primarily a disease of the body's connective tissue. Since connective tissue appears throughout the body, it's no surprise that lupus is so pervasive—and so stubborn. Not only the skin and joints can be affected but also vital organs such as the kidneys and brain, the circulatory system, and the sacs that surround the heart and lungs.

The rash that generally appears across the cheeks and nose is more likely to occur when the skin is exposed to strong sunlight, since another characteristic of the disease is that the skin becomes more sensitive to light.

Lupus is primarily a woman's disease; about 10 times as many women as men are affected. It is a chronic disease, and there is no known cure.

However, many people with lupus are able to enjoy long periods between flare-ups.

Treatment

The diagnosis for lupus is made by a blood test called FANA or lupus prep. If the test is positive and only the skin is affected, no systemic treatment is needed. Treatment of the rash will involve a combination of the corticosteroid medication prednisone and antiarthritic medication. However, if the disease affects the kidneys, brain, or other vital organs, treatment obviously requires a multidisciplinary approach depending on the organs involved.

RED, SCALY PATCHES

Description and Possible Medical Problems

Sometimes your skin may turn red due to nervousness or stress. The redness may last for a few minutes or a few hours.

However, if you develop solid red, scaly plaques on the trunk of your body that are very sharply defined and scaly in appearance, chances are you have psoriasis. Psoriasis is easy to diagnose because the borders between the normal and affected skin are usually very distinct.

Psoriasis can also affect your elbows, the palms of your hands, and the soles of your feet, but it usually does not provoke itching.

Treatment

The primary treatments for psoriasis have come a long way since my days in medical school. Back then, coal tar, special lamps, and steroid solutions were the norm. Today, these treatments do have their place, but when a small area of the body is affected, for instance, the elbows, a steroid cream such as Diprolene might be enough. If the psoriasis spreads across the trunk, however, you may need to schedule weekly sessions under special lamps that can help heal the lesions.

SKIN, BROKEN, ON
BUTTOCKS AND HEELS

Description and Possible Medical Problems

One of the biggest concerns of doctors who treat a large number of elderly patients is preventing the development of bedsores. The first sign of a bedsore is usually a break in the skin, so if an elderly relative is confined to bed, it's important that any break in the skin—especially on the buttocks or heels—receive medical attention. A bedsore can develop due to poor nutrition or immobility. If an area has constant friction and pressure on it—in the case of a person who is bedridden—the skin can become frail. The skin can then quickly break down and the sore can spread down to the bone and cause a bone infection called osteomyelitis. The infection can also spread into the bloodstream and cause a bloodborne infection of bacteria known as septicemia.

Treatment

The best treatment is prevention of the bedsore by helping a bedbound patient to move around and change position in bed several times a day.

For an existing bedsore, there are a variety of treatments. The most important treatment is excellent nursing care. An alert nurse will help keep pressure off the area; a special mattress made of foam or sheepskin or a special airflow bed can also help.

Once a bedsore develops, the area must be kept impeccably clean with saline solution and sterile packing materials. Bedsore care will also depend on the general health of the patient.

If the bedsore has caused an infection, your elderly relative will need to receive intravenous antibiotic therapy. If the bedsore contains areas of dead skin, the doctor will need to remove the dead skin surgically. This procedure, which is not painful, is called a debridment.

SKIN, BROKEN, ON THE LEG

See "Leg Ulcer (Open Sore)" in Chapter 16.

SKIN COLOR, CHANGE IN, ON A SMALL PATCH OF SKIN

Description and Possible Medical Problems

The fickle dictates of fashion tell us sometimes that it's in to be tan, while at other times it's better to be pale. In response, many people learn to manipulate the color of their skin with natural or artificial light and with tanning gels and lotions.

However, if the color of your skin disappears, it could be a loss of melanin or skin pigment known as vetiligo, a condition in which the melanocytes—the pigment-producing cells of your skin—lose their ability to produce pigment. The condition usually starts as a small patch and gradually grows larger. In recent years, it's come to be known as the Michael Jackson disease.

In addition to losing the color in the skin, some people with this condition also lose the color in their hair. They may begin to lose some of their hair, as well.

Treatment

While the depigmentation of your skin is not a health problem, it can be unaesthetic. Unfortunately, there is no satisfactory treatment for the condition, but many people use cosmetics and cover-up creams to make it less noticeable.

SKIN, ORANGE

Description and Possible Medical Problems

Every once in a while, I'm visited by a patient who has an orange hue to her skin, which is especially noticeable in the creases of the palms of her hands.

This is commonly seen in people in their twenties and early thirties and is called carotenemia. The most common cause of the syndrome is vegetarianism and an excessive intake of the vitamin beta-carotene, which is most commonly caused by eating too many carrots. As more people in their 40s and 50s become vegetarians, I am sure I'll be seeing more and more orange-colored patients walk through my door.

Treatment

Fortunately, carotenemia is not a serious condition, and there is no need for treatment. Just cut down on the number of carrots you eat.

BODY SIGNAL ALERT

SKIN, PALE

Description and Possible Medical Problems

I'll bet that when you were a child and not feeling well, your mother placed her hand on your forehead, announced that you were looking pale, and then sent you to bed. It's true that when we are young and become sick, it is not uncommon to become pale. In children and young adults, the pallor is usually a temporary condition that clears up once they start to feel better.

In adults, however, pallor is a different story. If other people have been telling you for a long time that you look pale, or if you've noticed it yourself, you should ask yourself the following questions:

1. Have I recently lost weight? Has my appetite changed?

2. Do I feel increasingly frail and afraid of falling down? Do I sometimes refuse to get out of bed?

3. Have my bowel habits recently changed? Has the color of my stool changed to black?

4. Am I taking aspirin or antiarthritic medications regularly?

5. Do I feel my health is slowly deteriorating?

Sometimes pallor occurs when you feel under the weather for a few days; your color returns when you feel better. At other times, however, a more serious medical condition can be the cause. When pallor is accompanied by weight loss, the cause can be gastrointestinal bleeding as the result of an ulcer, a benign lesion, or even cancer. If this is the case, your stool may have turned black or you may have recently vomited up a substance that resembles coffee grounds. In this case, because the symptoms are frightening, you usually seek medical attention immediately.

If you're taking a large amount of aspirin or antiarthritic medications, you may have a bleeding ulcer that is responsible for your pallor. If, however, you feel increasingly weak or frail and feel that your health is slowly deteriorating, your pallor may be caused by anemia. This is a problem more common in elderly people and can make them more prone to falling. Younger patients can adapt to the slow blood loss that typically occurs with anemia because, typically, their heart adjusts to the reduced blood supply by beating more quickly. In an elderly person, this can lead to a heart attack or heart failure.

Treatment

If the pallor is due to loss of blood from a bleeding ulcer or bleeding from the gastrointestinal tract, the doctor will treat these conditions (see Chapter 13, "Abdomen and Digestive System").

Pallor caused by anemia can also occur because of a reaction to a drug or a vitamin deficiency. In rare cases, it may also point to cancer. If the anemia is very severe, your doctor may order a blood transfusion. In an elderly patient, the transfusion will be done very slowly so as not to shock the system. The decision to give a transfusion will be based on all the information provided to the physician, and, as always, the risk of letting the illness proceed versus the benefits of the treatment will be considered.

SKIN, RED AND SWOLLEN

Description and Possible Medical Problems

As the skin ages, it becomes thinner and naturally less resistant to bacteria, viruses, and allergens that can irritate it, either on the surface or below, in the epidermis.

A variety of infections and allergens can cause the skin to appear red and swollen. Most are easy to treat.

Sometimes an insect bite, a scratch, or inflammation of a hair follicle can become infected and cause the surrounding skin to become red and swollen. This frequently occurs when bacteria enter the skin through the wound and then cause an infection. Frequently, however, an infection occurs when the skin has come into contact with a substance that has caused an allergic reaction—anything from poison ivy to a new brand of makeup.

Because older skin is also more sensitive to trauma, sometimes it may seem as though your skin is constantly red and irritated. Fortunately, this doesn't have to be the rule for you.

Treatment

First, try to determine the cause of the redness and swelling by asking yourself the following questions:

1. Have I recently eaten a new food?

2. Have I changed the brand of a cosmetic I normally use?

3. Have I recently been out in the woods and in contact with a variety of plants?

4. Did I recently scratch or injure the skin on my face in some way and neglect to clean and disinfect it properly?

You can treat the symptoms above yourself by (1) eliminating any suspect food from your diet; (2) not using any new cosmetic on your face; (3) treating the inflammation with calamine lotion and aspirin; and (4) cleaning the red, swollen area. You may also want to try an over-the-counter steroid cream such as Cortaid or an antihistamine such as Benadryl to relieve the itch. Never use alcohol, as it can dry out the skin and make the itch worse. Some people also find a cool bath to be helpful.

If you've taken these steps and your skin is still red and swollen, or the condition gets worse, see your doctor. You may have an underlying infection that will respond only to professional treatment and prescription medication.

SKIN TAGS

Description and Possible Medical Problems

The term "skin tag" is one of those things that sounds old-fashioned, like something your grandmother would talk about.

For those who prefer more up-to-date terms, a skin tag is also known as a cutaneous tag or an acrochordon. Skin tags are basically benign growths that protrude somewhat from your skin. They may be the same color as your skin or a bit darker, and they usually appear on the neck and torso. They are a normal part of aging and are nothing to worry about. Skin tags first start to appear in midlife and are especially common in people 60 and over.

Treatment

Though they are benign tumors, skin tags are not dangerous. Many people find them unsightly, however, and choose to have them removed by a physician. The usual method of removing a skin tag is cryotherapy or cauterization.

If you choose to leave the skin tag alone and its appearance later changes, it's a good idea to have it checked by your doctor since any changes in a benign skin tumor, from a mole to a skin tag, can be a sign of malignancy.

BODY SIGNAL ALERT

SKIN, YELLOW, WITH DARK URINE

Description and Possible Medical Problems

If your normally rosy complexion has recently taken on a yellowish tinge, and if the whites of your eyes also start to look somewhat yellow, you may have jaundice. Jaundice is caused by an accumulation of waste product from the bloodstream that collects in the liver. This waste product is called bilirubin. With jaundice, the body is unable to remove the excess bilirubin from the body, which then causes it to build up in the liver, turning your skin yellow and your urine dark. You might also have other symptoms such as weight loss and changes in your bowel habits, the color of your urine, and your appetite.

Jaundice is usually caused by a liver disease such as hepatitis or cirrhosis, but anything that blocks the flow of bile from the liver—such as a gallstone that becomes trapped in the bile duct—can also cause jaundice. Other causes may be an enlargement of the pancreas or a reaction to a medication.

Treatment

When you first notice your skin turning yellow, you should immediately call your doctor, who will base his treatment on the underlying condition. Also see "Liver Function Test, Abnormal" in Chapter 18 for treatment options.

I once had a patient who had developed a large hematoma—a mass of blood that collects under the skin—as a result of a car accident. When the hematoma began to break down, it released the bilirubin that had been stored up. The liver was not able to metabolize the bilirubin fast enough, so he developed jaundice. After a week or two, however, when the liver was able to process the extra bilirubin, his skin returned to its natural color.

SUNBURN

Description and Possible Medical Problems

I can't begin to tell you how many of my patients have had their vacations ruined by sunburn. They know the precautions to take—with high-SPF lotions and restricted exposure to the sun—but once they're on vacation, many disregard common sense completely.

A sunburn, a condition in which the skin becomes sore and red as a result of excessive sun exposure, is usually the result of an overzealous effort to become tan, often on the first day at the beach. The increased use of sun lamps at home and in tanning parlors has also increased the number of sunburn cases.

In extreme cases of sunburn, a person can develop sun poisoning, in which the skin actually is burned. Chills, fever, and swelling may also occur.

Treatment

To prevent a sunburn, try to restrict your exposure to the sun to 15 to 20 minutes at a time over the course of several days. Using a sunblock with a high SPF number will allow you to spend more time in the sun than if you were unprotected.

If you have become sunburned, use cool compresses and sunburn cream to soothe the pain and redness. Aloe vera seems to work quite well, as do many of the commercial aftersun preparations.

If you develop a fever or blisters, you should see your physician, who may prescribe a course of antibiotics.

WRINKLES

Description and Possible Medical Problems

Like gray hair, wrinkles are a normal part of aging. However, wrinkles tend to appear earlier than gray hair in most people and so are fought more rabidly and for a longer period of time.

One factor we can't control when it comes to wrinkles is the fact that skin becomes thinner as it ages, which hastens the appearance of wrinkles. Certain factors can speed up the initial appearance of wrinkles and make them worse once they do appear. Cigarette smoking and sun exposure are often cited as the two best friends a wrinkle can have. Failing to drink enough water every day is also a significant factor, since adequately hydrated skin tends to wrinkle later and less often.

Most of the expensive skin creams that supposedly "turn back the clock" on wrinkles help keep the skin moist—if you apply the cream to damp skin—but the most important thing you can do is to hydrate your skin from within by drinking 8 to 10 glasses of water a day. It's never too late to start. You should also stop smoking cigarettes and restrict your exposure to the sun.

Treatment

Wrinkles, of course, are irreversible, unless you decide to opt for cosmetic surgery.

Getting a face-lift has been a popular choice for both women and men for years, but the major drawback, besides the fact that any surgical procedure is dangerous, is the fact that it isn't permanent, which necessitates a repeat performance in a number of years—and at regular intervals afterward. For some people, however, a face-lift is definitely worth it.

Dermatologists have prescribed the use of certain preparations for years, though the side effects can sometimes be harsh (see sidebar on Retin-A).

Again, more and more people today are deciding to let nature take its course and to age with grace—which includes getting wrinkles.

A FEW WORDS ABOUT RETIN-A

The hot new product in skin care the past couple of years has been Retin-A, popularly called the "antiwrinkle cream." Retin-A is the brand name for tretinoin, a derivative of vitamin A, and it's been around for 20 years for the treatment of acne. Retin-A has been shown to reduce fine wrinkles and improve skin texture by smoothing out rough patches of skin, but this prescription drug has still not been approved by the FDA for the specific purpose of reversing the effects of photoaging.

It's not known exactly how Retin-A works, but it does stimulate new collagen growth in the dermis of the skin and help restore the epidermis to its natural, undamaged state. As with any medication, some individuals are sensitive to Retin-A and many people experience dryness, peeling, redness, and swelling when they use it. People who are prescribed this preparation by their physicians are also advised to use sunscreen regularly, as Retin-A increases sensitivity to the sun.

Although Retin-A may help make your skin look and feel younger, you shouldn't relax when it comes to monitoring any changes in your skin that could point to melanoma and other skin cancers.

Chapter 10

BACK AND SPINE

<table>
<tr><td colspan="2" align="center">BODY SIGNAL ALERT</td></tr>
<tr><td colspan="2">Call your doctor immediately if you experience any of the following symptoms:</td></tr>
<tr><td>SYMPTOM</td><td>POSSIBLE MEDICAL CONDITION</td></tr>
<tr><td>You have severe pain localized in one area of the spine or suddenly lose the use of a limb or the sphincter muscles</td><td>Osteoporotic fracture to or cancer of the spine</td></tr>
<tr><td>You feel pain in your lower back and numbness in your buttock and lower leg</td><td>Sciatica</td></tr>
<tr><td>You feel pain in your upper back and neck and numbness in your arms</td><td>Sciatica</td></tr>
<tr><td>You are unable to walk on your heels or toes, and you feel pain when you move from a sitting, lying, or standing position</td><td>Sciatica</td></tr>
<tr><td>You feel a pain on one side of your back that radiates to your genitalia</td><td>Kidney stone or infection</td></tr>
<tr><td>You feel a ripping pain in your back and are sweating and feel weak</td><td>Dissecting aneurysm</td></tr>
</table>

HOW THE BACK AND SPINE AGE

More than one observer has wryly noted that the moment we as a species stood up and began to walk on two legs instead of all fours, the need for back surgeons was born.

Truthfully, from the moment we learn to walk, we ask a lot of our backs. As children, we learn that it's impolite to slouch, so we sit up straight, which puts stress on the lower back. The physical risks many teenagers take in sports can cause back injuries and also create future problems for the back and spine. As midlife adults, we begin to pay the price for this cumulative abuse with chronic back pain, a limitation in physical activity, and even a loss in height. Back pain causes more days off from work and permanent disability than any other illness. Yet it's easy to prevent problems.

The back and spine provide the entire body with the support it needs to function. When your back hurts, you'll find that it's difficult to do anything that involves moving your body. When you examine the construction of the back and spine and its apparent fragility, it's easy to see why so many people are afflicted with back problems.

The spine is the main support column of the body. It consists of 33 bones, or vertebrae, that are interspaced with discs of cartilage that act as shock absorbers. The muscles of the back connect with the vertebral processes, tiny bone projections that hold the musculature fast. The spine adapts to the movement of the muscles, bending and twisting as we go about our everyday activities.

In fact, the structure of the spine can be compared to a highly unlikely combination: in truth, it's nothing more than a column of cinder blocks with a jelly donut wedged in between each two. The individual parts of the back, from the vertebrae to the discs to the muscles, are so intricate that problems and injuries tend to show up suddenly, rather than gradually. Most people have borderline problems with their backs, and a sneeze or cough can push them over the edge and straight to the doctor's office.

There are two types of back problems: mechanical and neurological. Ninety-nine percent of back complaints are mechanical in origin. Whether caused by a lack of muscle tone or by suddenly twisting or picking up a heavy load, mechanical back problems are due largely to the connective tissue being too tight. That tightness is caused and aggravated by an inherent inflexibility that occurs all through the body. This is true for most sedentary people, as well as many active people.

The various common diseases of the spine can cause pain and limit your ability to function. Besides osteoporosis, which is responsible for a majority of the structurally based back problems that are a result of age, the gradual loss of muscle mass and tone can contribute to back pain.

This weakened structure can create a situation in which long-forgotten back injuries can crop up again.

One reason why back pain is more common among midlife adults is that they tend to eat fewer foods that are rich in calcium. When dietary intake of calcium is insufficient, the body needs to get it from somewhere, so it turns to the vertebrae to leach out the calcium. This is the primary cause of osteoporosis. Over the years, the entire skeletal system weakens, and, as its strength decreases, the spinal cord becomes more prone to injury. As the spine loses bone mass, the vertebrae tend to compress onto one another, which can result in a loss of height and a hunchback, also known as a dowager's hump.

A healthy spine is essential to good health and posture. Fortunately, it is possible to slow down the effects of aging on the back and spine through exercise, weight management, and increasing your intake of calcium, either through your diet or with supplements. For postmenopausal women, hormonel therapy may also be necessary to prevent degeneration of the skeletal system that is due to the effects of the lack of estrogen, which causes bones to become brittle. It may sound too good to be true, but if you suffer from back pain, a daily walk and glass of milk may be all you need to prevent osteoporosis and other problems with your back and spine.

BACKACHE WITH WEAKNESS

Description and Possible Medical Problems

It's not uncommon for the muscles in your back and shoulders to ache after doing work where you have to hunch over, such as gardening or other work around the house. If you've also been twisting your body and bending over, your hips may be painful after any exertion that you don't do every day. As a result, there's a good chance that, the morning after, you may feel as though you don't have the strength to get out of bed.

Muscle ache that's accompanied by weakness is a common occurrence. But if you have a constant, dull ache in the muscles around your shoulders and/or the backs of your hips and you don't have the strength you once did, you may have a rare, progressive disease called polymyositis. This disorder is a variation of dermatomyositis, in which the muscle pain and lack of strength are frequently accompanied by a deep red rash that may be scaly. The rash most often appears around the eyes or on the neck, chest, hands, or elbows.

Both polymyositis and dermatomyositis are arthritic disorders, but they affect primarily the muscles, which become inflamed and swollen, not the joints, as do other forms of arthritis. Doctors believe that polymyositis and dermatomyositis occur due to a defect in the immune system. Two thirds of the people with polymyositis and dermatomyositis are women between the ages of 30 and 60.

Another disease that has some of the same symptoms as polymyositis and dermatomyositis is polymyalgia rheumatica. This disease affects mostly women over the age of 50. Polymyalgia rheumatica occurs when the blood vessels in the musculoskeletal system become inflamed. In addition to the muscular ache and weakness, you may also have a low-grade fever and weight loss. If you have polymyalgia rheumatica, you'll find that it tends to strike suddenly, whereas with polymyositis and dermatomyositis the onset of symptoms is more gradual; the pain is also usually more acute in the morning and wears off as the day progresses. Polymyalgia rheumatica primarily affects the muscles of the shoulders and neck, not the hips. In fact, polymyalgia rheumatica resembles the condition called temporal arteritis, in which the branches of the carotid arteries in your head become inflamed and painful.

If the muscles in your shoulders and/or hips ache and you have any of the other symptoms I've mentioned, it's important to see your doctor. If polymyositis, dermatomyositis, and polymyalgia rheumatica are left untreated, the muscular ache and weakness can spread into the muscles of the chest and even the heart.

In many cases, the disease will disappear within a few months of the initial flare-up; in others, they may last a few years. Fortunately, with regular treatment and checkups, all three diseases can be managed; in time, you may even forget you have the disease.

But polymyositis, dermatomyositis, and polymyalgia rheumatica are—fortunately—rare; it's likely that the muscular aches and weakness you're feeling are just a result of overdoing it on the weekends.

Treatment

If your doctor discovers you have polymyositis, dermatomyositis, or polymyalgia rheumatica, he will probably prescribe the corticosteroid prednisone to help reduce pain and inflammation. Prednisone will also help lessen the skin rash and inflammation that accompany dermatomyositis. Prednisone works by reducing inflammation in the blood vessels and tissues by increasing the body's tolerance to the inflammation, thus alleviating the symptoms.

The prednisone will be started at a high dose, usually about 40 to 60 milligrams daily. This will then gradually be decreased to a lower dose over a period of several weeks to several months. Side effects include bloating and a "moon face."

If your muscles remain weak and achy despite treatment, or they occasionally stiffen up, your doctor may recommend that you schedule regular sessions with a physical therapist to help keep your muscles flexible with range of motion exercises and the use of heat therapy. In any case, it's a good idea to participate in an exercise program after the initial pain and inflammation subside; regular activity should become part of your life in order to prevent future flare-ups.

HEIGHT, LOSS OF

Description and Possible Medical Problems

I recently saw a patient I hadn't seen for about a year. She seemed a little shorter than the last time she had visited me, and I asked her if she thought she had shrunk.

"Oh, yes," she replied. "My clothes fit differently, and when I stand at my kitchen sink, I can't see out the window anymore."

We measured her height, and sure enough, she had lost about ¾-inch since her last office visit. She was concerned about the possible causes of her loss of height and asked me if there was anything she could do. She was in good health, and I told her she had nothing to worry about.

Treatment

A slight loss of height each year is a normal part of the aging process. Since the vertebrae of the spine become more porous with age, they can gradually compress onto one another, decreasing the length of the spine and thus your height.

One way to prevent further height loss and even help reverse the bone degeneration is exercise. Walking is an excellent activity that will help replenish the bones with lost calcium because it is a weight-bearing exercise that strengthens the entire skeletal system. Walking will also strengthen your muscles, which will help to support your spine better.

Eating more calcium-rich foods such as low-fat dairy products and taking a 1000-milligram calcium supplement at least once a day can also help replace calcium in bones that have begun to deteriorate due to osteoporosis, which is a normal part of aging.

In postmenopausal women, estrogen replacement therapy can help the bones retain calcium and thus prevent future fractures and further deterioration.

HUNCHBACK

Description and Possible Medical Problems

If you've ever visited a public park where a lot of elderly people congregate, you've probably noticed that several of the women and a few of the men walk in a stooped manner and have a visible hunchback. It looks as though it must be difficult for them to get around, yet somehow they manage despite their altered posture.

A hunchback, also called a dowager's hump, is an advanced form of osteoporosis of the spine. The condition is very common in older women and in some elderly men. Since the bones become increasingly porous with age, the vertebrae begin to compress onto one another so that in time there is little or no space left between each two vertebrae. In addition, the bones can become so brittle that over a period of time, they may undergo a series of compression fractures that shrink the vertebrae even more.

You'll barely be able to notice a compression fracture if it's a hairline fracture; you might feel a slight twinge of pain when you twist your torso or bend over to pick something up. A more serious fracture will cause an overall backache that will gradually fade away in one or two months.

Whether the spine is compressed through a fracture or the loss of space between the vertebrae, over time the spine can become so compressed that it forces the head and neck to stoop forward, resulting in a dowager's hump.

Treatment

If you're healthy, get enough exercise, and supplement your diet with calcium-rich foods, your odds of developing a dowager's hump later in life are virtually nonexistent. But your older relatives who did not care for their health in midlife may not be so lucky. Once osteoporosis of the spine has advanced to the point where it creates a hunchback, there's not much anyone can do to make it disappear.

Since a weakened spine is one cause of the common problem of hip fractures among older adults, if one of your relatives has a hunchback, you should help him or her to take extra care when walking or going up and down stairs.

PAIN IN BACK AGGRAVATED BY MOVEMENT

Description and Possible Medical Problems

You may scoff at weekend athletes, those people who sit in the office all day from Monday to Friday and then act as though they're the star quarterback for their high school football team all weekend. "Come Monday morning, their backs are going to make them very sorry," you think before going back to your more sedate activities such as walking and gardening.

Don't laugh! Though Monday mornings may be difficult for the midlife adult who likes being a weekend athlete, any activity—from gardening to turning your head to reaching for a spoon—can cause the muscles in your back to spasm suddenly.

A muscle spasm can be caused by a number of conditions, both pre-existing and current:

• You may have strained a ligament or muscle in your back.

• You may have pulled a muscle.

• You may have made a sudden movement, such as a sneeze, that jarred your back or spine, or you may have injured your back previously.

• You may have fractured one of the vertebrae of the spine.

• You may be able to move your back easily, even though it hurts, or your back muscles may have stiffened up to the point where it's difficult to move at all.

The cause of a sharp pain in your back may be difficult to determine, though it is usually due to overuse of the muscles in the back in some way.

Treatment

The best treatment for back pain is the use of rest and Advil for a few days. If, however, your back pain doesn't subside after a few days of rest and aspirin, you should see your doctor, who will probably take some X rays to rule out the possibility of a slipped disc or vertebral fracture. He may prescribe a muscle relaxant such as Flexeril or Robaxin, taken three times a day. In severe cases, I'll prescribe a low-dose prescription for Valium. A nonsteroidal anti-inflammatory medication such as Naprosyn or Toradol will help reduce inflammation and muscle spasms. If they don't relieve the pain, I'll prescribe a stronger analgesic such as Tylenol with codeine.

To test for any damage to the vertebrae or misalignment of the spine, I like to take an X ray of the lumbosacral spine. Then, if I think a patient has slipped a disc, I'll want to do an MRI, or magnetic resonance imaging, which will offer a detailed image of the discs.

If you've already had back problems, which in most people tend to occur in the lower back, you've probably grown to expect occasional back trouble that, unfortunately, can recur anytime and without warning. While ice packs may help numb the pain, bed rest until the pain disappears is the best solution. Massage may feel great on aching muscles, but if you have a slipped disc, it can actually make it worse.

There are some preventive measures you can take to lessen your chances of recurring back pain. The first is to bend your knees—never your back—when you lift a heavy object. Increasing the amount of exercise you get is also important, though you should concentrate on activities that are kind to your back, such as walking and swimming, not running or weight lifting.

You can also make it a point to sleep on your back on a firm mattress. And excess body weight places a lot of strain on the back, especially in men—where a pot belly causes the back to arch forward, putting stress on the muscles and spine. If you're carrying more than a few extra pounds, you should plan to lose them to take some of the burden off your lower back.

If you need help getting out of bed, some of my patients have found a trapeze placed directly over the head of the bed to be helpful, especially when the back problem is severe.

PAIN IN BACK WITH INSOMNIA

Description and Possible Medical Problems

Even a mild form of back pain can interfere with most of your daily activities, including your ability to sleep. When the back pain doesn't go away despite rest and treatment, you may find that it's difficult to sleep through the night. This can quickly turn into a Catch-22 situation, because the accompanying lack of sleep makes it difficult for you to function during the day. You may then become stressed and frustrated, which only makes your back pain worse.

If you have chronic back pain that is interfering with your sleep, you may have a condition called fibromyalgia, or fibrositis, in which the tissues that connect the muscles to the bones and ligaments become inflamed. Fibromyalgia is common in midlife adults, and women are affected more often than men. It can flare up without warning if you strain or pull a muscle in your back or if you are under emotional stress.

Sometimes it's difficult to distinguish between fibromyalgia and the back pain that comes as a result of a muscle pull; here's some help. With fibromyalgia, you'll feel the back pain deep within the muscles of your back, not on the surface. The pain is likely to occur along the spine and perhaps the shoulder—anywhere muscle connects to the bones: the shoulder, the hip joint, and the back of the neck. Even though the pain originates in the connective tissue, any slight movement will cause pain to radiate throughout the rest of the back, frequently making the exact area hard to pinpoint.

Treatment

Fibromyalgia can sometimes be a difficult condition to treat because the pain is so generalized and occurs deep in the muscles of the back, making it hard to pinpoint. If you have chronic deep back pain and have trouble sleeping, you should see your doctor. If the pain doesn't gradually fade after a few days, you may have rheumatoid arthritis and not fibromyalgia. If the diagnosis is indeed fibromyalgia, there are certain things you can do to treat the symptoms yourself.

First, you should try to relax, both physically and emotionally, with exercise, listening to music, and reading. If your body tightens up in response to stress, the connective tissue will tighten up as well, which will just make the pain worse. Unfortunately, fibromyalgia is a chronic condition; the best you can do is try to control your lifestyle, which will help a lot.

Aspirin or another nonnarcotic painkiller will help whenever the pain flares up. If the pain occasionally becomes severe, your doctor may prescribe a corticosteroid medication such as prednisone, 20 mg. to be taken each day.

Learning how to manage stress with the use of biofeedback and relaxation exercises should help get your pain down to a level where it's almost unnoticeable. Regular exercise and hot baths will also help and make it easier for you to fall asleep at night. Some people also find it important to maintain good posture, which helps to place less stress on the connective tissue.

BODY SIGNAL ALERT

PAIN IN ONE SIDE OF HIP RUNNING TO GENITALIA

Description and Possible Medical Problems

Most of us know at least one person who has had kidney stones. With few exceptions, he will describe the process of passing the stone as one of the most painful things he has ever experienced. Those of us who haven't had kidney stones wonder how a tiny grain of crystal can create so much intense pain for such a long period of time.

The truth is, kidney stones are a common condition. Kidney stones fall into several categories, depending on their composition. More than three quarters of all stones are calcium stones, and these are the most likely to recur. One out of every 10 people has a uric acid stone, which is commonly caused by the disease gout. Other stones that occur more rarely are cystine stones and struvite stones, which arise due to a urinary tract infection.

Kidney stones are a common condition, and for the majority of people they pass through the urinary tract unnoticed. When one or more of the tiny crystals that form in the kidney cluster together, the stone becomes larger than the ureter tube it must pass through, and that's when trouble starts.

As the stone starts to move down the ureter, you may feel the pain first on your side just above your hip and down to your bladder directly above your genitalia. Then both the stone and the pain slowly make their way further south through the ureter. The entire process may take up to three weeks. Along with the acute pain, you might also suffer from a fever and bloody urine, signs that the stone has blocked the ureter, which can prevent urine from escaping. In some cases, these symptoms may be a sign of a severe kidney infection, which is much more common in women than in men.

Once the stone reaches the bladder, the pain stops and the stone is quickly eliminated from the body. Some people may pass several significant stones a year with no more than a backward glance. Others, for whom the pain is too fresh a memory, may embark on a plan of prevention while they're still passing the first stone.

Treatment

Surgical removal of the stone was once the rule in treating kidney stones; now it is the exception. The treatment for kidney stones depends on what type of stone it is.

For most people, prescription painkillers such as Tylenol with codeine every three or four hours, or even Demerol, will help decrease the pain without interfering with or prolonging the process of passing the stone. For others, whose pain is disabling because several stones are being passed at once, a process called lithotripsy is commonly used. Also known as a form of underwater shock-wave treatment, lithotripsy is a process in which a machine called a lithotripter is used to aim ultrasound waves directly toward the stone while the patient lies partially under water. The waves will not harm your body, but because the stones are so fragile, the waves will cause the stones to break up into smaller pieces, making them easy to pass. While the waves are emitted, your urologist watches the process on an X-ray monitor.

Because of the success of lithotripsy, surgery has largely become obsolete as a method of treating kidney stones. With particularly stubborn stones, a small version of the litrotripter is used to enter the body through a small incision on the abdomen. The surgeon inserts a tube called a cystoscope into the bladder to aim the ultrasound waves at the large stones. They break up, and when the surgeon removes the cystoscope, the remaining broken-up stones come out with it.

If your doctor determines that a kidney infection and not a stone is causing your pain, he will prescribe an antibiotic such as the sulfa medication Bactrim, to be taken twice daily for ten days or until the infection clears up.

Tips and Precautions

Once you've had one stone, the emphasis will be on the prevention of future stones. Though only 10% of kidney stones are due to a hereditary condition, most people will have to take preventive measures after they suffer through one episode.

The most important—and easiest—thing to do is to drink lots of water every day; I recommend from 8 to 10 8-ounce glasses. Adequate fluid intake will help prevent stones from forming and also help flush any existing stones from your system quickly.

Since some stones are a result of excess protein or calcium in the diet, your doctor may recommend that you cut your intake of foods that are high in these nutrients.

BODY SIGNAL ALERT

PAIN IN LOWER BACK WITH NUMBNESS IN BUTTOCK AND LEG

Description and Possible Medical Problems

I remember one patient recalling her battle with sciatica. Margo was healthy, active, and in her mid-40s. A few years earlier, she had told me that she sometimes felt a slight tingling run down her hamstring, but she had always just shrugged it off.

Three years after the tingling first started, Margo and her husband were on vacation 1000 miles away from home when she suddenly felt excruciating pain begin to shoot through her back and down her left leg. "I'd had back pain before," she told me later, "but it was never anything like this. It was so bad that sitting was all but impossible for me. The only thing that helped was walking."

She finally went to the emergency room several hours after the pain first appeared. By that time, her foot and ankle were totally numb. The neurologist told her it looked as though she had sciatica and thought it was caused by a herniated disk in her back. Sciatica is a condition in which the sciatic nerve, which runs the length of the hamstring and through to the foot, becomes swollen and leads to pain and numbness in the leg.

A slipped disc occurs when one of the discs in your back that serve as a cushion between vertebrae either ruptures or bulges out and presses on one of the nerves that originates in the spine. This can occur due to age, overexertion, or a sudden twist of your body.

A prolapsed disc is also known as a slipped disc, though the disc doesn't actually slip but instead protrudes. When sciatica occurs, the disc that is the most likely culprit is the fourth or fifth disc in the lumbar region, or the lower back. With sciatica, the disc presses on the sciatic nerve, the longest nerve in the body. The pain will run down your back into your buttock and down your leg. As Margo discovered, it may be difficult to walk on either your heels or your toes, and your range of motion will be severely limited.

To confirm the diagnosis, Margo underwent an MRI. An MRI, like a CAT scan, is a specialized radiological procedure. The patient is placed on a platform and wheeled into a huge cylinder. The machine causes claustrophobia in some people; you might need some mild sedation if you expect that you will feel anxious, even though the entire procedure takes less than an hour and, in some cases, only 20 minutes. Some MRI machines actually have music piped into them.

Margo's diagnosis for sciatica was positive, and since it was caused by a herniated disc in her back, surgery was scheduled for the next day. When she had fully recovered, Margo was able to enjoy all her old activities, with one important difference: she had no more back pain.

Treatment

Margo's case was especially severe, but not all people with sciatica caused by a herniated disc have to undergo surgery. In many instances, a prolapsed disc responsible for sciatic pain may heal on its own. Doctors recommend bed rest, aspirin, and patience. With the nonsurgical method, however, it is necessary for your physician to treat the pain. Muscle relaxants such as Robaxin 500 taken three times a day can help relieve the pain. Valium can also be used; it will relieve painful back spasms as well as reduce your anxiety. An anti-inflammatory medication such as Naprosyn may be prescribed as long as you have no prior history of an ulcer. The drug will be injected near the ruptured disc and will ease the pain and decrease the swelling. Total recuperation might take up to two weeks when medication is combined with the bed rest

Most herniated discs do heal themselves, but that doesn't mean you will be without pain. Unfortunately, after your first bout with a herniated disc, your back will never again be quite the same; however, surgeons today view surgery as the last resort, even though only surgery will completely ease the pain of a herniated disc. During the operation, the surgeon opens up the lower back and takes the pressure off the nerve by removing parts of the disc. The recovery period is usually one to three months; during this time, bed rest is about all you may be able to manage. After your back pain disappears, you will be able to do everything you did before.

Tips and Precautions

How do you know when to wait out a ruptured disc and when to have an operation? Your doctor will describe the pros and cons of each, but, as a general rule, if the pain is localized in your back and you feel it gradually decreasing over the course of a couple of days, it's a good idea to wait it out. If the pain starts to get worse and your leg and buttock begin to grow numb, or if your back still hurts while you're resting and aspirin doesn't help, you're a good candidate for surgery.

PAIN IN TAILBONE

Description and Possible Medical Problems

Though midlife adults who keep active by exercising regularly have stronger musculoskeletal systems than sedentary people, their activity makes them prone to injuries that people who are inactive rarely encounter.

While sedentary adults are prone to hip fractures because they have fragile bones and tend to carry themselves unsteadily, men and women who are active are more likely to injure their coccyx, or tailbone, which can be extremely painful. A swift kick in the rear by a playful son, daughter, or grandchild may cause a severe pain accompanied by a loud crack. A patient of mine had a chair pulled out on him in jest, which, of course, is a common trick. He heard a crack, felt a sharp pain, and had a severe ache in his tailbone for at least two months.

Treatment

If you've injured your tailbone in a fall, its discomfort will cause a limitation in your activity, which is necessary to the healing process. You'll probably find that sitting is altogether too uncomfortable or that only one position is possible.

Aspirin or acetaminophen will help ease your discomfort as the tailbone heals. If, however, you have a sharp pain in the bone that doesn't subside within a few days, it's important that you see your doctor; you may have fractured or cracked your tailbone, and medical attention is necessary. Your doctor will prescribe a nonsteroidal medication such as Motrin and may suggest bed rest of a few weeks or more.

BODY SIGNAL ALERT

PAIN IN UPPER BACK AND NECK WITH NUMBNESS IN ARMS

Description and Possible Medical Problems

If you feel pain in your back and numbness in one or both arms, it is probably caused by a ruptured disc and is similar to the sciatica described in "Pain in Lower Back with Numbness in Buttock and Leg" above, with one major difference: The affected disc is located between one of the cervical vertebrae in the spinal column of your neck, and not your lower back. Instead of numbness in the legs, you'll have no feeling or sensation in your arms instead.

BODY SIGNAL ALERT

PAIN LOCALIZED IN ONE AREA OF SPINE

Description and Possible Medical Problems

There's always the possibility that if you feel a pain in your spine that becomes sharp when you move, you may have fractured one of your vertebrae. But for women with a history of breast cancer and men who've had a bout with prostate cancer, it's possible that the cancer has metastasized, or spread, to the spine.

If you suddenly feel a sharp, stabbing pain in your spine that you haven't felt before and you have a history of cancer, it's essential you see your doctor immediately. A sudden loss of bladder or bowel control is another sign of bone cancer.

Unfortunately, half of women with breast cancer and men with prostate cancer initially discover that they have cancer only after it has already spread to other parts of the body, including the spine. Primary cancers that originate in the bone and haven't spread from another part of the body are rare; most are benign. However, bone cancer that has metastasized from a tumor elsewhere in the body is usually malignant, since it has spread from a tumor that is already malignant.

Sometimes a tumor that spreads to the vertebrae will press against the spine and its connecting nerves, which may cause you to lose the use of your limbs or control of your sphincter muscles. Though these symptoms are severe, I have seen only two people with this condition in the last five years.

Treatment

Your doctor or oncologist may prefer to treat a malignant tumor in a vertebra with chemotherapy, since any surgery involving the spine—especially removing a portion of it—may result in paralysis or another neurological disorder. Radiation therapy may also be used. However, if the pain in your spine has appeared recently and suddenly, surgery can be the best form of treatment, since it can reverse any damage to the nerves before it becomes permanent.

As with any form of cancer, early detection is the best way to prevent it from spreading to the spine or any other part of the body. See your doctor for regular checkups, and stay alert to any small changes in your body that could signal cancer.

RASH, PAINFUL, ON ONE SIDE
OF THE BACK

See "Pimples, Painful, on One Side of the Face" in Chapter 9.

BODY SIGNAL ALERT

RIPPING PAIN IN BACK WITH
WEAKNESS AND SWEATING

Description and Possible Medical Problems

If you have a history of hypertension and you suddenly feel a tearing sensation in your chest that then spreads to the back, you should see your doctor immediately. You may have what is called an aortic dissection, in which the aorta—the main body artery leading to the heart—has torn away from where it connects to the aortic valve on the heart.

In addition to the feeling that you've torn something inside your chest, you may start to sweat heavily, feel weak, and have a feeling of doom and futility.

An aortic dissection is most common among sedentary men and women over the age of 50 who have chronic high blood pressure and have done little to treat it.

Possible Medical Problems and Treatments

This is a medical emergency, and you will need to go to the emergency room immediately.

To treat a dissected aorta, your doctor will first stabilize your blood pressure with a beta-blocker. Surgery is usually necessary, using a series of grafts to repair the tear and the aortic valve. During and after your recovery, you will be monitored and prescribed a beta-blocker or another antihypertensive medication to regulate your blood pressure and help prevent another aortic dissection in the future.

HINTS FOR A HEALTHY BACK

It's easy to prevent back problems from occurring—and recurring—if you just start to pay attention to how you move your body. All that's needed is a little common sense.

Sitting: When you sit in a chair, always sit all the way back and keep your back erect. Adjust the chair so your feet reach the floor and rest flat.

Standing: When you must stand for a period of time, place one foot on a stool or small bench. Keep an erect posture; avoid sway-back. Tuck your pelvis forward to straighten your back. Try to walk and move around as much as possible.

Driving: In a car, keep your car seat back upright so that your body is erect. Adjust your seat position so that your legs reach the pedals comfortably without either having to stretch or getting cramped. Adjust the steering wheel, if possible, so your arms and shoulders are relaxed. On long trips, stop every hour or so and walk around to relieve tension and relax your muscles.

Lifting: When lifting any object from the floor, you should always bend your legs and keep your back straight. Don't bend over at the waist to lift something; instead, let your leg muscles do the lifting work.

Sleeping: Sleep on a firm mattress or put a ¾-inch plywood board under your mattress if it's a soft one. If you sleep on your back, put a pillow under your knees, not under your head. If you sleep on your side, keep your knees bent. Avoid sleeping on your stomach.

Get regular exercise and take some time to relax every day. If your back starts giving you problems, don't delay. See your doctor immediately.

Chapter 11

CHEST: HEART, LUNGS, AND CIRCULATION

BODY SIGNAL ALERT

Call your doctor immediately if you experience any of the following symptoms:

SYMPTOM	POSSIBLE MEDICAL CONDITION
You are coughing up blood or phlegm mixed with blood	*Infection, blood disease, or lung tumor*
You feel short of breath and have a productive cough	*Pneumonia or worsening emphysema*
You begin to wheeze severely	*Status asthmaticus or, in an elderly person, heart failure*
You have chest pain that moves into your jaw and down your left arm, with pallor and sweating	*Possible heart attack*
You are short of breath, are wheezing, and have pinkish sputum	*Acute pulmonary edema*
You have chest pain with shortness of breath that occurs upon physical activity	*Angina pectoris*
You are short of breath and feel sudden chest pain	*Collapsed lung*

HOW THE HEART AND LUNGS AGE

In a game of word association, if you mention the word "chest," most people will automatically think "heart." So much of the health and medical information around today concerns the heart, whether it's diet, exercise, or stress management, that this is not totally surprising.

However, the chest area of the body as I refer to it includes not only the rib cage but also the lungs, the major blood vessels, and the esophagus. Since all of these can send out a multitude of body signals when something goes wrong, it's especially important that you learn how to describe your symptoms specifically so your doctor can provide you with the appropriate diagnosis and treatment.

As with the rest of the body, the effect aging has on the organs, bones, and muscles in the chest cavity varies widely from one person to another. Lifestyle and personal habits—such as diet, exercise, and general outlook—are responsible for most of the difference.

The rib cage and spine begin to show signs of aging first, becoming less resilient and more porous. In addition, osteoporosis of the spine can cause deformities in the rib cage that can make breathing uncomfortable. Fortunately, however, the vast majority of the population is not affected by this condition, as it primarily shows up after the age of 70.

The lungs also lose some of their resiliency as we age, starting in our 40s, but this is usually minor. The amount of air the lungs normally hold decreases very little as we age. The ability of the lungs' lining to fight infection also decreases due to the normal loss of the body's immunological response to infection, but this doesn't usually show up until the 70s. Most lung disease and infection are caused by the ravages of years of cigarette smoking.

Of course, the heart also ages, along with the entire vascular system. The blood vessels tend to stiffen with time, and they start to narrow as a result of decades spent eating foods that are high in cholesterol and fat.

In the 40s, the heart starts to lose some of its strength; for example, it takes longer for the heart rate to return to normal after a bout with stress. But the more regularly one exercises, the stronger it will remain. The heart valves also become thicker with age, causing them to leak a little or not to open as much as before, but this usually has no effect on the body. Most people, however, will be able to live well into their 70s and 80s without any heart problems at all, since the effects aging has on the heart become an issue only if there is a serious underlying disease such as a preexisting heart condition or diabetes.

Of course, regular exercise consisting of three 20-minute sessions each week can be quite beneficial, not only for your heart but for your entire body. It has for me, since I have a tendency to be overweight. While I was in medical school, I led a largely sedentary lifestyle, which made it very easy for me to gain weight. After medical school and during my residency, I began to exercise regularly.

Today, at the age of 48, I'm still at it. I exercise for at least one hour three or four times a week; sometimes I even exercise for an hour and a half each day. I run either inside on a treadmill or outside, and I follow it up with a regimen of light weight lifting to maintain my strength. If I can make time, so can you. Of course, you should consult your doctor before you begin any exercise program for a medical evaluation.

CHEST PAIN: QUESTIONS TO ASK YOURSELF

No matter what your age is, if you feel a pain in your chest, you should be concerned, since chest pain is one of the most serious complaints people can bring to their doctor. Heart attacks can happen at any age, but over the age of 50 the risk increases. As most of you already know, your risk also increases if you answer yes to any of the following questions:

1. Do I have a strong family history of heart disease?

2. Do I smoke?

3. Do I have hypertension or diabetes?

4. Am I obese and leading a sedentary life?

5. Is my total cholesterol level high, above 200?

Nevertheless, not every pain in the chest signifies an impending heart attack. To alleviate some of your worries, answer the questions below. If you ever feel a pain in your chest, your answers will help determine the possible cause, which is listed after each question.

1. Where is the pain occurring: in the center of the chest, in the back, or on the left side? Does it move into the arm or jaw (heart problems)

2. Does the pain occur after eating or physical activity (heart)?

3. Does it last for a few seconds (not heart), several minutes (heart), or more than ten minutes (heart)?

4. Am I coughing, and do I feel short of breath (heart or lungs)?

5. Am I sweating (heart or esophageal spasm)?

6. Does it get worse when I inhale or move (muscular pain)?

7. Can I feel it in one small area (muscular), or do I feel it all through my chest (heart and/or lung)?

8. Is the pain burning and sharp (gastrointestinal problem) or heavy (heart)?

9. Am I belching (gastrointestinal problem or heart)?

10. Am I having heart palpitations (gastrointestinal problem or heart)?

11. Do I feel there is something seriously wrong (heart)?

Your answer to each of these questions will help your doctor to determine the cause. There is often tremendous overlap between symptoms that appear in the chest. For instance, if you are having palpitations along with sweating, belching, and a heavy feeling in your chest, it's probably due to a problem with the heart. However, if you are belching and having palpitations but no other Body Signals, the problem could be in the heart, but it could also be caused by an accumulation of gas in the stomach or a hiatal hernia. This is why it's important that you try to be as specific with the descriptions of your Body Signals as you can: your treatment will depend on it.

BELCHING, SWEATING, SHORTNESS OF BREATH

Description and Possible Medical Problems

When I first began my medical practice, one of the first patients I saw was an elderly gentleman who came into my office off the street because he couldn't stop belching; he was also mildly short of breath. He thought all he had was a severe case of indigestion. However, I admitted him to the emergency room because he was actually having a heart attack, though he didn't believe me. At times a person may have heart attack symptoms—such as belching—without any significant chest pain.

In fact, if you have been diagnosed with heart disease and show some of the risk factors for a heart attack, if you start belching and can't stop, go to the hospital immediately!

Treatment

See "Chest Heaviness with Pain That Moves into Jaw and Down Left Arm, with Sweating" below.

BODY SIGNAL ALERT

CHEST HEAVINESS WITH PAIN THAT MOVES INTO JAW AND DOWN LEFT ARM, WITH SWEATING

Description and Possible Medical Problems

Usually, if you are having any one of these symptoms by itself, the cause is probably not too severe. Heavy sweating can be the result of anxiety or fright, and a pain that runs down your left arm may be caused by a pinched nerve in your neck.

When the symptoms occur all at the same time, however, they are the classic signs of a heart attack, and you must get help immediately.

Certainly the body language of a person who's having a heart attack can be frightening. He or she will be pale in color, sweating heavily, and possibly vomiting. Heaviness in the chest can last for a minute or two to several hours, and the pain can radiate from the chest into the left arm but may stop at the shoulder. On rare occasions, the pain can radiate into the right arm, but don't let the fact that the pain is appearing in your right arm instead of your left change your opinion that you're having a heart attack. The pain usually causes a person to be quiet and not to move much.

A heart attack occurs when one of the coronary arteries that supplies the heart with blood becomes blocked, usually as a result of arteriosclerosis. The supply of blood to an area of the heart muscle is suddenly interrupted, which can result in permanent damage to the heart, since the interruption of blood causes the heart muscle supplied by that vessel to die; this is what initially causes the severe pain and the other Body Signals.

After a heart attack, a person will usually be able to recover fully, unless a major portion of the heart muscle is destroyed.

Treatment

What is and isn't done during the first hours after a heart attack is extremely important to contain the damage to the heart and to ensure future good health. Call 911. The most important thing you can do is not to waste time but go directly to the hospital. The use of modern declotting agents such as streptokinase, which is administered intravenously in the emergency room, will increase your chances for long-term survival after a heart attack since the medication can dislodge the blood clot before the heart muscle is destroyed. Once you're in the hospital, the coronary team can evaluate the extent of the damage to your heart with a thalium stress test as well as new cardiac imaging X-ray tests that can actually show the area of the heart that's been damaged. The doctors will also administer medications such as ACE inhibitors and beta-blockers to help stabilize your blood pressure and heart rhythm.

In the first few days and weeks after a heart attack, your doctor will primarily be concerned with controlling your heart rate and blood pressure and preventing any more damage to the heart. The high-tech coronary care units in most hospitals are well equipped to monitor your heart rate and blood pressure.

Once your condition has stabilized, the team will use an angiogram or another test, such as an echocardiogram (see pages 239–241 for a full description of these tests), to determine the extent of the damage and whether bypass surgery is necessary to open the clogged blood vessels that caused the heart attack. Bypass surgery is a course of last resort, to be used when an angioplasty—a nonsurgical technique that uses a tiny balloon to open up a blocked coronary artery—does not do the trick.

If you experience no complications, you will probably be released in a week. After you leave the hospital and recover fully from the heart attack—which takes about a month—your doctor and other medical professionals, such as an exercise physiologist, a dietitian, and a stress manager, will work with you to develop a long-term commitment to changing your lifestyle, which includes attention to a low-fat, low-cholesterol diet, regular exercise, quitting smoking, and perhaps job retraining if necessary, for instance, if your job involves severe physical or emotional stress. The diet plan I offer my post–heart attack patients is pretty simple: Limit your intake of animal protein, which includes chicken, fish, and meat, and try to eliminate red meat entirely. Substitute low-fat cheese, milk, and ice cream for high-fat dairy products, and refrain from eating fried foods. I also suggest that patients eat no more than two eggs a week, go easy on the butter and margarine—olive oil is better—and eliminate junk foods such as potato chips; pretzels are better.

Today, fortunately, if a patient has proper rehabilitation and makes the proper lifestyle changes, a heart attack does not mean the end of a productive life. I've seen many people, even in their 60s and 70s, use a heart attack as an excuse for a whole new—healthier—lease on life.

TESTS AND PROCEDURES USED TO INVESTIGATE AND ALLEVIATE PROBLEMS IN THE CHEST

TESTS

- An angiogram, which is usually done before bypass surgery; a special dye is injected into the coronary vessels to check the degree to which they've narrowed.

- Blood tests, including a skin test for tuberculosis.

- A bronchoscopy test, which allows the doctor to look directly into your lung to see if there are any lesions or tumors; this test is done in the hospital under sedation.

- A cardiac imaging test, which uses special X-ray equipment during a specific type of stress test to show the extent of heart damage and to evaluate if a blood vessel is blocked.

- A computerized axial tomography, or CAT, scan,

which is an X-ray procedure that provides extremely detailed pictures of the chest or other body parts.

- A chest X ray, which helps determine overall heart size as well as any incidence of heart failure by revealing fluid in the lungs.

- An echocardiogram, which is a sound-wave test that checks how your heart valves function and measures the output of your heart.

- An electrocardiogram, which shows the electrical activity of your heart and reveals any damage or the presence of an irregular heartbeat; can also show if a recent heart attack has affected the heart—or if there is an acute heart attack actually in progress.

- A full medical history and a physical exam.

- A Holtor monitor, which is a 24-hour electronic device that checks your heartbeat for any irregularity.

- An oximetry test, which is done with a simple monitor that's placed on your earlobe or finger to check the oxygen content of your blood.

- A spirometry test, which checks your lung function when you breathe into a tube; it measures the amount of air that is expelled from your lung and helps your doctor determine if asthma or another lung dysfunction is the reason for your cough.

- A stress test, which is an exercise session performed in a controlled environment; it can be conducted on either a treadmill or a bicycle or in one of the newer high-tech nuclear scans, to measure how the heart reacts to the stress of physical activity.

PROCEDURES

- An angioplasty, which is a nonsurgical technique that uses a balloon to open up a blocked area of the coronary artery; this is possible only if the blockage is small.

• Coronary bypass surgery, which is a surgical technique used to bypass a blocked artery; this is performed when an angioplasty won't achieve the desired results.

BODY SIGNAL ALERT

CHEST PAIN, SHARP, WITH SHORTNESS OF BREATH

Description and Possible Medical Problems

If you suddenly become short of breath and at the same time have a sharp pain in the chest that doesn't disappear, you should call your doctor immediately. These symptoms may mean that in the outer lining of one of your lungs you have an air bubble—called a pleb—that has burst, causing the lung to collapse in a matter of a minute or so.

Frequently, a burst air bubble and collapsed lung occur in people over 60 who have emphysema, since the disease causes plebs to form. At other times, especially in a person who's in the 40s or 50s, the lung can collapse because of a congenital defect in the lung.

Treatment

If your lung has collapsed due to a burst air bubble, you will be hospitalized, and your doctor will place a tube called a chest tube into the lung in order to expand it. The procedure is done under local anesthesia, and the tube will probably remain in place for several days. You will recover fully, and the chances are good that you won't be bothered by burst air bubbles again.

CHEST PAIN, STABBING, WORSENED BY DEEP BREATHING

Description and Possible Medical Problems

A new patient recently told me about his experience with pericarditis, a disease that can sometimes be difficult to diagnose because its symptoms are similar to those of other problems in the chest.

"It was early Sunday morning, and my wife and I had just gotten home from a night out on the town," he told me. "We went to sleep, and a couple of hours later I woke up feeling a pressure around my chest. Every time I took a breath, it felt like someone was stabbing me.

"I had just had a physical the week before and had a clean bill of health. I knew the signs of a heart attack, and what I was feeling didn't fit. I woke my wife, and for a few minutes we both hoped the pain would go away if I would lie back down. But it just made it worse.

"To make a long story short, I ended up in the emergency room, and they weren't sure what was wrong, so they put me on oxygen, ran some tests, and said it might be pleurisy [an inflammation of the lungs]. After a few hours, I was feeling better, so they sent me home.

"I slept most of the day and took the anti-inflammatory pills the doctor prescribed, but later that night the stabbing pain started up again. This time it was ten times worse than before. It almost felt like I couldn't breathe. So we headed back to the hospital.

"While the doctors were asking me all kinds of questions, they zeroed in on one in particular: Had I been feeling under the weather lately? My wife answered for me, saying that I had been complaining that I felt like I had some kind of virus for the last few weeks. They took an electrocardiogram and immediately diagnosed me with pericarditis and admitted me for a few days. I have to admit that I had never felt pain like that before."

Pericarditis is a condition in which the lining around the heart called the pericardium becomes inflamed. With one type of pericarditis, the only symptom is pain in the chest. Another form of the disease will show a buildup of fluid in the lining around the heart. In people up to the age of 50, the most common cause of pericarditis is a virus that causes an upper respiratory tract infection, as my patient found out. In people over 50, pericarditis is sometimes caused by a cancer in another part of the body that has spread to the heart. A number of other conditions can also cause pericarditis; these include rheumatoid arthritis, pneumonia, systemic lupus erythematosus, AIDS, a heart attack, and kidney failure. Occasionally pericarditis can be life-threatening because the buildup of fluid can constrict the heart and stop it from beating.

Treatment

If your doctor suspects you have pericarditis, he will confirm the condition with a chest X ray, echocardiogram, EKG, physical exam, and complete medical history. The treatment of pericarditis will depend on its cause. With a viral infection, the chest pain will probably clear up within a few days. If a bacterial infection is the cause, your doctor will prescribe a course of antibiotics for you to take for at least two weeks. You will probably be hospitalized if there is fluid buildup or an irregular heartbeat. In rare cases, the fluid will need to be removed from the cardiac sac with a minor operation if your doctor believes that it may stop the heart from beating.

CHEST PAIN UPON BREATHING

Description and Possible Medical Problems

If you feel a pain in your chest that's either located in one spot or spread out throughout your chest whenever you take a breath, I have two pieces of good news for you. The first is that it probably doesn't involve your heart. The second is that this kind of chest pain is easy to treat.

As with any type of chest pain, you should note if you've recently been injured, had an infection of some kind, or experienced any change in the state of your health.

It's possible that you may have fractured a rib or strained the muscles of the rib cage by lifting, pushing, or pulling a heavy object. The lining of one of your lungs may have become inflamed due to fluid in the lung; the pain in your chest may be sharp and occur at a rib or across the back part of the lung. If you're under 50, this is usually due to a respiratory infection like pneumonia. In an older person who is frail, the cause can be due to heart failure, a malignant tumor, or liver or kidney failure.

Treatment

Your doctor will determine the exact cause and treatment based on your medical history and whether you've experienced any recent or past lung infection or trauma. She will also conduct a physical exam with a stethoscope and the "tapping" test on the chest that is known as percussion. She will also probably take a chest X ray or an X ray of the ribs.

As mentioned earlier, having a pain in your chest on breathing is easy to treat. In most cases, all you need is time—about two weeks—and an analgesic such as Advil, Tylenol, or Naprosyn to relieve the pain. If, however, the pain is caused by fluid in the lung, the fluid will need to be removed with a small needle in a hospital. Your doctor will send the fluid to a lab for testing and will perform a complete medical work-up to determine the underlying cause of the chest pain.

CHEST PAIN WORSENED BY MOVEMENT

Description and Possible Medical Problems

If you've been reading this chapter from the beginning, you know by now that not every pain in the chest automatically means a cardiac problem is brewing. In fact, if you have a pain in your chest that is localized in one spot that is less than an inch in diameter and it occurs primarily when you're coughing or breathing, you probably have a small viral infection in your lung. This is probably the cause if you haven't been feeling well in recent weeks. Another possibility is that the muscles or bones of your rib cage have been injured in some way, especially if breathing or taking a deep breath makes the pain worse.

Treatment

If you think a viral infection is causing the pain in your chest, you should make an appointment to see your doctor. After a visual and physical examination and perhaps a chest X ray, the treatment your doctor will give you is an easy one: rest and an analgesic such as Motrin or Tylenol, two pills or capsules taken four times a day or as needed. If your doctor discovers that your pain is caused by a rib fracture, the treatment will be exactly the same as for a viral infection, since there is no other treatment than to relieve the pain.

BODY SIGNAL ALERT

CHEST PRESSURE WHEN WALKING WITH SWEATING OR SHORTNESS OF BREATH

Description and Possible Medical Problems

Maybe you lead a pretty sedentary life by default. You don't have the time or energy to exercise, or, frankly, you're just not interested. On those occasions when you do exert yourself, maybe walking up a flight of stairs, you might feel a generalized pressure in your chest, and you may start to sweat lightly and be short of breath. However, the pressure passes when you sit down and catch your breath again, and you probably figure it's due to your sedentary ways.

There's more to it than that. You may have a condition known as angina pectoris, a sign that you have an advanced case of arteriosclerosis. If the vessels to the heart are narrowed severely, even a mild form of exertion such as carrying a basket of laundry upstairs will make it difficult for sufficient blood to flow to the heart at a time when more blood is needed. If this occurs, this temporary lack of blood and oxygen will cause pressure in the chest that's usually accompanied by shortness of breath. You may also have other symptoms such as shoulder pain, jaw pain, and belching.

Treatment

If you think you have angina pectoris, you should see your doctor. She will give you a physical exam and ask you questions about the nature and occurrence of the pressure in your chest. If the pressure and your other symptoms have been occurring frequently, she may recommend that you be hospitalized to prevent an impending heart attack. Some medications that are commonly used to treat angina pectoris include beta-blockers such as Inderal and Lopressor and nitrates in a sublingual form to be taken under the tongue such as nitroglycerine or in an oral form such as isosorbide. Or perhaps your doctor will recommend that you wear a cardiac nitroglycerine patch during your waking hours. The patch is removed at night to prevent you from developing a tolerance to the medication.

COUGH: AN INTRODUCTION

A cough is a very common condition. Most of the time, the purpose of a cough is very simple: we cough to expel an irritant from the lungs or the throat, whether it's a piece of food, particle of dust, or an infection of the upper respiratory tract, such as a cold or flu. In these cases, a cough encourages the lungs to rid themselves of phlegm and irritating substances.

However, a cough can also be caused by emotions, as some

people cough when they get upset; it's almost as if they're trying to rid the body of the negative thoughts and feelings that are causing them to be upset.

These kinds of coughs are usually not serious and tend not to last for more than a week or so. Since most coughs are part of the body's infection-fighting system, they usually disappear without any specific treatment. However, if your cough lasts for more than a week or appears on and off over a period of a couple of months, you should see your doctor.

More uncommonly, a cough can be a sign of a serious disease. Asthma and heart disease can first show up as a simple cough. Likewise, many cancers of the lung begin with a cough as the only symptom. Therefore, the words you use to describe your cough to your doctor are very important. If you're not sure of the reason why you're coughing, ask yourself the following questions:

1.   How long have I been coughing? Hours, days, or weeks?

2.   Is it a productive cough? In other words, am I coughing up mucus, phlegm, or blood? If so, how much? Less than a tablespoon or more than that? And what is the color? Bright red, brown, grey, green, black, or clear?

3.   Do I start to cough when I'm in a certain position such as lying down?

4.   Do I start to cough when I increase my level of physical activity?

5.   Am I wheezing?

6.   Do I have other symptoms, such as weight loss, fever, or chills? Has my voice changed over a period of several months?

7.   Do I start coughing when I'm eating?

8.   Do I tend to cough when I become nervous?

Your answers to these questions will help your doctor diagnose your cough and prescribe appropriate treatment. If he thinks your cough is a sign of a serious underlying illness, he may order one or more of the tests listed earlier in this chapter that are used to investigate problems in the chest.

OVER-THE-COUNTER COUGH MEDICATIONS

When you go to the drugstore to select an over-the-counter preparation to treat your cold or flu, you'll encounter a dizzying array of liquids, lozenges, pills, and potions to choose from.

Buy a cough medication with an expectorant if your cough is thick and phlegmy. Drinking lots of fluids also helps, as does avoiding dairy products, as they seem to make secretions thicker. Cough suppressants are primarily for dry, hacking coughs that only irritate the throat and lungs more. In this case, it's also important to keep your throat well lubricated to cut down on the cough. When buying a cough syrup, you should also choose one that doesn't contain alcohol. If you're diabetic, you need to take a sugar-free formulation. If you need help, ask your pharmacist.

COUGH, NONPRODUCTIVE, PERSISTENT, BROUGHT ON BY PHYSICAL ACTIVITY

Description and Possible Medical Problems

You consider yourself to be quite active, but more often than not you find you start to cough whenever your heart rate gets above 80 during exercise. You may also find it hard to breathe and be short of breath at other times of the day.

Exercise-induced asthma occurs mainly in children and adults from their 20s through their 40s; I've rarely seen new onset exercise-induced asthma in people over the age of 30. The cough may be persistent and may last as long as you exercise or continue after the exercise session is over.

In people over 50, when a nonproductive cough is brought on by a short walk, it can be a sign of an underlying heart problem such as angina pectoris, in which narrowed vessels make it difficult for sufficient blood and oxygen to reach the heart.

Treatment

Even if a person has exercise-induced asthma, I'll almost never recommend that she stop exercising, since regular physical activity is so beneficial for your body and your general health. If you begin to cough and have trouble breathing during exercise, your doctor may recommend you carry a handheld inhaler such as Ventolin and take two puffs as needed. If you're over 50 and have exercise-induced asthma, I'll usually recommend that you undergo a complete cardiac work-up, including a stress test, to make sure that the condition is not an early sign of heart failure or angina.

See also "Wheezing" below.

COUGH, NONPRODUCTIVE, PERSISTENT, UNRELATED TO PHYSICAL ACTIVITY

Description and Possible Medical Problems

Sometimes you develop a hacking cough that wants to stay around for a while. You should first determine if it's due to a new item that's recently been introduced into your home. This could be a new piece of furniture, a different brand of floor wax, or a new pet. It's not unusual for adults to develop a new sensitivity to a substance or chemical. In the presence of a new irritant, the only symptom will likely be a nonproductive, persistent cough (see "Cough, Nonproductive, Single Episode of" below for more details).

If, however, you can't trace your cough to a likely irritant, there are a number of other possibilities. If you're under fifty, a nonproductive persistent cough can be caused by a scratchy throat or by an infection of the trachea; many times, this type of infection is caused by a virus. If this is the case, you might also have a low-grade fever, swollen glands, or a sinus infection. I have seen a chronic cough develop in people who tend to be very anxious; occasionally, they can develop a cough that can last for many months.

This type of cough can also occur in people who are taking the class of medications known as ACE inhibitors, such as Capoten, Accupril, or Zestril, for high blood pressure or heart failure.

Treatment

Before your doctor treats your nonproductive, persistent cough, he may take your full medical history and do a physical exam and conduct other tests, which may include a blood test, a chest X ray, a tuberculosis skin test, and a spirometry breathing test. If the cough persists, a bronchoscopy and possibly a biopsy will be performed. These tests will help to rule out any underlying illness, such as a lung malignancy.

Once your doctor determines that your health is fine except for your cough, he might prescribe an antibiotic such as erythromycin, to be taken by mouth four times a day for a week, plus a mild cough suppressant such as Robitussin. If your cough is due to a viral infection, he will recommend that you rest and take aspirin or Tylenol; if your sinuses are also acting up, there are plenty of over-the-counter sinus remedies such as Sinutab and Dristan to help you. If these don't do the trick, a prescription nasal inhaler such as Nasacort and/or a prescription antihistamine such as Claritin can be used.

If you're taking an ACE inhibitor, tell your doctor as it may be responsible for your frequent cough. Your doctor may switch you to another medication, like a calcium channel blocker such as Cardizem or verapamil.

COUGH, NONPRODUCTIVE, SINGLE EPISODE OF

Description and Possible Medical Problems

It's Saturday morning, and you've decided to do a little work around the house. Whether it's dusting the living room, painting a closet, or cutting a piece of wood to fix a kitchen drawer, you may suddenly begin to cough. When you move into another room or outside, the cough stops. Once you resume work, however, you start to cough again. What's wrong? Are you really allergic to work, as you've always maintained?

Sorry; try another excuse. When you develop a cough and have no other symptoms, it's probably caused by a particular irritant that's in the air. Dust, paint fumes, and sawdust are all possible causes.

Treatment

If you want to, you can get out of doing a certain chore because it makes you cough. Since most spouses and partners won't buy this, however, hardware stores sell a lot of those little white air filter masks so you can continue your work. Sucking on candy, chewing gum, and taking the work outside are other possible solutions.

BODY SIGNAL ALERT

COUGH, PRODUCTIVE AND ACUTE

Description and Possible Medical Problems

The first thing you should realize with a cough that has appeared suddenly and brings up mucus or phlegm is that this is the body's way of getting rid of an irritant that has entered the lungs. With an acute, non-productive cough, the cause is usually an inhaled irritant, like dust. A productive cough, however, is probably caused by an underlying illness that is irritating the lungs and causing them to produce more phlegm than usual.

If you have an acute, productive cough, ask yourself the following questions:

1. What color is the secretion: grey, brown, green, red, yellow, or clear?

2. Am I coughing up a lot of phlegm or mucus—more than about a teaspoon—and is it thick or thin?

3. Am I coughing only at night or all day long?

4. Do I have a fever, chills, body aches, or lethargy?

5. If an elderly relative has an acute, productive cough, has there been a change in his or her consciousness and mental acuity?

6. Have I recently lost weight?

7. Was I a heavy smoker in the past?

8. Do I have night sweats?

If you have thick, copious secretions that are grey, yellow, brown, or green, you probably have a bacterial infection, which means you could have pneumonia. Some other symptoms could be fever, chills, or fatigue. If you have these symptoms, you should see your doctor.

If you've recently lost weight and have night sweats along with an acute, productive cough, you may actually have tuberculosis.

Treatment

After a physical exam, blood test, and chest X ray, if your doctor determines that you have pneumonia, he will prescribe antibiotic treatment. Most midlife adults up to the age of about 65 are treated on an outpatient basis with an antibiotic such as penicillin, Cipro, Bactrim, or Keflex. The antibiotic your doctor chooses will depend on your age, as well as the usual antibiotics that are used in your area, depending on the particular organism that is suspected to have caused your infection.

Your doctor will also recommend that you take an expectorant, such as Robitussin or another over-the-counter product, three or four times a day. If the cough is especially bad, a cough suppressant with codeine can be taken. Two Tylenols every four hours will help reduce the fever, and drinking at least eight glasses of water a day will break up the secretions.

When your physician prescribes antibiotics, be sure to finish the medication. A severe case of pneumonia can take as long as a month to clear up completely. Although you may start to feel better, using antibiotics for only a couple of days will fail to knock the pneumonia out of your system.

If you smoke or drink alcohol, you will have a different course of treatment. A heavy smoker who has a case of pneumonia that recurs or never completely disappears might require a bronchoscopy, a procedure in which a lung specialist looks into your lungs to check for a possible obstruction. He may also decide to use a CAT scan of the chest as well as chest X rays to help find the cause.

If your doctor suspects you have tuberculosis, he will order a tuberculosis skin test to make a positive diagnosis. If you do have TB, you will probably need to be hospitalized and isolated and treated with antibiotics against tuberculosis for at least six to nine months.

Special Mention for the Elderly

If you have a frail elderly relative, living either at home or in a nursing home, and she comes down with pneumonia—though the only symptom of the disease may be confusion—she'll probably need to be hospitalized. She'll be treated with intravenous antibiotics, oxygen, and respiratory therapy, since a case of pneumonia that's easy to treat in a 40-year old can be life-threatening in an elderly patient.

I strongly believe that the Pneumovax vaccine, which helps prevent bacterial pneumonia, should be given to every man and woman over the age of 65, as well as people of any age who are smokers or diabetics or have had their spleens removed. Also, viral influenza can quickly turn into bacterial pneumonia in the elderly, so I recommend that all elderly persons should get a flu shot every year.

See also "Shortness of Breath with Cough, Pinkish Sputum, and Wheezing" below.

COUGH, PRODUCTIVE AND CHRONIC

Description and Possible Medical Problems

If you have been coughing for more than a few weeks and are coughing up mucus and/or phlegm, you have a chronic, productive cough. If you have no other symptoms of a cold or flu—in which a chronic, productive cough is common—and you're over 50 and are frequently short of breath, you may have emphysema. If you've been a heavy smoker for most of your life, the chances that you do have this lung disease are even greater.

Among my elderly patients, I often see frail older women who smoked two packs of cigarettes a day for many years and who now have a chronic productive cough. Many times, they will also be short of breath.

Emphysema is the most common cause of a chronic productive cough. The emphysema can occur as a result of either long-term cigarette smoking or long-term bouts with chronic bronchitis.

Treatment

If you have a chronic, productive cough and are diagnosed with emphysema, your doctor will treat you with a bronchodilator and various sprays. For a detailed discussion of the treatments I recommend, see "Shortness of Breath, Chronic, with Productive Cough" below.

COUGHING UP BLOOD OR PHLEGM MIXED WITH BLOOD

Description and Possible Medical Problems

Even if you normally don't dwell on the general state of your health, coughing up blood or phlegm mixed with blood is bound to get your attention and your doctor's as well.

It should. Whether you cough up blood or phlegm mixed with blood that is bright red, brownish red, or pink and bubbly, you must see your physician. It's usually the sign of a serious underlying disease. Anytime you cough up blood that is bright red in color, the cause can be a problem with your blood's ability to clot, a tumor in your lung, an aneurysm of the thoracic aorta, a low blood platelet count, or a burst blood vessel. When it's a frothy pink substance that's accompanied by wheezing and shortness of breath, it's a sign of heart failure. Another possible cause of coughing up blood is lung cancer or tuberculosis, especially if your cough has persisted for months and it hasn't been treated. However, when the blood is brownish and resembles coffee grounds, it's coming from the digestive tract and is a sign of a bleeding ulcer.

In addition to coughing up blood or phlegm mixed with blood, you may also have a fever, overall body aches, and a general feeling of malaise, all of which are signs of pneumonia.

It is also important to be aware of the amount coughed up. A small amount—a teaspoonful or less—can indicate that a small vessel in the trachea or upper airway has burst, which is a relatively minor occurrence. In fact, if you've had a cold or flu recently, it's highly likely that you have burst a blood vessel by frequent coughing. An amount larger than a teaspoonful can signify a serious medical condition requiring immediate medical attention.

Treatment

No matter the amount or color of blood or phlegm mixed with blood that you cough up, you need to call your doctor immediately. Many times, when the problem is a burst blood vessel caused by a frequent cough, your doctor will tell you to take it easy for a few days until the vessel heals. If, however, you've coughed up more than a teaspoonful and it's bright red, brown and coffee ground–like, or frothy pink, your doctor will usually suggest that you go to the hospital for further examination.

And if you have a relative or friend over the age of 60 who has any of these symptoms, even coughing up less than a teaspoonful of blood or phlegm mixed with blood, you should drive that person to the emergency room as soon as possible. The doctor will take a complete medical history and physical exam, including blood tests and sputum cultures, along with a chest X ray and bronchoscopy. The treatment will depend on the cause, though it will usually consist of antibiotic therapy.

COUGHING WHILE EATING

Description and Possible Medical Problems

We've all had a piece of food go down the "wrong pipe." Fortunately, for most of us, this kind of episode stops just short of requiring the Heimlich maneuver. While it may cause a temporary sore throat and loss of appetite, it's not a serious problem.

For people who are frail and elderly, however, it's another story. In fact, it's not uncommon for them to cough while they're eating or drinking. This especially tends to happen if a family member is feeding them, as the role reversal tends to make both parent and child tense.

In the elderly, the swallowing mechanism can become progressively weaker due to chronic illness, a stroke, or advanced dementia as caused by Alzheimer's disease. As a result, food can very easily go down into the windpipe, or trachea, which can potentially be very dangerous. Small amounts of food in the trachea can cause a lung infection called aspiration that can lead to aspiration pneumonia, a condition that can be lethal in a person whose immune system is already weakened by age and disease. Aspiration pneumonia requires hospitalization with intravenous antibiotics.

If an elderly relative often coughs while he's eating, his family should consult with his physician, who may contact an ear, nose, and throat specialist and/or even a speech language pathologist with expertise in swallowing disorders. Either of these specialists may perform special "dysphagia evaluations," which check a person's ability to swallow various types of food. These specialists may then recommend dietary adjustments (such as pureeing certain foods) to relieve the difficulties in swallowing.

Treatment

If your elderly relative has developed aspiration pneumonia, hospitalization is necessary. This will include a complete course of intravenous antibiotics. If feeding becomes a consistent problem despite treatment, it may become necessary to insert a feeding tube into the patient's stomach for a short time to make sure he gets the nutrition he needs.

HEART RATE GREATER THAN 100 BEATS PER MINUTE, WITH OCCASIONAL SHORTNESS OF BREATH

Description and Possible Medical Problems

If you occasionally feel your heart start to race for a minute or two and then return to normal, and you're under 50, you have nothing to worry about. Usually, this condition is the result of an excess of caffeine or stimulant medications, anxiety, or thyroid disease and is not an indication of heart trouble. Only if the rapid heartbeat lasts for more than several minutes should you call your doctor.

If you're over 50, however, and become short of breath when your heart rate goes above 100 beats per minute, and it lasts for several minutes, you should see your doctor; heart disease may be the cause (see also "Palpitations" below).

Treatment

If you're under 50 and your rapid heartbeat is caused by caffeine, anxiety, or a thyroid disease, your doctor will probably prescribe beta-blockers to slow your rapid heartbeat. Long-term medication will not be used.

If you're over 50 and develop a rapid heartbeat, your doctor will want to evaluate you for heart disease. An example of a rapid heartbeat that's the result of heart disease is atrial fibrillation, or atrial flutter; the underlying heart disease will then be monitored with an electrocardio-graph or a Holtor monitor and treated with medication such as vera-pamil, digoxin, or Inderal. In an elderly person, a rapid heartbeat will also be treated with these medications and requires close monitoring in a hospital to help slow the heartbeat. If the rapid heart rate is not slowed, heart failure can result. If an elderly person has had a series of small strokes and now exhibits a rapid heartbeat, the doctor will pre-scribe an anticoagulant medication such as Coumadin, which will require weekly blood tests after being discharged from the hospital to help determine the correct dosage. Since Coumadin is a potent medica-tion, side effects such as blood in the urine, a black stool, a nosebleed that won't go away, or any new symptoms that appear anywhere in your body require the immediate attention of a doctor.

HEART RATE, RAPID, THEN SLOW, WITH FAINTING

Description and Possible Medical Problems

Some elderly people have a condition in which the heart rate alter-nately speeds up and slows down, and it can vary back and forth sev-eral times a day. Sometimes the person may appear to be in normal spirits, but occasionally she may have chest pain, shortness of breath, or fainting.

The body's nervous system regulates many body functions that we take for granted. The stabilization of the heartbeat during stress, exer-cise, and sleep is controlled by a node in the carotid artery in the neck called the carotid sinus. If this node starts to malfunction due to aging, the heart can rapidly speed up and slow down for no particular reason. This is called sick sinus syndrome and can sometimes be exacerbated by tight collars or neckties.

Treatment

If you think that an elderly relative has sick sinus syndrome, she will need to be hospitalized and her heart closely monitored for 24 hours or more. Treatment will be with a beta-blocker such as Inderal, verapamil, or digoxin and/or a pacemaker, according to her overall health. Also, she will be prohibited from wearing tight collars.

HEART RATE, SLOWER THAN 50 BEATS PER MINUTE

Description and Possible Medical Problems

If you're under 50 with a heart rate to match, it means you're in excellent health and physically fit. If, however, you have a history of heart disease and you're taking beta-blockers—which deliberately slow the heart rate—as long as you have no other symptoms, you don't have to worry.

A slow heart rate in an elderly relative is cause for concern, however. Also, a slow heart rate may be discovered only in the course of an exam for possible heart failure, especially when it's accompanied by shortness of breath or a sudden fall.

Treatment

If an elderly relative has a heart rate under 50, her doctor will use an electrocardiogram and echocardiogram (see pages 239–241 for a description of these tests) to evaluate the health of her heart. If the slow heart rate is not caused by beta-blockers, she may need to have a pacemaker surgically placed.

A pacemaker is a small device that keeps the heart beating. After a pacemaker—a small generator that measures about four inches square—is placed under the collarbone with local anesthesia, it normally takes less than a week to fully recover from the procedure; the pain is usually minimal and can be treated with aspirin or Tylenol. Pacemakers are totally safe; their batteries almost never need to be replaced, and they have been responsible for saving thousands of lives. Contrary to popular belief, you don't have to have had a heart attack to require a pacemaker, though people who have had a heart attack still receive the majority of pacemakers to forestall potential problems with the rhythms of the heart.

PALPITATIONS

Description and Possible Medical Problems

Heart palpitations are common in people of all ages. Whether the palpitations are described as a skipped or extra heartbeat, a rapid heartbeat, or a rapid flutter, palpitations are usually nothing to worry about when they occur without other symptoms. If you have heart palpitations, either frequent ones—every day—or only occasionally, once or twice a year, it's a good idea to answer these questions so you can monitor your palpitations.

1. Do I also have shortness of breath?

2. Do I have chest pain?

3. Can I tap out the rhythm of the palpitations with my finger?

4. Which activities tend to bring on the irregularity?

If you sometimes feel as though you have an extra heartbeat, you probably shouldn't worry. An occasional extra beat is very common in people under 50. The most common cause is anxiety, caffeine, or smoking. If there are no other symptoms but the extra beat is appearing with greater frequency, you may be hospitalized for a few days and put under observation. A Holtor monitor, an electronic device that checks your heartbeat for irregularities, will record every heartbeat for 24 hours or more. Your doctor will also use an echocardiogram to see if you have any problems with the valves in your heart. He will check for mitral valve prolapse, which is a congenital condition in which blood leaks slowly through the mitral valve. The condition can cause a variety of symptoms; besides palpitations, they can include headaches and a vague chest pain. This condition is more common in women than men.

If you have mitral valve prolapse, your doctor's number one concern will be that you take antibiotics before any dental, urological, or gastrointestinal procedure, which will help to prevent infection of the heart valve by any bacteria that are loosened during these procedures.

Treatment

If you notice an extra heartbeat only once in a while and have no other symptoms, you don't need to do anything. If the palpitations occasionally become strong and upset you, your doctor may prescribe beta-blockers to help prevent the more severe episodes. If your doctor determines that you have a mitral valve prolapse, a medication such as Inderal or another beta-blocker may be prescribed to limit the episodes. I also recommend you increase your activity and go easy on caffeine.

RASH ON CHEST

See "Pimples, Painful, on One Side of the Face" in Chapter 9.

RASH UNDER BREAST

See "Rash Under Breast," in Chapter 12.

≡ SHORTNESS OF BREATH: READ THIS FIRST ≡

If you have shortness of breath, ask yourself the following questions. Then use your answers to look up information about shortness of breath in the individual sections according to your specific symptoms.

1. Is my shortness of breath an acute, isolated episode, or have I had it for a long time? (page 260)

2. Does it become worse during physical activity? (pages 261–262)

3. Does lying down make it worse? Are my ankles also swollen? (pages 266–267)

4. Do I have a cough? Is it productive or dry? (pages 262–265)

5. Have I been wheezing lately? (pages 269–271)

6. Do I have a history of smoking, drug use, or exposure to chemicals? (pages 264–265)

7. Do I have any other body signals, such as weight loss or fever? (pages 262–263)

8. Do I have shortness of breath after I've been exposed to an allergen? (pages 261)

9. Do I have chest pain? (pages 267–268)

10. Do I have palpitations or any irregularity of the heart? (pages 257–258)

11. Do I have other ailments that are currently being treated, such as heart disease or emphysema? (pages 262–263)

12. Is my color pale and ashen or blue, and am I sweating? (page 262)

SHORTNESS OF BREATH, ACUTE

Description and Possible Medical Problems

Acute shortness of breath can be a frightening event for people of any age. If you're under 50, or are older and in pretty good condition, and you don't have any other symptoms, your shortness of breath might not be serious. It could be the result of a sudden emotional shock, an anxiety attack, or recent exposure to a substance you're allergic to. When a person who is ordinarily in good health suddenly becomes short of breath, it can be a sign of acute pneumonia or bronchitis.

An anxiety attack can occur anywhere, but especially in a crowded area, in an elevator, or during a stressful situation. In addition to shortness of breath, you may have heart palpitations and numbness in your hands or feet.

Treatment

If you suddenly become short of breath due to an anxiety attack and you have no other symptoms, it's a good idea to rest quietly for a few hours. To prevent future attacks, biofeedback can be helpful.

Basically, biofeedback is an exercise that helps you learn how to relax. You are instructed in the technique by a physical therapist, a psychologist, or a biofeedback specialist. First, special electrodes are attached to your forehead. These electrodes, which are not painful, are hooked up to a machine that measures your muscle tension, which is reflected in sounds that are emitted by the machine or on a monitor that measures your tension in waves, much like an EKG does. For instance, if you are feeling stressed, the machine will respond by emitting a series of fast, high-pitched beeps; if you're relaxed, the beeps are slower. Once you relax your muscles—and therefore decrease your tension—the machine responds in kind. In essence, the machine teaches you how to relax by controlling the amount of tension that you're holding in your muscles. For a referral to a biofeedback specialist, you can look in the Yellow Pages or call your local hospital.

If you think your shortness of breath was caused by an allergen, make sure someone else removes it from your immediate vicinity. Relax until you can catch your breath.

If, however, your throat begins to close during an acute allergic response, you will need immediate medical attention. Your doctor may give you the drug epinephrine via injection.

Special Mention for the Elderly

In people who are frail and elderly, an acute case of shortness of breath can occur from a heart attack, an irregular heartbeat, heart failure, or emphysema. If you notice these signals in an elderly relative, call 911 or get her to the emergency room immediately.

BODY SIGNAL ALERT

SHORTNESS OF BREATH, ACUTE, UPON PHYSICAL ACTIVITY

Description and Possible Medical Problems

The body is a funny thing. It can accept a sedentary lifestyle for many years, usually with no ill effects. Then suddenly, as if to make up for decades of being taken for granted, it will rebel, almost as if to make you atone for the lack of attention you've paid it.

One of the signs it may send you is shortness of breath during activities that previously didn't stress you at all. If you're over 50 and suddenly have shortness of breath while climbing stairs or carrying packages, you'll need to heed your body's messages. Stop and rest! Especially if you begin to sweat heavily and experience chest pain during any physical activity and you've been ignoring these episodes for a while, you will need to see your doctor.

Along with the shortness of breath while exercising, if you're a heavy smoker and you wheeze occasionally, you could be experiencing the early signs of emphysema. By itself, shortness of breath can also be the first sign of an imminent heart attack or even a manifestation of a heart attack itself in a person who is elderly or diabetic. Even if you don't have the classic signs of a heart attack—chest pain, pallor, sweating, and pain that radiates to the shoulder and down the arm—you should still seek medical attention immediately. The cause may be heart disease or lung disease, or perhaps a combination of the two.

The shortness of breath might be caused not by a heart problem but by an underlying malignancy creating a buildup of fluid in one part of a lung. Again, a complete evaluation will be necessary.

Treatment

If the shortness of breath does not disappear with rest or quickly recurs during any kind of physical activity, it is a medical emergency and professional care should be sought.

Your doctor will perform a number of tests, including a complete medical history and physical exam, a blood test, a chest X ray, an electrocardiogram, an echocardiogram, a stress test, and/or an angiogram.

Once you've been admitted to the hospital, your heart will be constantly monitored with electronic monitoring and blood tests to see if the heart has been damaged. The treatment will depend on what shows up on the various tests. The problem could be angina pectoris (see "Chest Pressure When Walking, with Sweating or Shortness of Breath" above.) If you do have angina pectoris, your medication might include beta-blockers, nitrates, and calcium channel blockers, depending on your age, your health, and the condition of your heart. Your doctor might also recommend that you carry sublingual nitroglycerine tablets to place under your tongue whenever you experience chest pain or shortness of breath.

SHORTNESS OF BREATH, ACUTE, WITH PRODUCTIVE COUGH AND FEVER

Description and Possible Medical Problems

There may have been some occasions where you've suddenly been short of breath—it probably caught you off guard, but chances are you were able to trace it back to a specific cause. Maybe you haven't had a chance to exercise for a few days—that's just how long it takes for your body to begin to lose up to 10% of its conditioning—or maybe you'd been feeling under the weather.

If you don't fit into either of these categories and you are also coughing and have a fever, it could be something else entirely.

When these symptoms appear in a person over 50 who also has emphysema, acute shortness of breath accompanied by cough and fever can be the sign of an acute flare-up of the disease; frequently, this can be sparked by the flu or pneumonia or even a virus. However, these collective symptoms may also be a sign of bronchitis, heart failure, or lung cancer. People who have emphysema can live symptom free for long periods of time, even years, without problems except for a chronic cough and shortness of breath upon exertion.

When people over 70 complain of shortness of breath with a cough and fever, they may also be confused and disoriented. In rare cases, an elderly person might also experience heart failure.

Treatment

If you have acute pneumonia, your doctor will probably treat you with a combination of oxygen, respiratory therapy, and antibiotics. If you're under 50, the treatment can be done at home. If you're over 50, home-based treatment is still possible, although your doctor will first evaluate you closely to see if this is the best thing. If your doctor decides hospitalization would be best, you'll be given antibiotics intravenously.

If you have emphysema and get pneumonia, your doctor will conduct a complete examination, including a chest X ray, a CAT scan of the chest if needed, and a bronchoscopy or biopsy if a lesion is found. If your doctor determines that you do have lung cancer, a combination of radiation and chemotherapy will be used to treat your condition.

SHORTNESS OF BREATH, CHRONIC, WITH NONPRODUCTIVE COUGH

Description and Possible Medical Problems

If you have a history of angina pectoris or emphysema, you may find over the years that you have become increasingly short of breath, regardless of your physical activity, and have developed a nonproductive chronic cough. If you have emphysema, it may be due to a chronic lung spasm; if you have angina, use of the commonly prescribed ACE inhibitors may be the culprit.

Treatment

The treatment for chronic shortness of breath with a nonproductive cough will be based on whether you have angina or are in the early stages of emphysema. If it's emphysema, your doctor will recommend that you use bronchodilator inhaler sprays such as Ventolin or Proventil, especially if you're also wheezing. If your shortness of breath is caused by angina, nitroglycerine or other cardiac medications like diuretics will be prescribed to ease your shortness of breath and cough.

SHORTNESS OF BREATH, CHRONIC, WITH PRODUCTIVE COUGH

Description and Possible Medical Problems

Most of us know at least a couple of people who have emphysema and/or bronchitis. In almost every case, these two serious lung diseases occur in people who have been heavy smokers for most of their lives or have been exposed to excessive amounts of chemicals.

One of the hallmark symptoms of emphysema is chronic shortness of breath with a productive cough, sometimes accompanied by wheezing. These symptoms are a result of the loss of lung volume that is indicative of these diseases. It's normal for us to lose a small amount of lung tissue due to the aging process, but this loss accelerates in heavy smokers and during ongoing exposure to certain chemicals.

Emphysema is a disease in which the lungs lose their elasticity. Because the lungs are not working efficiently, it becomes difficult for the blood to receive enough oxygen and to give off its carbon dioxide since it does this through the lungs. As a result, the amount of oxygen in the blood goes down while the carbon dioxide content increases. If the carbon dioxide levels go too high, a person with emphysema will first start breathing very rapidly in an effort to get more oxygen into the lungs but may then stop breathing. He will then need to be placed on a ventilator, which will require that a tube be inserted through the mouth and into the lungs.

There are two types of emphysema. One is called blue bloater, and it appears most often in people who are overweight. They tend to have chronic bouts with bronchitis and produce large amounts of secretions from their lungs. The second group are referred to as pink puffers. They are people who are thin, small framed, and extremely frail. Ultimately, however, the blue bloaters will also lose weight since it requires so much effort to breathe, while the pink puffers will get even thinner.

Treatment

If you have emphysema, treatment will depend on which stage of the disease you're in. Your doctor will want to take a full medical history and do a physical exam plus run some tests that show the extent of the damage to the lung. She will also need to measure the amount of oxygen and carbon dioxide in your blood. Certainly, you'll need to stop smoking and increase the amount of exercise you get. Your doctor will prescribe certain medications, which may include a bronchodilator such as Serevent, Azmacort, Ventolin, or Theophylline in the form of inhalants, or oral medications and possibly a steroid such as prednisone, given by mouth, or Solu-Medrol, administered intravenously in the hospital.

Unfortunately, people with emphysema are never able to regain the amount of lung volume they've lost, even if they stop smoking or cut down on their exposure to chemicals. The end stage of emphysema is not pretty: large amounts of secretions slowly collect in a lung that already has a greatly reduced capacity. Often, a person with emphysema feels as if he is drowning. I once had a patient who described emphysema as a feeling of being plunged underwater and becoming short of breath, then taken out of the water just long enough to catch his breath. And as soon as he did, he felt as though he was plunged right back in. However, by using bronchodilators, steroid therapies, home oxygen treatments, and breathing exercises, many people with emphysema can live well into their 80s. To keep the disease under control, the most important thing you can do is to prohibit anyone from smoking around you.

BODY SIGNAL ALERT

SHORTNESS OF BREATH WITH COUGH, PINKISH SPUTUM, AND WHEEZING

Description and Possible Medical Problems

If you suddenly become short of breath and simultaneously begin to cough up a pinkish sputum, you need to call 911 for immediate medical attention. You may also be sweating, pale, and wheezing.

These are all signs of acute pulmonary edema, in which the lungs begin to fill with water. Acute pulmonary edema can be caused by a dietary change, a sudden change in or cessation of a medication, a reaction from mixing two or more kinds of medication, or a heart attack or change in heart rhythm. If you have phlebitis, acute pulmonary edema can also be the result of a clot that travels from the veins of the legs into the lung, a condition known as pulmonary embolus.

Treatment

Acute pulmonary edema is a life-and-death situation, and immediate medical attention is necessary. While waiting for medical help, the most important thing to do is to keep a sitting position. If you have any diuretics or water pills at home, there is no harm in taking two of these pills immediately.

Regardless of the cause of acute pulmonary edema, once professional help is on the scene, the treatment for acute pulmonary edema includes the injection of a diuretic, such as Lasix, which will remove excess fluid from your body, meaning the heart has to work less, and nitrates, which reduce the amount of effort the heart has to make. In severe cases, it will be necessary to put you on ventilator support.

SHORTNESS OF BREATH WORSENED BY LYING DOWN

Description and Possible Medical Problems

You'd think that if you had a tendency to become short of breath with slight exertion, sitting or lying down would allow you to catch your breath. Not so for some people; lying down can actually make breathing harder.

If you find yourself to be short of breath when lying down or sitting and you also often have the seemingly unrelated symptom of swollen ankles, you should see your doctor. This is important, especially if you have diabetes or a previous history of heart disease of any kind.

If your shortness of breath is accompanied by wheezing, coughing, and an inability to talk, you will need to seek immediate medical attention.

In the elderly population, shortness of breath that occurs while lying down is usually caused by heart failure. Other times, however, the cause can be as simple as a heavy intake of salt. When I was a young doctor, we saw a group of nursing home residents come to the emergency room with heart failure. They had recently eaten a meal of hot dogs, corned beef, and pastrami, provided as a generous gift by the local deli. These people, who usually ate low-salt diets, could not handle the sudden overload of sodium, and as a result several ended up in the emergency room.

Treatment

If you are short of breath whenever you lie down and your doctor suspects heart failure, he will perform a total medical evaluation, which will include an electrocardiogram and an echocardiogram, among other tests. The ensuing treatment will depend on the degree of the heart failure.

The condition might actually require only a simple change in diet—limiting salt intake. Fat consumption should be reduced, and, if you're overweight, you'll probably need to lose some weight.

If your condition requires it, your doctor may prescribe a diuretic such as hydrochlorothiazide to reduce your blood pressure and take some of the strain off your heart. The ACE inhibitors digoxin and Lasix may also be used on an individual basis.

See also "Shortness of Breath with Cough, Pinkish Sputum, and Wheezing" above.

STERNUM, PAIN IN

Description and Possible Medical Problems

If you exercise regularly and are in relatively good shape, and you feel a sharp pain in your sternum, or breastbone, which runs from just below your chin to a few inches above your navel, you may jump to the conclusion that you're having a heart attack.

Don't worry. Tenderness in the sternum is actually a merit badge given for your good health and is a very common condition in people in their 40s and 50s who are physically active. In addition to the pain in the sternum, you may also feel pain in your joints and between the ribs and the sternum.

If you feel pain and tenderness in your sternum, it's probably caused by a sprain that's the result of overactivity, especially on exercise machines, which can easily strain your joints, muscles, and sternum in ways they haven't been stressed before. In people over 60, a pain in the sternum can also be caused by osteoarthritis.

Treatment

The treatment for a pain in your sternum is easy: rest and analgesics like aspirin and Tylenol. If the pain lasts for more than a week, your doctor may suggest the injection of a stronger analgesic.

STERNUM, MASS OR LUMP ON THE END OF

Description and Possible Medical Problems

We've all been thoroughly trained to believe that any mass that suddenly appears anywhere on the body must be cancer, an attitude that often results in unnecessary visits to the doctor's office. The good news is that if a mass suddenly appears on your sternum, it's probably not a serious health problem.

This mass, called a xiphoid process, is actually a small area of the sternum that extends below the rib cage in the center. If you've recently lost a large amount of weight, you may suddenly feel a "mass" and think it's a tumor. However, it's actually been there all along. Others might become aware of it if they experience a trauma to the chest wall and the xiphoid process becomes bruised or inflamed.

Treatment

If you've recently discovered your xiphoid process, you have nothing to worry about. If it is painful, Tylenol or Advil, taken four times a day or as needed, will work just fine.

WHEEZING

Description and Possible Medical Problems

When I was growing up, there was a girl down the street who had asthma. She always carried an inhaler around with her, and whenever she felt an asthma attack coming on, she'd scream, "I'm wheezing! I'm wheezing!" Then she'd whip out her inhaler, take two puffs, and be fine.

Whenever I hear a patient complain of wheezing, I always think of two things: that girl who lived down the street and what a funny word "wheeze" is.

But if you have asthma and start to wheeze, of course it's not funny at all.

Wheezing occurs when there is a constriction in the bronchial tree. The bronchi are the passageways of air that lead from each lung to the windpipe. If these begin to narrow for whatever reason, you will start to wheeze; the wheeze usually comes on the exhalation. Since asthma can develop at any age, a simple test is to try to blow out a match at arm's length. If you can't blow it out, you may have asthma.

Treatment

Of course, anyone who's had asthma since childhood is familiar with its various medications, such as the Ventolin inhaler, which is used during an attack, and theophylline which is taken in pill form and provides longer-lasting relief.

If you have had asthma for many years but have kept it under control with medications, you are still prone to developing an occasional respiratory tract infection caused by a virus or bacterium or exposure to chemicals, paints, or insecticides. This can bring on an acute wheezing episode that's known as a bronchospasm. If you have such an infection, your doctor will prescribe antibiotics and a bronchodilator spray such as Ventolin. If you are 40 or older, you might also be given an injection of epinephrine as long as you don't have a history of cardiac disease. Epinephrine is a bronchodilator and decongestant that will help keep spasms from occurring in the lung and bronchial tissue.

But again, most asthmatics are comfortable with self-treatment, and their disease usually doesn't progress past the point where more serious treatment is necessary. If the usual inhalers and medication fail to work, however, or the wheezing is accompanied by shortness of breath, you should seek medical attention, especially if you're over 50.

During the initial exam, your doctor will do a physical exam and check your health history. He may also choose to take a chest X ray if he believes an infection is present. A handheld peak-flow meter, a device you exhale into that measures the volume of air you're able to exhale quickly, will also help your doctor to tailor your treatment.

Sometimes the wheezing is very pronounced and the typical therapies aren't effective. If this is the case, you may have to be hospitalized. You will be given oxygen, and the amount of oxygen in your blood will be monitored with either regular blood tests or an oximeter, a device that measures the blood oxygen level in your earlobe or finger without piercing the skin.

See also "Shortness of Breath, Chronic, with Productive Cough" above.

BODY SIGNAL ALERT

WHEEZING FOR PROLONGED PERIOD, WITH SHORTNESS OF BREATH AND COUGH

Description and Possible Medical Problems

If you have a history of asthma, whether it's been stable or not, if you begin to wheeze and can't stop and you are also coughing and feeling short of breath, you are experiencing a series of severe bronchospasms, and you need immediate medical attention. This is a condition known as status asthmaticus, and you should call 911 right away.

Many people who have lived for years with their asthma remaining relatively stable are angry and confused when it suddenly becomes worse. They try to look for a reason and can't find one, and some may attribute it to the aging process.

Nope. It's probably caused by a viral infection or a medication such as an antihistamine or even an over-the-counter anti-inflammatory preparation such as Advil or aspirin. And some people can eventually trace the cause to an increase in the local air pollution.

Treatment

If you are having severe bronchospasms, you will be treated with a bronchodilator spray such as Ventolin or Proventil or a Maxair Autohaler, which works especially well in elderly asthmatics. After an acute attack, you will be observed for a couple of days to help prevent a repeat episode. If the severe wheezing was caused by an infection, you may be hospitalized until the infection clears up. If it's the result of an allergy medication, your allergist will need to switch your medication to a spray such as Intal or Atrovent to cut down on allergic reactions. A steroid spray such as Vanceril may also be used to prevent status asthmaticus in the long term.

As for pollution, the best prevention is to stay indoors when the air quality index shows that it would be dangerous for you to go out.

Chapter 12

BREASTS

BODY SIGNAL ALERT

Call your doctor immediately if you experience any of the following symptoms:

SYMPTOM	POSSIBLE MEDICAL CONDITION
You have a discharge from one or both of your breasts	*Hypothyroidism, side effect of medication, pituitary or breast tumor*
You feel a mass or see a change in the texture of the skin of your breasts	*Cancer, fibrocystic disease, fibroadenoma*
The skin of your breasts has taken on a dimpled, pitted look, resulting in a change in the contour of your breasts	*Cancer*

HOW THE BREASTS AGE

Though some of the effects aging has on a woman's body may largely pass unnoticed, it's the rare woman who doesn't measure the passage of time by the noticeable changes in her breasts. Because the breasts lose both fat and glandular tissue as they age, they may begin to sag and flatten a bit when a woman reaches her early 30s. The ratio of fat to glandular tissue actually increases as the functionality and size of the milk glands decrease with age.

You can prevent flabby muscles with regular exercise, but in the past there wasn't anything a woman could do to stave off the appearance of the aging process in her breasts—that is, until the advent of breast implants and reconstructive surgery. In the wake of the ban on silicone breast implants that became law in 1992, I'm curious to see how most women will regard their aging breasts. Even with the wide availability of saline-filled implants, which are supposedly safer, because of the dangers of the silicone implants, I'm finding that many women have been spooked by the thought of putting something into their body that wasn't there in the first place.

A SPECIAL WORD ABOUT BREAST CANCER

Another way in which aging influences the breasts is that a woman's odds of getting breast cancer increase once she turns 40. In fact, breast cancer is the most common form of cancer in women aged 40 to 55. One in eight women—or roughly 12%—of the female population in this age group will develop breast cancer at some point in her life. Seven in 10 of these women will be cured of the disease.

A monthly self-exam is the most important thing any woman can do to detect breast cancer early, no matter what her age. Fortunately, it's also simple to do. As with most cancers, the earlier the cancer is caught, the better the chances for a cure. Early detection is also important to prevent the cancer from spreading to other parts of the body, where it can become lethal. Despite a general phobia among American women concerning their breasts and anything that might disfigure them, many women still do not take the time to examine their breasts each month—or else they might do it every few months or whenever they remember. A monthly self-exam is vital to maintaining your good health; I'll provide you with full instructions on how to do it.

Interestingly, after the age of 55, a woman's chances of getting breast cancer actually decrease. In recent years, there has been some controversy about how often women aged 55 and over should be screened for cancer with a mammographam, due to its sometimes inaccurate readings, a slightly increased health risk from the radiation in the test, and the fact that women in this age group get breast cancer less often than younger women. This lessened risk may be due to the fact that with menopause, as the production of the hormone estrogen decreases, their stores of the hormone are gradually depleted, and thus their risk of breast cancer; some studies have detected a link between high estrogen levels and breast cancer. I should note, however, that in almost 20 years of working with women from midlife to their 90s, I have seen very few elderly patients who have died of breast cancer.

Your risk of having breast cancer increases if you fall into one or more of the following categories:

• You have a close female relative who has had breast cancer.

• You've already had breast cancer in one breast.

• You have not given birth, or else had your first child after the age of 35.

• Your first period came before the age of 12; menopause came after the age of 55.

• You've been exposed to excessive amounts of radiation.

Unfortunately, these risk factors are etched in stone; there's nothing you can do to change the fact that your chances of getting breast cancer are increased if you answer yes to one or more of the above statements.

Whether or not you are at risk, however, there are some things you can actively do to cut your chances of developing breast cancer. Being overweight, drinking more than a moderate amount of alcohol—more than three drinks a week—and using estrogen replacement therapy for hormonal problems during and after menopause can all increase your risk slightly. However, I feel that the benefits the hormone provides to the cardiovascular system and in treating osteoporosis outweigh this slightly increased risk. Contrary to popular belief, however, breast-feeding does not lower the risk of contracting breast cancer.

In recent years, there has been a question of whether or not the presence of fibrocystic disease in your 20s and 30s will increase your risk of breast cancer later on. The conclusion has been that the disease itself does not significantly increase your risk; however, if some of the cells involved in the disease turn out to be abnormal upon testing, your risk does increase slightly.

In very rare cases, where a woman's chances of getting breast cancer are almost certain, she may choose to prevent any tumors from ever forming by undergoing a bilateral mastectomy—the removal of both breasts—before a tumor has a chance to grow.

In recent years, researchers have discovered that a low-fat diet helps to decrease a woman's risk of breast cancer. So does taking antioxidants—nutritional supplements such as vitamins A, C, and E—which promote healthy cell growth by giving a boost to cells that are at risk.

As mentioned previously, the one preventive measure you can take whether or not you are at risk for breast cancer is doing a monthly self-exam. I recommend the following, depending upon your age:

- If you're between 40 and 50, it's important to examine your breasts monthly, get a complete physical exam every year, and have a mammogram every year or two, depending whether you fall into one or more of the high-risk categories.

- If you're 50 or over, you should follow the same guidelines, except you should definitely have a mammogram once a year.

- If you're under 40, you should have a mammogram only if you're specifically at risk for breast cancer. Your own doctor will help you to determine the frequency. You should also be in the habit of performing a breast self-exam every month.

BREAST SELF-EXAMINATION

Because many women are afraid of what they might find, or because they don't think they can get cancer, they may continually postpone doing a breast exam. But it takes less than five minutes to examine your breasts thoroughly. It's important to check your breasts every month because early lumps and tumors usually cannot be detected just by visual examination. In addition, by the time you notice a lump, it may be too late and the cancer may already have spread to other parts of your body.

When examining your breasts, it will help to ask yourself the following questions:

1. Do I feel a change in the size of one breast, as compared to the other?

2. Do I feel a lump in my breast?

3. Does my partner feel a lump in my breast?

4. Is the lump painful?

5. Is there a discharge from the breast?

6. Has the appearance of the skin of the breast changed?

It's a good idea to perform the self-exam the week after your menstrual period has ended. Your breasts will be less congested at this time, and any new growths will be easy to detect. Some women do their self-exam in the shower, because moist skin makes it easier to massage the breast in a circular motion, which is the best way to detect a lump.

First, stand before a mirror and check the nipples and skin of your breasts for any visible changes. Have the nipples or areola changed color since your exam last month? Does any portion of the skin of the breast appear puckered like an orange peel? Is there any noticeable swelling?

Next, raise your arms above your head. Do you notice any difference in the symmetry or appearance of your breasts?

The next, most important step can be done either in the shower or lying on your back. Start with your right breast. Raise your right arm above your head, and, holding your fingertips closely together, start at the top of the breast, at what would be twelve o'clock. Gently move your fingers in a circular motion while you check for any lumps. Next, move to one o'clock, and so on, until you have checked for lumps at the position of every hour on your breast. Next, follow the same motion for the area of the breast that lies under the nipple. Then, gently squeeze the nipple to check for any abnormal discharge. It's also important to check the area under your armpit, where lymph nodes are located.

Repeat the procedure for your left breast.

If you discover a lump in your breast, you should see your doctor. A regular monthly self-exam can be helpful because it helps you to become familiar with lumps or masses that appear in your breasts and are non-cancerous, and also to be aware of changes in your breasts that might indicate the presence of a malignancy. If you have trouble distinguishing between normal breast tissue, glands, and a lump, ask your gynecologist if she has a breast prosthesis that you can feel so you know what a lump feels like. Normal breast tissue can have masses and stringy tissue, but a lump is usually hard and starts out the size of a small pebble.

If you detect a lump, immediately see your doctor, who will then determine the status of the mass. Most lumps are not cancerous, but any new masses that you may find and that your doctor deems suspicious will require further examination. She may choose a mammogram, ultrasound, or biopsy.

A monthly self-exam can mean the difference between successful treatment and a fatal illness. Get in the habit of checking your breasts every month without fail.

BREASTS, TENDER AND SWOLLEN

Description and Possible Medical Problems

Just about every woman has experienced the feeling of tender, swollen breasts just before her menstrual period begins. A few days before the first day of your period each month, your breasts swell slightly as they become engorged with some of the fluid that the body normally retains to prepare for the beginning of each cycle.

For some women, the discomfort is mild; for others, the pain and tenderness is so severe that they have to apply an ice pack to their swollen breasts several times a day for three or four days a month, take aspirin or a prescription painkiller, and spend a good deal of time in bed, since even the slightest movement can cause excruciating pain. Some women with larger breasts find they are affected more than smaller-breasted women.

Treatment

No matter what your degree of discomfort, there are a number of things you can do to lessen the pain. Though some women deal with the pain and tenderness by gritting their teeth through it all, others take an active stance.

Taking a diuretic—either prescription or over-the-counter—will help cut down on the amount of fluid your body retains during your premenstrual cycle and thus on the amount of fluid in your breasts, which will reduce the swelling. I usually recommend a mild diuretic such as Dyazide, which is taken for two or three days before your menstrual period begins; it's not a good idea to take a diuretic every day, since it can interfere with the levels of sodium and potassium in your body. Cutting down on the amount of salt in your diet will also prevent your body from holding on to excess fluid. Some women also find some relief if they cut down on or eliminate caffeine, fat, sugar, and/or alcohol from their diet.

During their premenstrual periods, some women wear a bra that's tighter than usual, so the swollen breasts are held closer to the body and movement is restricted. This, however, can be even more painful to engorged breasts. Many women have found that wearing a bra with less support than normal helps relieve some of the pain; some even wear one while they sleep during the nights when their breasts are painful.

BODY SIGNAL ALERT

CHANGES IN THE CONTOUR OF THE BREAST WITH DIMPLED OR PITTED SKIN

Description and Possible Medical Problems

As your body ages, your breasts flatten out slightly and start to droop as gravity continues its long-range plans. Since you are probably already aware of these changes, you might not know that other changes in the contour of the breast—such as dimpled or pitted skin—might signal a serious medical problem. Some women might just associate these changes in the shape of their breasts as another sign of aging.

This is a big mistake.

When the shape of the outside of your breast changes, it usually means that something on the inside has changed to affect the shape. In fact, if you feel your breast where the skin has changed, you'll probably be able to feel a small lump beneath the skin. Whether it's a slight bulge or a small caved-in area, a change in the contour of one or both of your breasts usually means that a malignant tumor is affecting the tissue of the breast itself.

If you're diligent about your monthly exam, you should be able to detect a lump in your breast long before the skin of your breasts begins to look pitted or dimpled. However, if you've just recently noticed the dimpled or pitted skin that then led you to discover the lump, you need to see your doctor immediately.

If you notice that the skin of your breasts has changed, see your doctor immediately.

Treatment

If the skin of your breasts appears dimpled or pitted, changing the contour of your breasts, your doctor will examine your breasts, first visually, then manually. Since the major cause of dimpled, pitted skin is a lump in the breast, your doctor will probably perform a biopsy to determine whether or not the lump is a benign or malignant tumor.

If the lump is benign, your doctor will determine if it is a cyst or a fibroadenoma, a benign tumor. If, however, the lump is malignant, your doctor will have several treatment options. These include a lumpectomy, in which only the lump is removed; a mastectomy, in which the breast is removed, or a modified radical mastectomy, in which the breast is removed along with some of the lymph nodes that extend into the armpit. A radical mastectomy was common up until the early 1980s; today, it is relatively rare. In this procedure, the breast, lymph nodes, and pectoral muscles were typically removed, which resulted in a loss of range of motion for the arm on that side of the body. Today, a radical mastectomy is considered only when the cancerous cells have metastasized, or spread, to the pectoral muscles. Otherwise, a modified radical mastectomy leaves the pectoral muscles intact.

After surgery, because the cancer may have spread to the lymph nodes, many women who have had a lumpectomy or mastectomy may also be treated with radiation therapy. Chemotherapy may also be an option, though it is most often recommended for women who have not gone through menopause. It is also most often prescribed for use before and/or during the surgery, but not after, when the drug tamoxifen is usually prescribed. Tamoxifen is the most commonly prescribed drug for breast cancer because it has almost no side effects, which is unusual for an anticancer drug. In fact, tamoxifen is actually a hormone that is often prescribed in combination with other hormonal therapy. It can slow or reverse the spread of breast cancer when a tumor has not responded to other treatment methods.

Tamoxifen works by depleting the estrogen receptors in breast cancer cells, which, in essence, starves the cells, since they thrive on estrogen. The side effects of tamoxifen include mild pain in the bones, an increased need for calcium, and hot flashes in postmenopausal women. Because estrogen naturally strengthens bones, there is some concern that tamoxifen, an antiestrogen hormone, may increase a woman's risk of developing osteoporosis after treatment, but usually this can be offset by increased intake of calcium and exercise. The advantages of using tamoxifen to treat breast cancer are that these side effects are minor compared to those of other anticancer drugs and that it reduces the risk of a recurrence of the cancer.

However, breast cancer can be fickle in the way it responds to treatment. Some tumors will shrink and go into remission in response to estrogen hormones, while others will completely disappear with antiestrogen hormones such as androgens and progesterone. Because it is difficult to predict how a tumor will respond to a given hormone, if your doctor is treating you with chemotherapy, you may feel like a guinea pig at times. But tumors are fickle, and what may have worked successfully to shrink a tumor once may not succeed on the next go-round. So your doctor will keep trying, with the final goal being complete remission. If hormonal therapy fails to work, your doctor may try a corticosteroid such as prednisone, which can also be effective in treating breast cancer.

If you have undergone a modified radical mastectomy and would still like your breasts to look like new, one of your options—silicone breast implants—is no longer available. There are always breast prostheses to be worn with specially designed bras, but if you find this to be insufficient and you don't want saline implants, you may consider breast reconstruction, in which a new breast is "made" from muscle or fatty tissue that's been taken from the abdomen, the buttocks, or the outside of your upper thigh. It is formed into the shape of a breast with a layer of skin covering it before it is surgically set into place. The skin that's used to cover the new breast is often taken from the remaining breast or from another part of the body. If you should choose this option, you should be aware that you are still vulnerable to breast cancer, either in the remaining breast or in the reconstructed one, so you'll still need to rely on mammography and self-exams.

BODY SIGNAL ALERT

DISCHARGE FROM BREAST

Description and Possible Medical Problems

The only time in a woman's life when her breasts produce milk is obviously immediately after giving birth. However, a very small percentage of women will sometimes have a milky discharge from their breasts that is not associated with pregnancy or childbirth. Even less often a man will have a discharge from his nipples.

Anytime the body produces milk when a woman is not pregnant—or at any time in a man—the condition is called galactorrhea. The discharge may be whitish or greenish in color, and it usually comes out of both breasts.

Galactorrhea may appear for a variety of reasons. Sometimes it is caused by too much estrogen in the bloodstream; an oral contraceptive or another estrogen-based medication could be the culprit. Or the hormone prolactin—which stimulates the production of breast milk—might have been activated by the presence of a tumor on the pituitary gland, which controls growth in the body and produces the hormone.

Certain drugs—antihypertensive medications such as Aldomet or tricyclic antidepressants such as amitriptyline—can also cause the breasts to produce milk in the absence of pregnancy or childbirth. Phenothiazine—a tranquilizer—and amphetamines can also stimulate the production of prolactin. If you have hypothyroidism, you may also be prone to galactorrhea.

However, in about half the cases, there is no traceable cause.

Treatment

Your doctor's diagnosis depends on the color of the discharge, along with a recent history of your health practices, though in the women and men who get galactorrhea with no clear cause, the condition will usually clear up on its own without treatment. However, your doctor may want to order a test that will check the levels of thyroid hormones and prolactin in your blood. She may also want to conduct an MRI or CAT scan of your brain to check for a pituitary tumor.

If you've given birth in the past year, your discharge is white, and your doctor can find no reason for the galactorrhea, it's probably not serious. If, however, you've never had children and you have a whitish discharge from your nipples, your doctor will look for medication to be the culprit; the discharge might also be a sign of an underlying endocrine disorder. To see if this is the case, she will run blood tests and perhaps a CAT scan to see if your hypothalamus—a gland that regulates your endocrine system—or your pituitary gland is damaged in some way. If the cause of your galactorrhea is found to be hypothyroidism, she will prescribe a thyroxine replacement medication such as Synthroid. The dosage of this medication depends on the results of blood tests that are taken over the course of several weeks or months and will be adjusted slowly when your doctor determines how your body is tolerating the medication.

If the condition is determined to be a side effect of a medication you're taking, your doctor will recommend you stop taking the drug and may switch you to another type of medication.

If the discharge is greenish or brown—indicating a bloody tinge—you should see your doctor immediately. Your galactorrhea may be caused by cancer or another kind of tumor in the breasts.

If your doctor decides that a pituitary tumor is causing the galactorrhea, she may suggest you take a drug called bromocriptine, which will attack the tumor and reduce the gland's production of prolactin. If the tumor has grown too large to treat with bromocriptine, he will probably want to remove it surgically. To ensure that the pituitary gland stays tumor free after surgery, your doctor will probably recommend that you take bromocriptine for several months after the operation.

Bromocriptine is typically prescribed to treat some of the symptoms of Parkinson's disease; however, it also serves to suppress the production of prolactin.

LUMP IN BREAST AFTER MINOR INJURY

Description and Possible Medical Problems

In my practice, I have seen that it is not uncommon for a woman to develop a mass in her breast after a fall or a minor car accident. In fact, she may not even notice the mass or lump in her breast until several weeks after the initial trauma, when other more obvious symptoms have subsided.

It's likely that a hematoma has formed in her breast as a reaction to the impact. A hematoma is a swollen mass or lump like a cyst—except that the mass contains clotted blood, not pus. A hematoma forms when a blood vessel breaks, even slightly, and the blood seeps out and becomes trapped in tissue. The hematoma will often cause a large area of the breast to become black and blue. Fortunately, it usually looks much worse than it actually is.

If a lump suddenly appears in your breast, the surrounding area is or has recently been bruised, and you have recently experienced a severe blow to your breast, you probably have a hematoma. I've treated several women who discovered lumps in their breasts and were convinced they had breast cancer; instead, they had hematomas.

Treatment

Sometimes a hematoma will clear up on its own without treatment. To ease the pain, you should apply an ice pack to the swollen area several times a day and take Tylenol to help reduce the swelling, since aspirin might cause more bleeding.

If this doesn't heal the hematoma, your doctor may recommend that the lump be drained, much like a cyst in your breast would be. Though some doctors suggest that you wait to see if a hematoma clears up on its own, others feel that if it is relatively large, it should be drained immediately.

BODY SIGNAL ALERT

MASS IN BREAST

Description and Possible Medical Problems

Contrary to sociological expections, the *Playboy* centerfold's breasts are rarely found in nature. Most likely, they've benefited from silicone implants, heavy makeup, and airbrushing. Yet many women think there's something wrong with their own breasts because they don't resemble this unrealistic ideal.

That also goes for the various glands and fat tissue that make up the breast. Some women find it hard to distinguish between the various irregularities that normally appear in the breast as part of the mammary and lymphatic systems and those that need immediate attention.

The main purpose of a woman's breasts is producing milk. The milk glands are located throughout the breast tissue, but all of them meet in the nipple. The majority of breast tissue is fat, and behind the fat lies muscle.

It is important for every woman to recognize what the typical irregularities in her breasts are, both during her menstrual periods and between them, since the breast itself changes according to what stage of her cycle she's in. After menopause, the breast shrinks due to a loss of fat. Even in menopause, it's important to recognize the changes in your breasts, even though the changes are no longer as frequent.

I consider any change that occurs in the breast to be an abnormal mass or lump. I use these words interchangeably, though it may sometimes lead to confusion. If you feel a mass in your breast of any kind—whether it's a new growth or a smaller mass that has recently begun to grow—you should see your doctor. If it's a hard, small mass that has recently appeared, it may be a tumor. However, if the growth is spongy and you feel more than one mass, then you may have fibrocystic disease. The cysts may appear with some regularity and are usually painful to the touch.

Cysts are bits of tissue that have filled with fluid. They are usually soft and spongy to the touch and move around under the skin when you palpate them. They may occur singly or in clusters. Women who drink a lot of coffee and/or caffeinated soda are more likely to have fibrocystic disease than women who don't.

Fibrocystic disease tends to be more common in women aged 40 and over. As your body prepares for menstruation, there is a buildup of fluid in the body, particularly in the breasts. After menstruation ends, the excess fluid is usually excreted and absorbed into the body. In older women, it's sometimes difficult for the fluid to be reabsorbed into the lymphatic system, and some of the excess fluid may remain in the breast tissue, where it becomes trapped and forms cysts.

If the mass feels firm, has a well-defined shape, and is mobile underneath the skin, you probably have a fibroadenoma, which is a benign tumor. A fibroadenoma contains both fibrous and glandular tissue, which causes it to be rubbery in texture.

If you feel a mass in your breast that might be a cyst or a fibroadenoma, and you have PMS or are currently menstruating, you may decide to wait until you've finished your period to call your doctor, since many cysts become swollen and painful during menstruation. If the pain and size of the cysts recede after your period, the cyst is probably harmless.

Treatment

If you're concerned about a mass in your breast and you call your doctor, he will use one or more of several diagnostic tools to determine what the mass is.

If he suspects the mass is a cyst, he will use a needle to drain the fluid from the cyst, causing the cyst to fade away. If you have a family history of breast cancer, the fluid will probably be analyzed to see if it contains cancerous cells.

If the mass is thought to be a fibroadenoma, your physician will perform a biopsy to make a positive diagnosis, and then, based on the results, may recommend that the tumor be removed.

The fibroadenomatous tumor doesn't always need to be removed, however. Sometimes it can be left intact if it causes no pain. It should be checked every so often, however, to make sure it does not become malignant.

For fibroadenomas, there is no specific preventive technique you can use. Your physician may advise you to take hormonal treatment to correct a hormonal imbalance, which is thought to be the cause of fibroadenomas.

To improve your chances of preventing a recurrence of fibrocystic disease, your doctor may recommend you cut down or eliminate your caffeine intake. Taking extra vitamin E has also been found to be helpful.

To treat both fibrocystic disease and fibroadenomas, if you decide against having the masses surgically removed, aspirin will help relieve the pain when the cysts make your breasts feel swollen and tender. Also, a bra with firm support will also help reduce the pain.

See also "Changes in the Contour of the Breast with Dimpled or Pitted Skin" above.

NIPPLE, RETRACTION OF

Description and Possible Medical Problems

A health columnist at a popular women's magazine has said that two of the most commonly asked questions from readers are (1) Why do I have hairs growing around my nipples? and (2) What can I do about my inverted nipples?

Although she could answer the same two questions in her column every month, making her readers happy, she limits the appearance of each question to once a year. Her answers: (1) They're perfectly normal—pull them out with tweezers and (2) They're perfectly normal—ignore them.

Inverted or retracted nipples are perfectly normal if you've had them since puberty. Only if the inverted nipples have developed recently could they be a sign of trouble—that is, cancer.

Treatment

If your nipples have recently turned inward, see your doctor right away. Any change in the skin of the nipple—whether a color change or an inversion—could be a sign of cancer. She will do a routine breast exam and a mammogram if she suspects you have a tumor.

Otherwise, if you've had them all your life, you have nothing to worry about.

See also "Changes in the Contour of the Breast with Dimpled or Pitted Skin" above.

PAIN IN BREAST

Description and Possible Medical Problems

If you have a sore area in your breast that may or may not be characterized by a bruise marking the spot, you may have experienced a blow to the breast or bumped into something. Some women bruise so easily that they might not even be aware they've undergone a trauma to one of their breasts. The affected breast may also be swollen.

Treatment

If you think you've injured your breast, apply an ice pack to the sore spot several times a day. Aspirin, Tylenol, or Advil will also help relieve the tenderness.

If the pain has not subsided after a few days, see your doctor.

See also "Lump in Breast After Minor Injury" above.

RASH UNDER BREAST

Description and Possible Medical Problems

Common skin problems that can occur elsewhere on the body can also appear the breasts. Acne, an infection of the hair follicles called folliculitis, and even a close cousin of athlete's foot, a fungal infection that appears mostly between your toes, can also show up in the skin under your breasts. Your skin will probably itch and be red and moist in the affected areas.

A rash under the breasts can be common in women who have large breasts or are obese, but it can also occur in thin, small-breasted women as well as in diabetics. The rash is caused by a fungus called dermatophytes, which, like other breeds of fungus, is found all over your body. But it's in warm, moist areas that it especially thrives; that's why a rash under the breasts is especially common in the summertime.

Treatment

A fungus-based rash under your breasts is easy to treat, but without constant attention the rash will have a tendency to reappear.

To treat the rash, buy an over-the-counter antifungal ointment like Zeabsorb, or even cornstarch, to use until the rash disappears. If the rash doesn't respond to this preparation, see your doctor, who may prescribe a prescription antifungal drug such as Lotrimin or Mycelex cream applied two or three times a day for at least two weeks. If the area is also itchy, your doctor may prescribe a cortisone preparation such as Lotrisone cream two or three times a day for two weeks.

Once the rash has been cleared up with the medication, it's important to pay special attention to the area so that it does not recur. To prevent future outbreaks, wash the rash-prone area with soap and water at least once a day. Dry well. Then apply talc or baby powder to help keep the area dry as you go about your day.

SORE ON BREAST

Description and Possible Medical Problems

If you are currently breast-feeding or have recently stopped nursing a child, and you have what appears to be a reddened, swollen, localized patch on your breast, you probably have mastitis, an infection of the breast. Mastitis occurs when bacteria enter through a crack in the nipple and enter the fatty tissue in the breast. Cracked nipples are common in women who are nursing.

Because there are many women in their 40s who are having children and who are choosing to breast-feed, they are more prone to developing mastitis because aging can lower the effectiveness of their immune systems slightly.

The bacteria start an infection, which will grow into an abscess if left untreated. If your breast becomes infected, one small area will redden and become painful. The infection may be accompanied by fever and swelling in the armpit on the same side as the infected breast.

If a breast infection appears in a woman who is not nursing, she should see her physician immediately, as it might actually be a sign of underlying cancer. And if you get a skin infection for which the cause is not immediately clear, you should see your doctor and ask her to check for diabetes, since diabetics are especially prone to contracting both bacterial and fungal skin infections. In fact, I once saw a woman with a breast infection whose mastitis turned out to be a symptom of diabetes.

Treatment

If you are breast-feeding and you think you have an infection, see your doctor. He will give you a prescription for an oral antibiotic such as a penicillin derivative or erythromycin that should clear up the infection in one to two weeks. You can continue to nurse your baby, since the antibiotic won't affect your milk. Aspirin will help relieve the pain and tenderness. You should, however, refrain from nursing your baby with the infected breast until it heals.

It's a good idea to keep your nipples clean and dry between feedings. You might want to apply a soothing ointment to your nipples to keep them from drying out and cracking—and thus encouraging another infection.

If an abscess forms in your breasts, even after taking the antibiotic, your doctor will want to drain it of fluid. If one of your breasts becomes infected and you aren't currently breast-feeding—or haven't for some time, if ever—see your doctor immediately. A breast infection in a non-nursing woman is rare—except when breast cancer is present.

Chapter 13

ABDOMEN AND DIGESTIVE SYSTEM

BODY SIGNAL ALERT

Call your doctor immediately if you experience any of the following symptoms:

SYMPTOM	POSSIBLE MEDICAL CONDITION
You have bloody diarrhea	*Bacterial or viral infection, diverticulosis, internal bleeding*
You suddenly have diarrhea	*Food poisoning, viral infection*
You have had diarrhea for a week or longer	*Malabsorption of food, medication, dietary changes, lactose or gluten intolerance*
You notice that your abdomen has suddenly increased in size	*Tumor*
You are vomiting blood or a substance that resembles coffee grounds	*Bleeding ulcer*
You have a severe pain in your abdomen	*Gallbladder disease, ulcer, diverticulitis, appendicitis*
You notice a lump in your abdomen	*Enlarged spleen or liver, fibroid mass, tumor, distended bladder*
You feel a pain in your left lower belly	*Diverticulitis, appendicitis, tumor, gynecological problem*
You have a fever, and your bowel habits have changed. You notice a change in your bowel habits with weight loss and a change in appetite	*Cancer*

HOW THE DIGESTIVE SYSTEM AGES

Though there are hundreds of body parts that are involved in the digestive process, in this chapter I'm going to focus on the digestive system, which includes the esophagus, stomach, intestines, liver, and pancreas. If you're having a problem with chewing, see Chapter 7, "Mouth, Teeth, and Gums." Here, I'll cover the area from below the diaphragm, at midchest level, down to the hips.

The human digestive system is an extraordinary machine, as it continually paves the way for nutrients to enter our bodies over the course of a lifetime. The intestine especially stands the test of time since it's constantly exposed to a wide variety of foods, toxins, and chemicals and is able to process them, usually without any problem. Surprisingly enough, as you become older, some of the digestive problems that may have plagued you in your 20s and 30s may actually disappear, irritable bowel syndrome and certain types of colitis among them. Ulcers, however, will tend to trouble a person throughout life, though the specific causes can vary from one year to the next.

The three most common minor digestive complaints of midlife adults are heartburn, constipation, and hemorrhoids. However, for most of us, they remain only minor disturbances. In fact, as a general rule, except for a slight decrease in the time it takes the digestive system to absorb and process food, age has very little effect on the digestive tract at all. I've seen many people in their 90s who have never had any problems with their bowels.

On the other hand, I am always amazed at how many of my patients are worried that they'll get bowel cancer. I tell them that they probably have nothing to worry about, since bowel cancer is relatively rare until after the age of 50. And, as with many forms of cancer, unless you have a family member who has had the condition, you might just as well relax.

A routine yearly exam will include a physical examination as well as your personal health history. Some of the tests your physician may run include a blood test, a sigmoidoscopy, a colonoscopy, and a stool occult blood card. During this exam, many kinds of undetected cancers—or precancerous masses in the form of benign polyps—can be detected and removed. Colon cancer is the third most common form of cancer in this country, and since early detection is essential to the successful treatment, an annual exam is essential.

If you notice that your digestive system isn't working as smoothly as it usually does, you should ask yourself the following questions and relay the answers to your doctor. This will help you to articulate your Body Signals and your doctor to make an accurate diagnosis and treatment.

1. How long have I had the discomfort? Hours, days, weeks, years?

2. How would I describe the pain very specifically? Does it move or rumble? Is it sharp or dull?

3. If my stomach hurts, exactly where do I feel the pain the most? Point to the area.

4. Does the pain prevent me from sleeping or wake me up in the middle of the night?

5. Do I have other symptoms, such as fever, diarrhea, or constipation?

6. Have I noticed that a particular food makes the pain better or worse?

7. Do I have friends or family members with complaints that are similar to mine?

8. Have I recently changed my diet or medications?

9. Have I increased the time I spent traveling? Have I recently been to an area I haven't visited before?

10. Do I have a family history of gastrointestinal disease?

WHERE EXACTLY ARE THESE INTERNAL ORGANS, ANYWAY?

I usually tell my patients to divide the abdomen into four quadrants, which will help them to describe their symptoms more accurately to the doctor. Using a cross, make a vertical line from the belly button up to below the diaphragm. Cross this line with a horizontal line at the belly button.

On your right side, above the horizontal line, is the upper right quadrant, which includes the liver, gallbladder, and part of the intestines. The upper left quadrant includes part of the large intestine and the spleen. Your stomach lies within the space of both upper quadrants. Your left lower quadrant includes the intestines, and, in a woman, the left ovary. The right lower quadrant contains the lower large intestine and the right ovary. The bladder and the uterus lie within both of the lower quadrants. The kidneys are found in all four quadrants toward the back of the body.

BODY SIGNAL ALERT

ABDOMEN, INCREASE IN SIZE OF

Description and Possible Medical Problems

Of course, we know that the most common reason your abdomen would suddenly increase in girth over the course of several months is either weight gain or, if you're a woman, pregnancy.

However, there are a number of serious medical problems that can cause the abdomen to increase in size. Sometimes the amount of water in the abdominal cavity can build up due to cancer or to failure of the heart, liver, or kidneys. This condition is called ascites. Another reason for the increase in girth could be a bowel obstruction or a tumor in the digestive or gynecological tract. You may also be jaundiced, vomiting, or constipated, or you may have experienced a recent loss in weight.

Treatment

If you notice that the size of your abdomen has increased over the course of several months and your dietary or exercise habits haven't changed, you should see your doctor. If he suspects you have ascites, you will most likely be hospitalized in order to undergo a series of lab tests to analyze the fluid in your abdomen. If your doctor believes you have a tumor in your abdomen, he will use a CAT scan, a sonogram, and perhaps a colonoscopy to determine its size and whether it is benign or malignant.

ABDOMEN, LUMPS OR MASSES IN

Description and Possible Medical Problems

Anytime you notice a lump or other mass in your abdomen that wasn't there before, you should consult your doctor.

First, ask yourself these questions:

1. Does the mass disappear with a bowel movement? Does it appear after a meal?

2. When I change position, does the mass change as well?

3. Have I noticed any change in my urination habits lately?

4. Is the mass painful?

A new lump or mass in the abdomen could actually be an enlarged internal organ. If it appears under your left rib cage and feels smooth, it may be an enlargement of your spleen. If you notice a painful mass that is either smooth or bumpy under your right rib cage, your liver may be enlarged.

The most common cause of a lump or mass that appears suddenly, however, is a stool that stays in the bowel longer than usual due to constipation; it will feel like a sausagelike mass. You'll also be gassy. In older men who have prostate problems, the bladder can enlarge and become distended if an enlarged prostate makes it difficult to urinate.

In women, a mass that appears below the navel may be fibroid masses in the uterus. In some cases, a mass can actually be a harmless lipoma, or mass of fat, in the belly that might be present for years.

Treatment

If you detect a mass in your intestine, either by feeling it physically or by noticing that your abdomen is distended, if the mass does not go away after a bowel movement or if it has been present for more than a few days, you should see your doctor. He will conduct a physical exam and health history to help him determine the cause. Your descriptions of other Body Signals, whether a recent fever or cold or prostate problems, will help him make the diagnosis and determine treatment.

BELCHING AFTER A MEAL

Description and Possible Medical Problems

If you've spent any amount of time around kids, you've probably noticed that children, especially young boys, take great pleasure in learning how to belch and then showing others what they've accomplished. Though our society frowns on public belching, whether it comes from someone who's 9 years old or 90, there are societies that consider a belch to be a sign of appreciation of a good meal.

However, it could also be caused by swallowing too much air while you're eating, which happens in people who eat fast and/or talk while they're eating.

Treatment

When belching occurs during and after eating with no other symptoms, it's a totally harmless activity. If you belch a lot and it bothers you and the people around you, you may want to try to eat less food at one sitting. Some people also find that if they eat more slowly or try to keep their conversation to a minimum, their problem with belching will disappear.

BELCHING, FREQUENT, NOT NECESSARILY AT MEALS

Description and Possible Medical Problems

I believe it would be close to impossible to eat a meal without belching at least once, even if no one else hears you.

If, however, you notice that you're belching a lot during the day, there are several surprising reasons. The most common cause is due to constantly chewing gum, especially if the gum contains sorbitol or xylitol as a sweetener; these are sugar-free products that can cause gas and stomach pains. Frequent belching may also be caused by lying down after a meal or by eating gassy foods, such as raw vegetables or beans and legumes.

Treatment

For most people, eliminating the culprit—whether it's sugar-free gum or the crudité platter for lunch—will help take care of the problem. If, however, you don't want to change your diet, you can take an antigas formula that contains the ingredient simethicone, such as Mylanta or Gas Plus, after each meal.

BELCHING WITH HEARTBURN, AN ACID TASTE IN THE MOUTH, AND A SORE THROAT

Description and Possible Medical Problems

Heartburn is probably the most common digestive complaint among people in their 40s and 50s—witness the sizable industry that offers pills and liquids in all shapes, sizes, and colors that profess to treat the condition. Most often, heartburn is a sign of stress and/or culinary overindulgence. To help determine the cause of your heartburn, ask yourself the following questions:

1. Do I have heartburn after every meal?

2. Do I sometimes find it difficult to sleep?

3. Does the pain occur in the middle of my abdomen between the upper left and right quadrants?

4. Do I frequently take over-the-counter heartburn remedies?

5. Is the heartburn painful?

Fortunately, heartburn is rarely a sign of a serious underlying illness. If you have persistent heartburn with a bad taste in your mouth and bad breath, then you may have a hiatal hernia, a physiological condition in which the valve between the esophagus and the stomach is not working right. With a faulty valve, the stomach breaches the area directly below the diaphragm and actually rises up into the chest area. This allows stomach acids to enter the esophagus and the mouth. The high acid content of the stomach juices can irritate the esophagus, and this is known as heartburn.

If you have a hiatal hernia, it's probably a by-product of too many years of eating rich food and leading a sedentary lifestyle. The obesity that usually results can also cause the stomach to push up into the esophagus. In addition, eating heavy meals just before you lie down to go to sleep can cause the valve to malfunction. And alcohol, cigarettes, spicy foods, and antibiotics can aggravate heartburn even more. When belching occurs in combination with sweating and a general malaise, it can be a sign of heart disease.

Treatment

If you have heartburn, your physician will consider your past history and conduct a physical exam. He may choose to order an upper GI test, consisting of X rays of the upper digestive system—the esophagus, stomach, and duodenum—which will help determine the cause of your heartburn.

If you have a hiatal hernia, you will need to lose weight, eat smaller meals, and cut down on spicy foods. If you smoke, you should stop. If your heartburn is preventing you from sleeping at night, you should take a couple of phone books and put them under the head of your bed. This will raise the level of your head, which will make it difficult for the stomach acid to back up into the esophagus, since it would have to work against gravity. Eating dinner several hours before you go to sleep and eating your largest meal of the day at lunch can also be helpful. Some people with a hiatal hernia find that a walk after dinner can help prevent heartburn later on that night.

If these methods don't work, try taking an over-the-counter antacid such as Maalox or Mylanta after each meal. You might also want to take them before you go to sleep. And if these don't work, your doctor might give you a medication that will speed up the rate at which your stomach empties, making it less likely to push up past the esophagal valve. Pepcid, Tagamet, and Propulsid are some of the medications I recommend in the short term. Again, however, the most important part of the treatment for hiatal hernia—and heartburn—is losing weight, quitting smoking, and eliminating the foods that make your heartburn worse.

BLOATING AND GAS

Description and Possible Medical Problems

The issue of abdominal gas and flatulence is a topic of humor from elementary school on. In people who are under age 50, gas is rarely a serious problem. However, if you're over 50 and become constantly bloated and gassy for the first time in your life, you should see your doctor.

Part of the problem is that in our society the expulsion of gas, whether through belching or flatulence, is not acceptable. However, with the popularity of high-fiber diets and an increased intake of beans, raw fruits, and vegetables, many of us are considerably more gassy than we were just a few years ago.

If you just have gas, the change in your diet is probably responsible. If, however, you have abdominal cramps in addition to the gas, you may actually have lactose intolerance. In addition, some women find that they become gassy and bloated right before their periods. Chewing gum and smoking cigarettes can also be the cause, since you're swallowing more air, which then travels to your intestine. You should also be aware that many sugar-free candies and gums use a sorbitol- or xylitol-based sugar substitute, which can cause severe bloating and gas pains, especially if you eat or chew more than three pieces a day.

Treatment

If you're bloated and gassy, there are several things you can try.

Getting more exercise and using Mylanta or another over-the-counter antacid product that contains simethicone several times a day may be helpful. Quitting smoking and cutting down on the chewing gum, especially sugar-free gum, and other sugar-free candies that contain sorbitol or xylitol should also help to eliminate gas.

If you're over 50, however, and suddenly become gassy, in addition to losing weight, becoming nauseous, or even vomiting, it's possible you have an obstruction in your intestine. This obstruction can be due to a stool impaction, cancer, or a condition in which the intestinal walls adhere to each other; this is usually a result of intestinal surgery that was performed a number of years ago. If this is the case, you need to see your doctor; the treatment may include surgery.

BOWEL MOVEMENT WITH BLOOD

Description and Possible Medical Problems

The topic of hemorrhoids is not a pleasant one. However, they seem to make their way onto the nightly news programs via commercials for Preparation H and other hemorrhoid treatments with great regularity.

The truth is that hemorrhoids are pretty common among Americans aged 40 and up. If you have hemorrhoids, you'll notice that the stool itself is well formed and that the blood usually appears around the stool.

Hemorrhoids are the distended veins that appear on the edge of the rectum. If they appear outside the anus, they are external hemorrhoids; if they remain inside the rectum, they are internal hemorrhoids. Many people with hemorrhoids have a combination of the two. In young women, hemorrhoids are most often due to pregnancy and childbirth. And in any age group, they can be caused by eating a diet that's low in fiber or by having hard stools. Many people get hemorrhoids from sitting on the john for long periods of time while reading. A general lack of exercise—which decreases the frequency of bowel movements as well as making the stool harder—and spending a lot of time sitting, which creates more pressure on the rectal veins, also increases the risk of hemorrhoids.

Treatment

The main course of treatment for hemorrhoids is getting off your butt—both literally and figuratively. You should start exercising, and don't sit for more than an hour at a time if you can help it. You should also eat a diet that is high in digestible fiber such as cereals and bran but low in nondigestible fiber such as nuts and popcorn. You can also use a stool softener such as Colace two or three times a day, especially if the stool is hard, and use premoistened Tucks pads after a bowel movement to help soothe the area. Preparation H or Anusol in cream form or suppositories will help shrink the hemorrhoids. Your doctor may also give you a prescription for a suppository containing cortisone, which will help reduce the swelling.

If your hemorrhoids tend to recur, your doctor may want to remove them surgically with a laser or by rubber banding them, a procedure in which a band is placed around the hemorrhoid, cutting off its blood supply so that it falls off. Or he may opt for traditional surgery.

THE TRUTH ABOUT COLON CANCER

Even though many midlife adults worry about getting colon cancer, the truth is that it is actually a treatable disease if it's discovered early. However, because it is so serious, you should be attuned to the signs of colon cancer and know the risks.

First of all, if you or someone in your family has a history of colon disease—not necessarily cancer, but perhaps colitis or polyps—or if you are over 50 and have chronic constipation, you should be monitored regularly by your doctor.

Besides chronic constipation, some of the other signs of colon cancer include a slow change in bowel habits that occurs over the course of several weeks or months. Diarrhea might also be present, as well as bloating, gas, weight loss, a change in appetite, anemia, and depression. These, however, are what I call "soft" signals; people might think they are appearing due to a change in lifestyle or another health problem. When they do seek help and recognize that it may be colon cancer, they will do so when their intestines become blocked by the tumor or they experience a serious blood loss from a tumor that begins to bleed.

Researchers have been studying the possible causes of colon cancer for years; in most cases, colon cancer occurs in the lower part of the intestine. Some say it is due to genetics, while others blame the typical sedentary American lifestyle and high-fat, low-fiber diet. However, they have found that the risk of colon cancer increases in families that have a history of intestinal polyps. If you are at risk for colon cancer and have shown signs of a change in appetite, weight loss, depression, or chronic diarrhea, your doctor will conduct one or more of the following common tests:

• *A complete history and physical exam.* This will help your doctor discover a possible genetic link or a recent change in your bowel habits.

• *Lab tests.* These may include a blood test, a liver test, and a hemocult test, which is a simple at-home test to help you check for hidden blood in the stool, which is often the first sign of cancer.

• *A digital exam.* Your doctor will use a gloved finger to check

for growths in your rectum, since many cancers are within
the reach of the finger.

• *An anuscope.* This is a device used to check the lower part of
the rectum

• *A sigmoidoscope.* This is a small, flexible tube your doctor can
use to look into the lower part of the large intestine.

• *A colonoscope.* This is similar to a sigmoidoscope, but it is
longer to enable your doctor to examine the entire large
intestine. If your doctor wants to perform a colonoscopy, you
will need to be mildly sedated.

• *A barium enema.* This is an X-ray exam that is usually performed on an outpatient basis. A barium enema is usually
used when your doctor suspects you have diverticular disease
or polyps or a mechanical problem with the intestine.

• *An upper GI series.* This is another kind of X-ray exam in
which you swallow barium on an empty stomach to allow
your doctor to view your intestine more closely.

After the diagnosis of colon cancer is confirmed by some or all
of these tests, along with, possibly, a CAT scan to see if the cancer has spread, the usual treatment is surgical removal of the
tumor, although chemotherapy and radiation may also be used.
The bowel will also need to be reattached; the procedure involves
a hospitalization period of about two weeks.

Before the tumor is removed, however, your doctor will administer a blood test called the CEA antigen test, which will be used
not as a screening tool but as a benchmark for future CEA tests
after the tumor has been removed to check that the cancer has
not reappeared.

If the tumor was located in the lower part of the intestine,
close to the rectum, reattachment of the bowel may not be possible. In this case, a colostomy bag will be necessary. This does not
carry the stigma that it once did, even a few years ago. People
who wear a colostomy bag can lead active, productive lives without anyone else knowing they have had a colostomy, since the
new appliances have no leakage and no smell.

CONSTIPATION, ACUTE

Description and Possible Medical Problems

Like a crick in the neck or a headache that won't go away no matter how many aspirins you take, if you become constipated, it tends to affect everything you do. Constipation that appears all of a sudden or over the course of several days is usually due to a recent change in your lifestyle.

The most common cause of acute constipation is a sudden change in your diet, such as going on a strict weight-loss plan, or sudden inactivity, which often occurs after an injury or accident for which your doctor prescribes bed rest. Pain medication such as codeine can also cause constipation. I've seen weekend athletes who get hit in the chest playing basketball, fracture a rib or two, and take Tylenol with codeine for the pain. The combination of sudden inactivity and medication results in a severe case of constipation.

Treatment

If you become constipated and suspect that it's due to a sudden change in your lifestyle, you can try one of the many laxative preparations that are on the market, such as Ex-Lax, taken several times a day, until your constipation clears up.

This should help relieve your constipation. If, however, your lifestyle change is going to continue, whether it's enforced bed rest, a change in diet, or continuation of a medication, you should ask your doctor for advice.

CONSTIPATION ALTERNATING WITH DIARRHEA

Description and Possible Medical Problems

Although they are polar opposites, it's not uncommon to have diarrhea that's followed by constipation and returns to diarrhea again a few days later. In fact, I see this back-and-forth syndrome occur with some frequency in men and women in their 40s. Besides diarrhea and constipation, you may also have abdominal cramping, bloating, and flatulence.

This condition is generally known as irritable bowel syndrome, or functional colitis.

If you think you have irritable bowel syndrome, you shouldn't worry that there's something wrong with your digestive system, because most often stress and particular foods such as dairy products and those that are high in fat are the culprit, especially if you have a history of abdominal problems that dates from your late teens and early 20s.

Generally, irritable bowel syndrome is an annoying condition that can be treated. If, however, you notice a sudden loss of weight or your health in general begins to deteriorate, you should see your doctor.

Treatment

If you think you have irritable bowel syndrome, your doctor will want to make a positive diagnosis with a battery of tests, which may include a GI series, a barium enema, and, in some cases, a colonoscopy to rule out a possible lesion on or polyp of the bowel. If you do have irritable bowel syndrome, you should know that your condition will improve as time goes on. The treatment for irritable bowel syndrome will start with you keeping a record of everything you eat in order to identify any foods that might be causing the problem, such as dairy products and high-fat foods—especially chocolate—and caffeine. You can experiment by limiting these foods to see if your irritable bowel syndrome clears up. Next, your doctor will recommend that you increase your intake of fiber with a product such as Metamucil or Fibercon. This increase in fiber will help regulate the water content of the stool. If the stool is loose, the increase in fiber will help make it more solid, and if your bowel is acting slowly and sluggishly, it will help regulate the transit time of your bowel movements. The amount needed will vary from one person to the next, but a good start is to take one to two tablespoons of Metamucil four times a day—at breakfast, lunch, and dinner and an hour before going to sleep at night. Exercise is also very effective, as it will help reduce your stress and regulate the bowel.

If you have diarrhea, I don't suggest you treat it with an antidiarrheal medication, since this will cause you to become constipated. Some of my patients have used Kaopectate alternating with Metamucil, which I feel is unhealthy since your intestine never really has a chance to work on its own and creates a chronic condition of constipation alternating with diarrhea.

There are certain prescription medications you can take for irritable bowel syndrome. These include Donnatal, Levsin, and Levsinex in pill or liquid form. Levsin is also available in a sublingual pill that's placed under the tongue to provide you with immediate relief. For most people, increasing the amount of high-fiber foods they eat as well as the amount of exercise they get, while reducing stress, can be very helpful.

CONSTIPATION, CHRONIC

Description and Possible Medical Problems

I don't know of anyone who hasn't been constipated at some point in his or her life. The problem, however, is that we all have a different definition of what constipation is. Some people say they have a bowel movement once or twice a day and think that's typical, while others think a bowel movement once or twice a week is perfectly normal. Although as a rule we don't make an issue of talking about bowel movements, on the other hand, we get bombarded by laxative manufacturers who advertise that regularity is one of the God-given rights of every American, regardless of age. What is considered normal? I tend to use the patient's own standards to determine what is normal.

The only normal thing that we all have in common is that as we get older the mobility of the bowel slows down, resulting in less frequent bowel movements. And the lack of fiber in the diet that is common among many older Americans will decrease the motility even more.

In most cases, the cause of constipation is easily identified, whether it's a long car trip, a change in diet, or new medication. If you are constipated, you should ask yourself a few basic questions and relay your answers to your doctor.

1. What do I consider to be a normal bowel movement?

2. Have I noticed a change in my bowel movements over the past few weeks or months?

3. Have I lost or gained weight recently?

4. Has my diet changed in any way?

5. Have I either added or dropped a medication lately?

6. Have I recently cut down on the amount of exercise I get?

7. Have I been using over-the-counter laxatives or antidiarrheal medications lately?

8. Is my stool hard and pelletlike?

9. Has my appetite changed? Have I been nauseous or vomiting lately?

10. Do I have constipation that alternates with diarrhea?

Treatment

If you are constipated only once in a while, you probably have nothing to worry about. If you are under 50 and you have had no lifestyle changes, as reflected in your answers to the questions above, you should simply try to increase the amount of exercise you get, the amount of fiber in your diet, and the amount of water you drink. I've found exercise to be the best cure for constipation. If you use laxatives, you should use them for only a few days. If you find that your constipation worsens without laxatives and you use them regularly, you should see your doctor, who will help wean you from them.

There are a number of preparations that can help ease the discomfort of constipation. In the laxative category, there are bulk agents such as Metamucil. They help ease constipation and can also help regulate a sluggish bowel. I suggest one tablespoon of Metamucil in eight ounces of water three times a day. A high-fiber cereal such as All Bran can also do the trick. Some people prefer to mix plain bran flakes into a glass of water in the morning. If you find that powders like Metamucil are difficult to swallow, you can try a product in pill form such as FiberCon, which can be taken four times a day. Bran muffins are not a good way to increase your fiber intake, as they are actually low in fiber and high in fat.

A stool softener such as Colace will help if the stool is very hard and especially if you also have hemorrhoids. Stool softeners are not laxatives, however, so once the stool has softened, you should stop taking the medication.

Preparations such as milk of magnesia and Dulcolax work by irritating the lower rectum so that the stool can be evacuated; they come in suppository form or in a pill or liquid. A suppository will provide quick relief, while one tablespoon of milk of magnesia taken at night before sleep should ensure a bowel movement in the morning. They can, however, cause permanent damage if they're used for many years.

Glycerine suppositories provide immediate relief when the stool is stuck at the bottom of the rectum and are safe when used occasionally. In fact, glycerine suppositories are commonly used in young children since they don't irritate the lining of the bowel.

Enemas should be used only on rare occasions, for example, for cleaning out the bowel for a test of the large intestine or following major surgery. I remember one patient who fractured his leg in a car accident. During his hospital stay, he refused the bedpan and eventually needed an enema. For most people, however, I do not believe in using enemas as a way to clean out the bowel, since with routine use, they can eventually destroy the rectal reflex that normally initiates evacuation of the bowel.

BODY SIGNAL ALERT

DIARRHEA, ACUTE AND BLOODY

Description and Possible Medical Problems

If you have diarrhea and notice that it has become bloody, you should see your doctor right away, especially if you have a fever and feel weak along with a general malaise.

Bloody diarrhea can be a sign of a viral or bacterial infection that is becoming more severe. It can also occur if you have a long history of ulcer disease or as the first indication of a bleeding ulcer. In this case, you will probably have a stool that is black and tarry or resembles the consistency of putty. If blood appears on the surface of the stool, it is probably due to hemorrhoids.

If bloody diarrhea occurs in a person in his 40s or 50s, it's possible that a condition known as diverticulitis, a sudden infection in the lower left-hand part of the intestine, may be the cause. Diverticulitis appears when the small pockets in the large intestine—called diverticula—become inflamed because small particles of food, especially seeds, get caught in them, resulting in inflammation and infection. Diverticulitis occurs most often among sedentary people who eat a high-fat, low-fiber diet. If you have diverticulitis, you may also have a fever. If you have a history of irritable bowel syndrome or colitis, you're more likely to develop diverticulitis. People with irritable bowel syndrome become used to living with an unpredictable bowel, but if diverticulitis develops, you will find that the pain is worse than usual and occurs over the entire abdomen.

Treatment

If you have bloody diarrhea, the doctor will do a physical exam, a blood test, and a digital rectal exam to help determine the cause. He may also need to use a sigmoidoscope in order to examine the intestine visually.

Sometimes, however, bloody diarrhea can be caused by bacteria, a virus, or a parasite, frequently resulting from foreign travel and strange food and water. If your doctor suspects that this is the case, he will probably run a series of blood tests as well as a stool test. If the bloody diarrhea is caused by a viral infection, your doctor will advise you to drink plenty of fluids; I advise soup, with additional salt to replace the potassium lost in diarrhea, or Gatorade. For a bacterial infection, he will prescribe antibiotics.

If you have a bleeding ulcer, see "Pain in Upper Midabdomen" below.

If you have diverticulitis, see "Pain in Lower Left Quadrant, with Fever and Change in Bowels" below.

Special Mention for the Elderly

In elderly people, if the blood supply to the bowel is suddenly reduced or even cut off completely, a condition known as ischemic colitis can develop. In this case, the stool will be foul, smelly, and maroon in color. An elderly person with ischemic colitis will also have a fever, and she may quickly go into a state of shock. However, diarrhea can also be caused by a course of antibiotic therapy that has lasted for several weeks, usually after a period of hospitalization, since it can be spread quite easily in hospital wards and nursing homes. This type of diarrhea is caused by the *C. difficile* bacterium, and requires another course of specialized antibiotic therapy.

For this reason, if the bowel habits of an elderly person suddenly change, it's essential that she see her doctor immediately.

See also "Diarrhea, Acute, Nonbloody" below.

BODY SIGNAL ALERT

DIARRHEA, ACUTE, NONBLOODY

Description and Possible Medical Problems

When you were a kid and you had diarrhea, you'd probably do anything else but admit to it. And now that you're an adult, you're probably the same way. Some people act as though they're ashamed when they have diarrhea.

Diarrhea is a sudden change in your usual pattern of elimination that usually results in more than three soft bowel movements a day. You may also have a sense of urgency and discomfort in your bowel.

Food poisoning is the most common cause of diarrhea that appears suddenly. If you have food poisoning, you will also probably be vomiting and have fever and cramps. Food poisoning results when staphylococcus bacteria in contaminated food—most often dairy products, pastries, or mayonnaise-based foods—form a toxin in the digestive system. The symptoms first appear about two to six hours after eating a contaminated food. Summertime picnics and barbecues are the number one cause of food poisoning; you should always keep salads and other foods covered and on ice, since staphylococcus bacteria can grow very quickly on a picnic table on a hot summer day.

A more severe type of food poisoning occurs when food is tainted with salmonella, a bacteria that is found most often in raw chicken.

A sudden case of diarrhea may also be due to traveling to another area of the country; this is known as traveler's diarrhea and is caused by bacteria in the water supply. Traveler's diarrhea usually occurs 24 to 72 hours after drinking the water, and you may also have fever, vomiting, and pain for up to a week. This form of diarrhea is seen especially in people who travel to Mexico; it is frequently referred to as Montezuma's Revenge.

Another common cause of diarrhea is a virus; the condition called gastroenteritis, an inflammation of the digestive system, is a form of viral diarrhea, and you will have some of the same symptoms as traveler's diarrhea, such as muscle aches, fever, and cough, as well as an upset stomach that lasts for a few days. There is usually no blood in the stools.

Acute diarrhea can also be caused by a change in medication; most often, it's the result of taking too many laxatives. In addition, antibiotics and antacids can cause diarrhea.

If you have diarrhea, ask yourself the following questions and be sure to communicate your answers to your doctor:

1. Do I have a fever?

2. Have I been vomiting?

3. Do I notice any blood in the stool?

4. Have I recently started or stopping taking a medication?

5. Have I changed my diet lately?

6. Have I been spending time in a different location, especially a foreign country?

Treatment

If you come down with a sudden case of diarrhea, you should take Pepto-Bismol, two tablets or tablespoons four times a day, until the diarrhea clears up. In severe cases, your doctor may prescribe an antibiotic called Bactrim, which you'll take in pill form twice a day for three to five days. A newer antibiotic known as Cipro, which is usually taken in 500-milligram doses twice a day for five days, can also be effective.

Viral diarrhea usually responds to over-the-counter measures such as Kaopectate, taken in doses of one or two tablespoons three or four times a day.

Whenever you cook chicken, it is very important to wash the chicken before you cook it. You should also be careful that any utensils or plates that have touched the raw chicken don't touch the cooked chicken; this is how salmonella spreads. You should also wash your hands after cleaning the chicken and make sure you cook it all the way through.

When you're traveling to a foreign country that's known for traveler's diarrhea, you shouldn't drink the water or use ice in drinks unless you are sure it is pure. Also, don't drink or eat from any of the food stands, since there is a high risk of contracting parasites that might strike in your digestive system weeks or months later.

If you've recently begun a new medication and have had no other changes in your lifestyle that I've described, ask your doctor if you can stop taking the medication and request an alternate. If your diarrhea clears up within a day or two, the medication was the cause of your diarrhea.

Special Mention for the Elderly

I once treated an elderly patient whose family always left him a plate of cooked chicken in his refrigerator. One day, his power was out for several hours, which gave the salmonella bacteria on the chicken a great opportunity to multiply. The man didn't eat the chicken until a week later, and he developed acute salmonella poisoning from the tainted chicken and unfortunately died from the attack.

If you regularly provide food—especially chicken—for an elderly relative or friend, make sure that the refrigerator is working properly, that the chicken is cooked all the way through, and that it is thrown out after a few days if it goes uneaten.

DIARRHEA ALTERNATING WITH CONSTIPATION

See "Constipation Alternating with Diarrhea" above.

BODY SIGNAL ALERT

DIARRHEA, CHRONIC, NONBLOODY

Description and Possible Medical Problems

Sometimes diarrhea can be the body's way of ridding itself of a harmful substance, such as the bacteria that cause food poisoning or contaminate water. However, when you have diarrhea that lasts for more than a few days, it's usually due to another reason.

Whenever a patient complains to me about chronic diarrhea, the first thing I look for is a change in his diet. Juice diets or diets that are high in fruit can cause chronic diarrhea when you first start the new regimen. A new medication, especially blood pressure medication, can also cause chronic diarrhea (see "Blood Pressure, Elevated [Hypertension]" in Chapter 18). Obviously, the continuing use of laxatives, stool softeners, and antacids can cause chronic diarrhea, as can new vitamin regimens, especially when they contain yeast.

If you have lost weight during your bout with diarrhea, it's probably because your intestines are not absorbing most of the food you eat; the most common cause of this malabsorption is lactose intolerance. Lactose is found in dairy products such as milk, ice cream, yogurt, and cheese.

A more serious kind of malabsorption is caused by an intolerance to gluten, which is found in all bread products and cereals made with wheat. If you have a gluten intolerance, you probably have a long history of diarrhea and weight loss, in addition to hair loss, mild anemia, and abnormalities in any liver function tests you take.

Treatment

Changing your diet or your medication will often correct chronic diarrhea.

If you think you have lactose intolerance, try eating some ice cream or drinking a large glass of milk. If you begin to have diarrhea an hour or two later, and you also feel pain and bloating in your abdomen, you probably have a lactose intolerance. You should then eliminate dairy products from your diet as much as you can. This, however, can be a problem, since you still need to get some calcium in your diet, especially if you are a woman. Fortunately, you can take calcium supplements, 1000 milligrams a day for premenopausal women and 1500 milligrams for postmenopausal women daily. You can also buy a lactose-free milk such as Lactaid in the supermarket or add Lactaid drops to your milk or take pills whenever you eat or drink foods that contain lactose.

If you have a gluten intolerance, your doctor will take an X ray of your small intestine to show the typical pattern of gluten malabsorption. An endoscope may also be used to take a biopsy to confirm the diagnosis. One of my patients came to me a few years back complaining of chronic weight loss, and we gave him every test in the book and came up empty-handed. Then I ordered an X ray of his small intestine, which immediately showed all the signs of gluten malabsorption. With the help of a dietitian, we changed his diet to avoid all gluten, and he recovered quickly.

If you have an intolerance to gluten, a gluten-free diet is easy to achieve, even though gluten is found in almost all bread products and cereals. You can eat rice cakes and buy gluten-free products at the health food store.

INDIGESTION

See "Belching with Heartburn, an Acid Taste in the Mouth, and a Sore Throat" above.

NAUSEA

See "Vomiting" below.

PAIN IN FLANKS
GOING DOWN TO GENITALIA

See "Pain in One Side of Hip Running to Genitalia" in Chapter 10.

BODY SIGNAL ALERT

PAIN IN LOWER LEFT QUADRANT WITH
FEVER AND CHANGE IN BOWELS

Description and Possible Medical Problems

With many medical problems, we never notice that anything's wrong until it's too late. It can flare up—either a new condition or a familiar one we thought we were all through with—and then it's all we think about. A problem with the intestine called diverticulitis is like that. If you have a fever and pain in your lower left quadrant and find that your bowel movements have changed—resulting in either severe, painful constipation or diarrhea—it's possible that you have this disease.

In order to understand diverticulitis, you should first understand how the intestine works. The intestine is responsible for both the absorption of food and the disposal of the body's metabolic waste. Since the feces can sit in the last part of the intestine for a while before being eliminated, the intestine can absorb a wide variety of toxins from the foods we eat. Our modern high-fat, low-fiber diet is frequently the cause of this disease; because the intestinal muscles don't have to work very hard with this kind of diet, they can become weak. As a result, the intestinal wall in the lower large intestine can also become weak and form small pockets or sacs called diverticula. Diverticula usually cause no problem until they become inflamed or, infected, a condition called diverticulitis. It's believed that seeds or indigestible items such as nuts or popcorn can become stuck in these diverticula and cause an infection. If diverticulitis goes untreated, the diverticula can actually rupture like a bubble on a tire, and the contents of the intestine can spill into the sterile area of the belly, causing a severe infection similar to that caused by a ruptured appendix.

Treatment

If your doctor determines that you have diverticulitis, you will need to be hospitalized. In addition, you will not be able to eat solid food or drink liquids for several days, since you will need to rest the bowel to clear up the condition. You will be given intravenous antibiotics and fluids, and a CAT scan will be done with a modified barium enema. This will serve two purposes. First, it will empty out your intestines, which will allow them to rest. Second, the barium will enable your intestines to show up on an X ray so that your doctor can examine the diverticula and determine if the infection is limited to a few diverticular pockets or has spread to form an infectious abscess. When your fever and pain disappear after about five days, you will be able to drink liquids again, and within a few days you will be able to eat solid food.

In most cases, surgery is not necessary to treat diverticulitis; only when an abscess has formed will surgery be considered. And, contrary to popular opinion, diverticulitis is not a preindication of cancer.

To prevent a recurrence of diverticulitis, you will need to exercise regularly and follow a high-fiber, low-fat diet, since a diet that's high in fat slows the bowel transit time, as does a diet low in fiber, which aggravates the diverticula. The combination of exercise, high fiber, and low fat seems to speed up the bowel transit time and helps to eliminate the problem. You should also avoid eating nuts, seeds, popcorn, and foods with an indigestable hull such as corn.

PAIN IN LOWER MIDABDOMEN WITH CHANGE IN URINATION

Women, see "Pain on Urination, Foul-smelling and Cloudy Urine, Pre- and Postmenopausal" in Chapter 14.

Men, see "Urination, Difficulty in" in Chapter 15.

BODY SIGNAL ALERT

PAIN IN LOWER RIGHT QUADRANT, ACUTE, WITH FEVER

Description and Possible Medical Problems

Here's another geographic biological quiz for you. When you feel a sudden pain in your lower right quadrant, what does it mean? Oh yes, you may also have a fever.

Time's up. Of course, if you ask most mothers about a pain on the lower right belly, she will immediately start to worry about appendicitis, a condition in which the appendix becomes infected either spontaneously or due to a virus. As we age, appendicitis appears less frequently, but still the possibility of contracting it never really goes away.

The most important thing to know about appendicitis is that if you feel a severe pain in the lower right quadrant of your abdomen and it lasts for more than a few minutes, you need to see your doctor right away.

Treatment

The first thing your physician will do is to press down on your lower right quadrant. If you feel a severe pain, you probably have appendicitis. But your doctor may want to make sure with a digital rectal exam or, for in a woman, a gynecological exam as well as a blood test. If all the tests for appendicitis are positive, he will probably schedule immediate surgery to take out the appendix. However, each case is different, and your doctor and surgeon will work together to decide the best course of therapy for you. In most cases, surgery is almost always necessary with a period of hospitalization that lasts about a week.

If your appendix has ruptured, your doctor will use antibiotics to quiet the inflammation, postponing surgery until the risk of infection is lower. If, however, a ruptured appendix does not respond to antibiotic therapy, the surgery will be performed anyway.

PAIN IN UPPER MIDABDOMEN

Description and Possible Medical Problems

One of the common benchmarks of success in corporate America is the news that you have an ulcer. "Ah, welcome to the club!" your colleagues will say, raising their bottles of Mylanta in a toast.

Although the stress and anxiety of the modern world are something that we all accept, the truth is that if you feel a burning pain in the middle of your abdomen just below the rib cage, your first instinct is probably not going to be "I've arrived!" no matter what your position is at the office. An ulcer occurs when the lining of the stomach begins to break down because the stomach acid is eating away at it.

However, sometimes what you think is an ulcer really isn't. You might be experiencing a high output of acid in your stomach or a condition called gastritis, an irritation of the stomach lining that is considered by many physicians to be a precursor of an actual ulcer.

Some people find that their ulcers get worse when the seasons change, as well as during times of stress. Certain foods—especially spicy ones—can also trigger the pain. The pain of an ulcer can wake a person from sleep, which can result in a feverish rush to the refrigerator to quickly eat some food and quell it. And I've seen a few patients who developed ulcers because of their prodigious intake of vitamin C—in excess of 5 grams per day.

A bleeding ulcer can cause vomiting of a substance that resembles coffee grounds as well as a stool that is black, tarry, and puttylike in its consistency. A bleeding ulcer is a major cause of anemia, and it can make an elderly person more prone to falls and passing out because of the low blood count. And in recent years, we've discovered that a strain of bacteria called *H. pylori* can actually be responsible for causing an ulcer.

Ulcers occur most often in men between the ages of 45 and 64, and in women who are 55 and older. Twice as many men as women have ulcers. People who have emphysema, liver disease, coronary disease, or rheumatoid arthritis are more prone to developing an ulcer. Unfortunately, once you have an ulcer and it clears up, you are always prone to developing another.

In people who are over 60, medication is the primary cause of an ulcer. In fact, I frequently receive calls from a family member telling me that an elderly relative is weak and has just vomited blood. This is quite common, since my older patients take more aspirin, Motrin, and Advil than younger people do because of their arthritic pain. Working like stomach acid, these medications can start to break down the stomach lining.

Treatment

If you think you have an ulcer, you should see your doctor, who will conduct a complete health history and physical exam, which may include a digital rectal exam to detect any blood in the stool. He will also ask you a series of questions to find out about your diet and any medications you take, especially aspirin or other antiarthritic medications.

If you are vomiting blood, your doctor will recommend that you head for the emergency room, where a nasogastric tube will be inserted to help confirm the diagnosis of a bleeding ulcer in addition to helping remove the blood clots from the stomach. Intravenous fluids will be administered, and, in the case of extensive blood loss, a transfusion will be done. An endoscopy may also be used to find the source of the bleeding, and a biopsy may be done to check for cancer. If *H. pylori* bacteria are determined to be the cause of your ulcer, your doctor will prescribe a course of an antibiotic such as Flagyl or ampicillin that will last several weeks.

To treat your ulcer or gastritis on a long-term basis, the first thing you should do is to eliminate the food, alcohol, cigarette smoking, or medication that is causing it. If stress is also the culprit, your doctor will tell you how to use biofeedback, exercise, and other relaxation techniques to ease your stress and soothe your stomach.

I also suggest using an antacid such as Mylanta or Maalox to ease the pain of the ulcer. Take a tablespoon of the liquid a half hour after eating and before going to sleep. Your doctor may want to prescribe an antiulcer medication such as Tagamet to be taken in 300-milligram doses four times a day and before going to sleep. Other antiulcer medications called H2 antagonists are available; they include Zantac, which should be taken in 150-milligram doses twice a day, and Pepcid, which should be taken in 20-milligram doses twice a day. You'll probably take these medications at their full dosage for a month and then cut back to once a day as maintenance for several months after that.

There is also a medication called Carafate that is taken in 1-gram doses four times a day in pill or liquid form. This coats the stomach lining and prevents acid from getting through. Carafate is often prescribed for older people who need to take a large amount of antiarthritis medications; taking aspirin or Motrin on a full stomach can also cut down on the ulcer pain.

PAIN IN UPPER RIGHT QUADRANT WITH VOMITING, NAUSEA, AND FEVER

Description and Possible Medical Problems

Like the appendix and the spleen, the gallbladder is one of those organs we've all heard of. But whenever I ask a patient to describe its function and location, I always get a blank stare.

Okay, function first. The gallbladder is a sac that stores bile, a substance secreted by the liver that helps to absorb fat. It is located directly under the liver, and if you feel a pain in your upper right quadrant under your rib cage, it's likely your gallbladder is acting up. You may also feel a pain in your right shoulder.

If your diet is high in fat, you may develop gallstones in your gallbladder, and there are two situations where they can cause problems: one is serious, the other isn't. Here's the less serious one: Whenever you eat a fatty meal, the gallbladder secretes bile. As it secretes the bile, the stones are swept away with the bile, and they can get caught in the channel that leads from the gallbladder to the intestines, causing pain. You may also feel nauseous. This is known as gallbladder colic.

A more serious condition is called cholecystitis, which can appear whether you're eating or not. The benchmark Body Signals are fever, an elevated white blood cell count, nausea, severe pain in the upper right quadrant, and vomiting.

Although gallbladder disease has traditionally been thought of as an illness that occurs in women in their 30s and over who are overweight, it has become a growing problem for anyone who eats a diet that's high in fat. Ironically, gallbladder problems are especially common in people who are overweight and who decide to follow a low-fat diet in order to lose weight. With a low-fat diet, the gallbladder is pretty much at rest. During a binge on high-fat foods, however, the gallbladder will start to contract severely in order to produce the necessary bile, and either the stone that is blocking the channel or the contraction of the gallbladder itself may suddenly cause severe pain.

If you think you have a problem with your gallbladder, your doctor will be able to tell by pushing down on the upper right quadrant underneath the rib cage. If it's painful, you probably have gallbladder disease. It's also likely that you have the condition if you find that you frequently have severe indigestion and bloating after eating a high-fat food, such as French fries, cheese, or a candy bar.

Treatment

If your doctor suspects that you have gallbladder disease, based on a physical exam and your health history, he'll do a sonogram to check for the location and size of the gallstone. If, you are under 50 and have the symptoms of gallbladder colic but not cholecystitis, you'll need to eat a low-fat diet for the time being. That should keep your symptoms in check.

In time, however, you may need to have a laparoscopic cholecystectomy performed. In this procedure, a small incision is made in the abdominal wall and a special camera-directed instrument cuts the gallbladder and removes it through the incision. This procedure will probably entail a hospital stay of no more than two days.

If your doctor determines that you have cholecystitis, you will probably need to have a laparoscopic cholecystectomy right away.

STOOL LACED WITH BLOOD, WELL-FORMED, BROWN

See "Bowel Movement with Blood" in Chapter 13.

STOOL, LOSS OF

Description and Possible Medical Problems

While many people—especially women—worry about becoming incontinent as they get older, some people worry about losing control of their bowels. In some cases, a person's stool might seep constantly. In others, a person might lose control of a bowel movement.

Losing control of a bowel movement is common if you have irritable bowel syndrome or colitis. The overuse of laxatives and stool softeners may also cause the problem.

Treatment

If you are taking laxatives or a stool softener several times a day and find that your stool is constantly leaking, you need to gradually cut down and then cut out your intake while increasing the amount of dietary fiber you eat. You can also take Metamucil or FiberCon three or four times a day.

See also "Constipation Alternating with Diarrhea" above.

Special Mention for the Elderly

Frequently, an impacted stool can lead to a condition known as pseudo-diarrhea in which the stool begins to leak around the impacted area. If a doctor determines that an elderly person has this problem, he will order an X ray of the abdomen to make a positive diagnosis and then administer an enema to clear up the impaction.

BODY SIGNAL ALERT

VOMITING

Description and Possible Medical Problems

In this chapter, there are a lot of symptoms and illnesses that are not suited to polite conversation. Vomiting is one of them. But the fact is that you need to evaluate the symptoms that accompany vomiting in order to know if you should contact your doctor or just rest until you start to feel better.

Though vomiting is most often the result of eating a food that doesn't agree with you, or dizziness or nausea, it may also occur because you're nervous or anxious about, say, an upcoming speech you have to give, or you're facing another big event.

If, however, you continue to vomit and a particular food or dizziness is not the cause, you should see your doctor. When vomiting continues, it could be a sign of gallbladder disease, an ulcer, a gynecological problem, or a bowel obstruction.

If you have been vomiting, ask yourself the following:

1. Is there blood in the vomit?

2. Is the vomit foul-smelling? Does it resemble coffee grounds in its appearance?

3. Do I have a fever?

4. Am I frequently nauseous?

5. Have I been anxious or upset lately?

6. Have I started chemotherapy or a new medication recently?

7. Do I get motion sickness?

Treatment

Most cases of vomiting last for only a day or two. If you are vomiting what looks like coffee grounds, which are actually partially digested blood, you may have a bleeding ulcer and should see your doctor immediately. You may also be sweating and start to go into shock. You or a family member will need to call 911. See "Pain in Upper Midabdomen" above for details about treating a bleeding ulcer.

The medication Compazine in pill form, taken in 10-milligram doses three times a day, is frequently effective in stopping vomiting episodes. Either Compazine or another medication called Reglan will be prescribed for people who are receiving chemotherapy.

If you tend to become nauseous and vomit due to motion sickness, ask your doctor if you can try a scopolamine patch, which is worn behind the ear. The "scope patch" usually prevents nausea and vomiting when it's worn before and during a trip to prevent car- and seasickness. Some of my patients swear by a bracelet that places pressure on their wrist that they say helps prevent motion sickness.

To determine the cause of vomiting accurately, your doctor will need to take a complete health history and perform a physical exam and a series of lab tests if the vomiting lasts for more than 24 hours and there is no obvious cause.

Chapter 14

FOR WOMEN ONLY: REPRODUCTIVE AND UROLOGICAL SYSTEMS

BODY SIGNAL ALERT

Call your doctor immediately if you experience any of the following symptoms:

SYMPTOM	POSSIBLE MEDICAL CONDITION
You are postmenopausal and have vaginal bleeding	*Cancer*
You are premenopausal and are experiencing irregular vaginal bleeding	*Fibroid inflammation, cancer*
You feel pain in your lower pelvis on the side	*Appendicitis, ovarian cyst, pelvic inflammatory disease*
You feel pain when urinating and your urine is cloudy or foul-smelling	*Urinary tract infection*
You have urinary incontinence	*Urinary tract infection, reaction to medication, fallen uterus*
You have a vaginal discharge and feel bloated and fatigued	*Ovarian cancer*
You feel an abrasion or lesion on the lips of your vagina	*Sexually transmitted disease*

HOW A WOMAN'S REPRODUCTIVE SYSTEM AGES

Compared to a man's, a woman's reproductive system is much more complex, physiologically speaking. Once she reaches puberty, a woman will experience three distinct stages of her reproductive cycle. First, she will have menstrual periods for 30 to 40 years. Of course, during this long stretch of time, she is physically able to bear children. The second stage of a woman's reproductive cycle consists of the premenopausal years, during which her body begins to adapt to the reality of not having children. The third stage is menopause, when her body ceases to be able to bear children. Each of these stages has its own sets of advantages and disadvantages. For this reason, when you look up a particular symptom in this chapter, you should understand that a Body Signal that occurs in one stage might mean something totally different when it occurs in another.

As a woman ages, she will experience a multitude of physiological changes that are caused by the shifts in the hormonal balance of her body—namely in estrogen. When she first begins to menstruate as a teenager, the level of estrogen in her body starts to increase. It rises gradually until she reaches her early 30s, when the production of estrogen is believed to be at its peak. From there, it slowly declines through the premenopausal years until menopause, when her body no longer produces estrogen.

The period of time between premenopause and menopause usually takes a few years. One sign that you're about to enter your premenopausal stage is that the regularity of your cycle changes. You might experience bleeding more frequently, less frequently, or in unpredictable patterns. Instead of 28 days between periods, for instance, you may have your period every five weeks or more.

When you enter the premenopausal stage, which is also known as the climacteric stage of a woman's reproductive cycle, your estrogen level starts to decrease, but your level of follicle-stimulating hormone, or FSH, starts to rise. When this happens, the elevated levels of FSH will cause the leftover egg follicles to mature, which may result in irregular vaginal bleeding. The symptoms in the second stage—hot flashes, cold sweats, and mood swings, among others—are usually what people think of when they hear the word "menopause." Once these symptoms disappear, which can take anywhere from six months to a year or more, you have officially entered menopause.

When you read through this chapter, it's important to realize that every woman experiences premenopause and menopause differently, whether it's in the severity of symptoms or the period of time that elapses between the cessation of menstruation and the onset of menopause.

When you're describing your symptoms to your doctor, you should try to be as specific as you can. You should also remember that even though there are many symptoms that are attributed to the premenopausal stage, you may actually have another medical problem that has similar Body Signals.

Regardless of which stage you're in, the changes you'll experience during premenopause and menopause will have no bearing on your sexuality.

Also, no matter whether you're in the menstrual, premenopausal, or menopausal stage, it's important that you have a yearly gynecological exam. Here are some of the tests you may have during your examination.

In a routine exam, your doctor or gynecologist will first conduct a visual and physical exam, including using a speculum to examine your vaginal walls and cervix. She will take a Pap smear, which is a sample of cells taken from your cervix, place it on a slide, and send it to a lab for testing. A Pap smear should be performed yearly on all sexually active women until the age of 65, since it serves as a screening device for cervical and other gynecological cancers. Your doctor may also do a pelvic sonogram, which is a sound-wave test that allows your doctor to look at your ovaries and uterus. If an area appears irregular, your doctor will use a culposcope, an instrument that allows her to examine the uterus closely, and take a tissue sample for biopsy if necessary.

She will also examine your breasts and ask you if you've noticed any irregularities in them during your monthly exam (see "Breast Self-Examination" Chapter 12). She will take your height and weight, measure your blood pressure, and ask you if your partner or form of contraception has changed since your last exam.

No matter what stage of your reproductive cycle you're in, an annual gynecological exam is a must for staying healthy.

ESTROGEN REPLACEMENT THERAPY, OR ERT:
THE CONTROVERSY CONTINUES

Traditionally, doctors have prescribed estrogen replacement therapy to women who have entered menopause to ease the physical and emotional discomforts that are caused because the body is no longer producing estrogen.

When ERT was first initiated on a widespread basis in the 1950s, women pretty much believed that their doctor and the medical establishment knew what was best for them. However, times have changed. ERT is no longer the panacea it was once purported to be, and the fact is that there are some women who shouldn't take estrogen medication at all.

Here are the facts about estrogen replacement therapy for menopausal woman.

Estrogen replacement therapy comes in four different forms. You can take it orally, in tablets in dosages ranging from 0.3 milligrams to 2.5 milligrams, though the typical dosage is one 0.625-milligram tablet taken once a day for three weeks. A vaginal cream called Premarin is also available, as is a transdermal patch called an Estraderm patch; the latter is worn on the skin and changed twice a week and allows a steady stream of estrogen to be absorbed through the skin. Make sure that it is changed at the same times each week.

One of the main advantages of estrogen replacement therapy is that it helps prevent osteoporosis, since estrogen helps keep bones strong. Estrogen also helps keep the genitals and reproductive organs from atrophying and losing their elasticity and support; this helps prevent the uterus from falling, which is a common condition among postmenopausal women. ERT also helps reduce the risk of heart disease because it increases the amount of the "good" HDL cholesterol in the system while lowering the level of "bad" LDL cholesterol. Estrogen is also frequently used during premenopause to reduce the severity of symptoms such as hot flashes and mood swings.

The disadvantages of estrogen replacement therapy, however, are as numerous as its advantages. Side effects can include nausea, headaches, breast swelling, and mood swings. ERT may increase the risk of uterine and/or ovarian cancer as well as the chances of developing gallbladder disease and high blood pressure, although in some cases the hormone may actually result in lowered blood pressure.

As I've mentioned, some women should never use estrogen because it can aggravate an existing medical condition. For instance, women with a history of clotting problems, liver disease, breast or uterine cancer, or high blood pressure should refrain from ERT.

Progesterone is a hormone that is frequently used in conjunction with estrogen replacement therapy, though it is sometimes prescribed by itself to treat hot flashes in women who cannot tolerate estrogen because of a preexisting health problem. When it is used in combination with estrogen, progesterone can help reduce the side effects of estrogen. Progesterone is available in pills and capsules as well as intramuscular injections. The side effects of progesterone include breast swelling, abdominal bloating, acne, headaches, and mood swings. And while estrogen reduces the risk of coronary disease, progesterone actually increases it because it decreases HDL cholesterol in the body and increases the LDL cholesterol.

Before prescribing estrogen, progesterone, or a combination of the two, your doctor or gynecologist will give you a complete medical and gynecological exam. This will include a blood test to check your cholesterol level, a breast exam, which may include a mammography, and a Pap smear.

If you've had a hysterectomy and you opt for ERT, you will be treated with estrogen alone; if your uterus is intact, you will be given estrogen, possibly combined with some progesterone. For example, you may take estrogen on days 1 to 25 and progesterone on days 13 to 25. In some cases, your doctor might prescribe a continuous program of estrogen with progesterone, especially if the side effects caused by taking estrogen alone are severe.

Although some women feel they should accept whatever their bodies dish out, there are others who want to be physically comfortable with the changes that occur during menopause. Because of the side effects, the decision to start ERT should not be taken lightly. Be sure to discuss the pros and cons with your doctor before you start.

GENITAL DRYNESS AND IRRITATION, PAIN DURING INTERCOURSE, POSTMENOPAUSAL

Description and Possible Medical Problems

When a woman's body ceases to produce estrogen in the menopausal stage, the genitalia start to lose some of their elasticity, and the tissues begin to dry out. As a result, many women who have entered menopause frequently experience pain or irritation during intercourse. Unfortunately, this can increase your chances of contracting a urinary tract infection and experiencing incontinence. Because of this discomfort, many menopausal women start to lose their sexual desire.

Treatment

One of the major benefits of estrogen replacement therapy is that it prevents the genital dryness, irritation, and pain that are common to menopause. If you don't want to start a full course of ERT because of the risk factors, you'll probably be able to use an estrogen cream such as Premarin to help ease your symptoms. You can apply either a half dose or a full dose with the applicator that comes with the cream, once a day for three weeks. You should then stop using the cream for one week before you start another three-week cycle. Premarin should not be used for more than six months. If the medication has no effect on your genital dryness, you should discontinue its use.

MENSTRUAL CHANGES, HOT FLASHES, DEPRESSION, INSOMNIA, FATIGUE

Description and Possible Medical Problems

For several decades, your menstrual cycle probably ran like clockwork. Except for during pregnancy and times of stress, you usually knew when to expect your period, you were more than a little familiar with your symptoms, and you even knew when to anticipate them.

Now it seems as though nothing about your cycle is predictable. Hot flashes appear out of nowhere, and you may feel depressed and tired and yet be unable to sleep at times. Plus, you've gone from being able to set your clock by your period to never knowing when it will start—or stop.

All these changes are due to the hormonal fluctuations that occur as your body prepares for menopause, when your periods will cease. Hot flashes and these other Body Signals occur in about 70% of women who are in the premenopausal stage, which usually starts when in the late 40s. Every woman will experience premenopause differently, however, depending on the severity of symptoms as well as one's degree of tolerance for pain and/or discomfort.

Treatment

Though many women choose to treat their premenopausal symptoms with estrogen replacement therapy, others decide to wait them out. Though hot flashes, depression, and fatigue can be eased by the use of progesterone or estrogen replacement therapy, the risks and benefits of hormonal therapy have to be considered carefully by both you and your doctor.

My advice is that you see your gynecologist and have both a mammogram and a Pap smear before you consider estrogen replacement therapy. Discuss the pros and cons with your doctor, taking into consideration your family's history of disease as well as your own risk factors. However, I do feel that if you have a high risk of coronary disease and/or osteoporosis, you will benefit from the protective effect hormonal therapy provides against both of these diseases.

BODY SIGNAL ALERT

PAIN IN LOWER PELVIS ON ONE SIDE

Description and Possible Medical Problems

Though we've all heard of the appendix and know that it basically serves no useful function except to be removed, many people would be hard pressed to pinpoint its exact location in the body. Even though pain in the lower pelvis alerts people to the possibility of appendicitis, it actually occurs on the right side and is frequently accompanied by vomiting, fever, and pain.

But appendicitis is by no means the sole cause of pain on the right side. Other causes of pain in the lower right side of the pelvis could be due to an ovarian cyst that has ruptured or pelvic inflammatory disease, an infection that can occur in any part of the female reproductive system. The most common form of PID is caused by gonorrhea. When the pain occurs on the lower left side of the abdomen, cysts, a PID, or an intestinal problem such as irritable bowel syndrome may be the cause. If you are still menstruating and the pain on either side occurs in the middle of your cycle, you could have a condition called mittelschmertz, when pain is caused by an egg in one of your ovaries maturing.

Treatment

If you feel pain in the lower part of your pelvis, you should see your gynecologist or internist, who will consider your past medical history, do a physical exam, and run some blood tests to check for an elevated white cell count, which is a sign of infection. A pelvic exam and a pelvic sonogram will also be performed.

If an ovarian cyst has ruptured, you will need to have surgery to remove the cyst, which will require a hospital stay of about four days. Your doctor will make a small incision in your abdomen and remove the cyst, while attempting to preserve the ovary, especially if you've never had a child and you plan to do so in the future.

If the diagnosis is appendicitis, you will immediately be sent to see a surgeon to have an appendectomy, which is usually performed as soon as possible, before the appendix has a chance to burst and cause an infection. Irritable bowel syndrome will be treated with a change in diet, an increase in fiber, and possibly a prescription medication such as Levsinex, which will relieve the bowel spasms (see also "Constipation Alternating with Diarrhea" in Chapter 13). And if your pain is caused by pelvic inflammatory disease, you will be given a course of an antibiotic, such as Floxin 400, taken twice a day for two weeks, or Flagyl 500, also taken twice a day for two weeks. If you think you have a PID, you'll need to inform all your sex partners and seek treatment immediately, since a PID can cause sterility if it's not treated.

BODY SIGNAL ALERT

PAIN ON URINATION, FOUL-SMELLING AND CLOUDY URINE, PRE- AND POSTMENOPAUSAL

Description and Possible Medical Problems

For some reason, Mother Nature had it in for women when she designed their external genitalia. I once heard someone compare the urethra, vagina, and rectum to a highway where the exit ramps are all too close together.

A fourth physical flaw can be added: the woman's urethra, or the tube that leads from the bladder to the outside of the body, is very short compared to a man's. This shortness is what helps create urinary tract infections, since the bacteria don't have very far to travel before they start to cause an infection in the urethra. The major symptoms of a urinary tract infection are a burning pain during urination and foul-smelling urine. A urinary tract infection can occur in different parts of the urinary tract. An infection of the urethra is called urethritis; if it spreads to the bladder, a bladder infection can occur. An infection of either the bladder or the urethra can be quite painful. Because urethritis is often caused by intercourse, when bacteria are pushed up into the urethra, it is often called honeymoon cystitis.

Rarely, the infection will proceed to the kidney; this condition is called pyelonephritis. This can cause permanent kidney damage, so it's important to treat urethritis in the early stages before it has a chance to spread.

Treatment

To determine if you have a urinary tract infection, your doctor will send a sample of your urine to the lab for a culture. If the sample comes back positive and the infection is found to be caused by a bowel bacterium such as *Escherichia coli*, you will be treated with a short course of antibiotics of the sulfa or penicillin variety. Your doctor may want you to come back in a week to make sure that the infection has cleared up.

Tips and Precautions

If you have had urinary tract infections in the past, it's a good idea to urinate after intercourse; this can help flush out any bacteria that may have entered the urethra during intercourse. Some women take 1000 milligrams of vitamin C each day to keep the urine in an acid state, which will help prevent bacteria from growing. And others swear by cranberry juice—which is high in acid—to help cut down on frequent urinary tract infections.

Hygiene is also important. After a bowel movement, you should always wipe *away* from the urethra so that *E. coli* bacteria don't have a chance to reach the urethra.

PERIOD, CESSATION OF

Description and Possible Medical Problems

If your periods suddenly stop, it's probably not a reason for worry; you're actually in good company. The temporary cessation of your menstrual periods, also known as amenorrhea, is actually a common occurrence that could be caused by one of a number of factors.

If your periods stop, and you're in your childbearing years and you're sexually active, the first thing to do is to eliminate the possibility that you're pregnant. I've seen many 40-year-old women who come to see me when their periods stop. They think they have a serious health problem but are surprised to discover that they are pregnant.

However, if you're not pregnant and you're nowhere near menopause, you should see your gynecologist, who will do a physical exam and run a blood test to determine the cause. Amenorrhea is common if you've recently lost a lot of weight. If you're on the contraceptive known as Depo-Provera, you may be one of the 50% of women who suffer from amenorrhea while receiving the quarterly injections. Chemotherapy can also be responsible, as can thyroid disease.

Treatment

If your periods have stopped because you've lost weight, increasing your daily calorie allotment will help maintain your new weight and will probably cause your periods to return as well. If your doctor can't find a specific cause, she will conduct a complete physical exam and take some blood tests. Other diagnostic tests may include an internal vaginal exam, a sonogram of the pelvic area, and a CAT scan of the abdomen and/or the brain. Your doctor will also look for a hormonal problem, such as a pituitary disease or a thyroid disorder, as a possible cause.

Of course, some women are happy that their periods have stopped. In fact, even if the cause is a serious disease, some are reluctant to be treated if it means that their periods will return. Whatever the cause, however, if your periods have stopped, it's important to know why and treat the cause.

URINARY INCONTINENCE IN WOMEN OVER 50

Description and Possible Medical Problems

Even though women of all ages have had the experience of losing control of their bladder due to coughing, sneezing, or even laughing, you'd be hard pressed to find a woman who would admit to incontinence. Losing control of the bladder is a medical condition tinged with shame. As a result, it often goes untreated; usually, this only makes it worse.

Urinary incontinence is so common in women over 50 because of several factors. First, the distance from the external part of the urethra to the bladder is so short that when a cough or a laugh causes loss of control of the bladder for even a second, urine doesn't have very far to go to make it to the outside of the body. Childbirth and the aging process can also cause the lower pelvic muscles to weaken; and when a woman reaches menopause, if she doesn't take estrogen or progesterone, the lack of the hormone causes the genitals to lose their tone and elasticity, weakening the urinary tract even more.

Urinary incontinence is a serious problem because it can cripple a person both emotionally and psychologically. When an elderly woman becomes incontinent, especially if she's living with her family, her family may decide that she needs to be placed in a nursing home. In my office, women will rarely volunteer information about incontinence, even when I ask them directly. However, I know that the adult diaper business is booming.

There are several types of incontinence that are common among women over 50:

- *Stress incontinence* occurs when you temporarily lose control of your bladder while laughing, coughing, or sneezing. The primary cause of stress incontinence is weakness of the pelvic muscles.

- *Urge incontinence* occurs when you suddenly become incontinent for no clear reason. It can be caused by either a urinary tract infection or nerve damage.

- With *overflow incontinence,* the bladder "overfills" because it never completely empties. Overflow incontinence is usually due to nerve damage in the bladder. The major symptom is constant dripping of urine.

- *Mixed incontinence* is a combination of stress incontinence and urge incontinence and is the most common cause of urinary incontinence in women over 50.

If you have any type of urinary incontinence, you can use the acronym DIAPPERS—"diapers" with an extra P—to check for the cause:

D: Delirium that may be caused by pneumonia, irregular heartbeat, or a small stroke

I: Infection of the urinary tract

A: Atrophic vaginitis or urethritis, dropped bladder, prolapsed uterus, and loss of pelvic floor tone and muscle strength

P: Pharmaceuticals, such as diuretics, sedatives, cold preparations, psychotropic medications, or blood pressure pills

P: Psychological agitation or depression

E: Excessive fluid intake

R: Restricted ability to get to the bathroom—is the bathroom on a different floor, or does arthritis prevent you from reaching it on time?

S: Stool impaction, another overlooked common cause of loss of urine

Treatment

If you have one or more of the problems listed in DIAPPERS, be sure to tell your doctor about all of them, as well as when you first noticed them. All of the conditions listed in DIAPPERS are treatable. For instance, if you are taking a "P"—a pharmaceutical such as a diuretic or other medication that is responsible for your incontinence, your doctor will suggest that you switch to another brand. And sometimes more than one of the causes of DIAPPERS can contribute to the problem.

Here's the treatment:

D (Delirium caused by pneumonia): Once the pneumonia is treated, the incontinence will disappear. Very often, urinary incontinence in an elderly woman is the first sign of pneumonia, a stroke, or an irregular heartbeat.

I (Infection of the urinary tract): For a urinary tract infection, a urine sample and culture are always the first step toward treatment. The most common cause of a urinary tract infection is *E. coli* bacteria, which will respond to the antibiotic Bactrim or Noroxin taken twice a day for one week.

A (Atrophic vaginitis, prolapsed uterus, dropped bladder): To treat atrophic vaginitis, your doctor may prescribe a vaginal Premarin cream (see "Genital Dryness and Irritation, Pain During Intercourse, Postmenopausal" above). To treat a prolapsed uterus or a dropped bladder, your doctor may want to use a pessary, a ring that is inserted into the vagina; this will raise the bladder and support the pelvic wall, adjusting the angle of the bladder so as to help you retain control. Reconstructive surgery to lift the bladder or vaginal Premarin cream may also be used.

P (Pharmaceuticals): A patient who takes a high dose of the laxative called Lasix only once a day may benefit if she takes a half dose in the morning and the other half in the afternoon or evening. If you plan to be away from home for the day, you should not take the medication until you are back home.

P (Psychological problems): People who become depressed often find that they lose interest in maintaining their personal hygiene. A mild antidepressant such as Zoloft, taken at night, can be helpful.

E (Excessive fluid intake): Many people believe they must drink eight glasses of water a day in order to maintain good health. While this is true for most people, in an older woman, the high water intake combined with a dropped bladder will make it almost impossible for her to hold her urine, especially if she also takes diuretics. With the help of your doctor, cut back on the amount of water you drink and the diuretics. A pessary can also help. (See the treatment for "A" above.)

R (Restricted ability to get to the bathroom): If activity is restricted, you should get a commode and keep it near the bed.

S (Stool impaction): Using FiberCon or Metamucil on a regular basis and increasing the amount of exercise you get will help relieve stool impaction.

Sometimes, however, the cause can't be found on the DIAPPERS list. For instance, if you have a chronic cough because you're a heavy smoker, the smoking can be directly responsible for your urinary incontinence. If you stop smoking, your cough will gradually disappear along with your urinary incontinence.

In addition to your doctor's treatments, Kegel exercises can be helpful for treating incontinence. These exercises involve contracting and releasing the pelvic muscles in the same way as you control the flow of urine. Try to do these exercises several times a day, starting at holding for 10 seconds and working up to as long as possible.

If you have urge incontinence or mixed incontinence, retraining your bladder can be helpful. Try to hold your urine for at least an hour before urinating; or, if you tend to wait too long before urinating, try to urinate every hour, which will help to reduce accidents.

For women with urge or mixed incontinence, certain medications, such as antidepressants and bladder antispasmodics, can be helpful in preventing incontinence.

Every woman has to become educated about incontinence and stop being ashamed so that the proper treatment can be found—or at least the proper way to cope and live well with the problem. Here's how one woman did it.

One of my patients is an active 60-year-old woman who stopped going to church and to places like Atlantic City because she was embarrassed that she might become incontinent. She began wearing a diaper, but she remained self-conscious.

Whenever she saw me for her yearly checkup, she never mentioned the incontinence even when I asked her. One time, she was waiting in the examination room for me. As I came in, she darted past me to the bathroom down the hall. When she reached the bathroom, she accidentally urinated on the floor and herself. She started to cry and told me and my nurse how ashamed she felt. She even offered to clean the bathroom.

My examination revealed that she had a urinary tract infection. She was also taking a diuretic every day to reduce swelling in her ankles, and she had had six children, which had left her pelvic floor quite weak. I referred her to a urologist, and together we decided that taking a different diuretic medication, getting her urinary tract infection treated, doing regular Kegel exercises, and keeping a urination diary was all she needed to do.

Two weeks later she returned to my office and told me that she wasn't having any more accidents, that I was the best doctor in the world and that—by the way—she had hit the jackpot on the slot machines in Atlantic City.

Tips and Precautions

If you have urinary incontinence, keep a diary. Here's how it works.

In a journal, each day for a week, you write down every time you urinate, the approximate amount, and the circumstances. For instance, did you drink a glass of water an hour earlier, or did you have to urinate in the middle of the night? Each entry will include whether the urination was normal or involuntary. This will help your physician to determine the exact cause(s) and help him decide on your treatment. A consultation with a urologist will also be very important in helping to discover the source of your incontinence.

URINARY INCONTINENCE IN WOMEN UNDER 50

Description and Possible Medical Problems

Though urinary incontinence affects women of all ages, it's rarely a problem in women who are still menstruating. Most often, the cause is a simple urinary tract infection, although many women report that they have a problem with urinary incontinence during pregnancy. This is caused by the pressure that's exerted on the bladder by the fetus.

Treatment

In the younger woman, occasional urinary incontinence is not a serious problem, and it requires no special treatment. If the problem starts to occur on a regular basis, however, or if you feel pain or burning when you urinate, you should see your doctor. If you have a urinary tract infection, you will be treated with antibiotics and told to drink more fluids.

See also "Pain on Urination, Foul-smelling and Cloudy Urine, Pre- and Postmenopausal" above.

BODY SIGNAL ALERT

VAGINAL BLEEDING, POSTMENOPAUSAL

Description and Possible Medical Problems

If you've entered menopause and you notice any amount of vaginal bleeding, whether light or heavy, you need to see your doctor immediately, since vaginal bleeding in a woman who's gone through menopause is a serious matter. If you've been taking estrogen and/or progesterone and you're either cutting down or stopping the medication completely, the bleeding might be due to withdrawal from the hormones. If you're not taking estrogen or progesterone, the bleeding may be due to cancer of the uterus, which is the second most common form of cancer in women but the most common in postmenopausal women. Your risk for cancer is increased if you are taking estrogen without progesterone or are diabetic and/or obese. And if you've never had children, your risk also goes up.

If you're postmenopausal and are experiencing vaginal bleeding, ask yourself the following questions:

1. Is the blood definitely coming from the vagina or from the urinary tract or rectal area? For instance, do I primarily see the blood when urinating or during a bowel movement, or does it also appear at other times?

2. How much blood do I see? Is it just a streak, or is it heavy enough that I have to use a pad or a tampon?

Treatment

Postmenopausal women who are experiencing vaginal bleeding will need to have a complete gynecological exam, including a physical exam, a Pap smear, and a biopsy that's done with a D and C, or dilation and curettage.

If the initial diagnosis confirms uterine cancer—and there's no easy way to say this—you will need to have a total abdominal hysterectomy. The uterus and ovaries will be removed; the vagina will remain in place. The total recuperation time in an otherwise healthy woman is three to four weeks. Your gynecological oncologist may also want to treat you with radiation or chemotherapy, if she believes the cancer has spread. If uterine cancer is caught early, it can be cured.

VAGINAL BLEEDING, PREMENOPAUSAL

Description and Possible Medical Problems

If you are in the second stage of your reproductive cycle, also known as the premenopausal stage, you may notice that your periods have become less regular with different amounts of bleeding.

If you are premenopausal and experiencing a change in pattern of bleeding or time of periods, ask yourself the following questions:

1. When did my periods start to change?

2. Are my periods more or less frequent than they used to be?

3. Do I have a smaller or larger amount of bleeding than usual? For instance, how many pads or tampons am I using?

4. Have I started to take a new medication or stopped taking one?

5. Do I have vaginal bleeding during or after intercourse?

Vaginal bleeding during the premenopausal stage can range from mild spotting to a flow that approaches what you experienced during the heavy days of your period. It's important that you see your doctor if you're spotting and head for the emergency room if the bleeding is heavy. It's not certain what causes premenopausal bleeding, but it's likely that it's related to the sudden and extreme hormonal changes that occur as the body prepares for menopause.

In some cases, usually in younger women who are sexually active, polyps and/or cervical lesions may be the reason for vaginal bleeding. Even though they are still menstruating, they may confuse the bleeding with the spotting that sometimes occurs between periods and delay seeking medical treatment because they don't think anything is wrong.

Fibroid tumors, which are growths on the uterine wall, are another common cause of irregular bleeding episodes in premenopausal women. They can be responsible for pain during intercourse, a sensation of abdominal fullness, and overall discomfort. In my practice, I have seen women with fibroid tumors who looked as though they were four months pregnant.

Treatment

If you are bleeding from the vagina, your gynecologist will perform a complete gynecological exam during which she will look for lesions or cancers of the gynecological tract. If your doctor suspects you have a cervical lesion, she will perform a culposcopy, a test that will allow her to view the cervix directly to check for lesions that might be cancerous. If you're premenopausal and not currently on ERT and are experiencing vaginal bleeding, your gynecologist may recommend that you start taking estrogen and/or progesterone. This will usually stop the bleeding.

If a fibroid tumor is causing your bleeding, your gynecologist may recommend that only the tumor be removed, especially if you want to have children. However, in many cases, you may be advised to have a hysterectomy since a complicated surgical procedure is required to remove just the tumor. The hysterectomy can be total, in which both ovaries and the uterus are removed, or it can be partial in which one ovary is left in place. The latter is often done when the patient is premenopausal in order to conserve her natural hormone supply.

VAGINAL DISCHARGE, MILKY, WITH SEVERE ITCHING

Description and Possible Medical Problems

In the last decade or so, vaginal yeast infections have come out of the closet, so to speak, as one of the most common gynecological problems around, and they can affect women of any age. If you notice a milky white, nonbloody vaginal discharge and your genital area itches, you probably have a yeast infection.

Small amounts of a fungus known as *Candida albicans* are normally present in the vagina. Bacteria also live in the vagina, and both the bacteria and the fungus usually maintain a healthy balance. However, when something occurs to create an imbalance between the bacteria and the fungus, the fungus can proliferate, resulting in a yeast infection. The most common cause of a yeast infection is use of antibiotics, especially penicillin. Stress, hormonal changes, or a lowered immune system can also cause a yeast infection. Therefore, the presence of a yeast infection does not necessarily mean a woman is allergic to antibiotics.

A yeast infection may also be a sign of diabetes. In fact, in my experience, I would say that about 10% of my female diabetic patients have a yeast infection as the first sign of the disease.

Treatment

If you have a yeast infection, you should first try to treat it with an over-the-counter remedy such as Tinactin vaginal cream, which is applied directly into the vagina at bedtime.

If none of these measures is effective, you should see your doctor, who will do a blood test to rule out diabetes as the cause. To prevent future yeast infections, some women swear by a daily dose of acidophilus pills or yogurt culture as a preventive measure; these products are available in health food stores.

BODY SIGNAL ALERT

VAGINAL DISCHARGE WITH
BLOATING AND GENERAL MALAISE

Description and Possible Medical Problems

It's easy to ignore some Body Signals, especially when they're vague. For instance, if you have a mild vaginal discharge and have had yeast infections in the past, you might dismiss this symptom because it usually clears up in a day or two anyway. If you also feel a bit bloated and experience malaise, you may just figure that it's "that time of the month," even if it isn't, and wait for it to pass.

The fact is, if you have a vaginal discharge that is accompanied by bloating and a general feeling of discontent and malaise, you need to see your doctor immediately. These are signs of ovarian cancer, which is the third most common form of gynecological cancer but also the most deadly.

The reason why ovarian cancer is so deadly is that many times a woman will show no symptoms of the disease until the cancer has spread. And if you're obese, have gone through menopause early, and eat a high-fat diet, you're more at risk. Using a hormone-based contraceptive such as the Pill or Depo-Provera and having had children decrease your risk of contracting this disease.

Treatment

If your doctor suspects you have ovarian cancer, he will use a sonogram, a CAT scan of the pelvis, and a physical examination to make a positive diagnosis. There is also a blood test that can detect the presence of ovarian cancer and also track its progression. However, this test isn't a standard part of a regular gynecological exam because it is very expensive. In addition, the test is not 100% accurate: in other words, a negative result does not mean you are free from cancer, and a positive doesn't necessarily mean you have cancer.

If you do have ovarian cancer, you will need surgery to remove the cancer and help determine whether the cancer is in an early or advanced stage. In addition to your ovaries, your fallopian tubes, uterus, and lymph glands will also probably be removed to make sure that the cancer has not spread. After surgery, you will likely be treated with radiation or chemotherapy to keep the cancer in check.

VAGINAL ITCH

See "Vaginal Discharge, Milky, with Severe Itch" above.

BODY SIGNAL ALERT

VAGINAL LESIONS

Description and Possible Medical Problems

Sometimes, the day after a particularly intense lovemaking session, you may notice that your genitals, particularly your vaginal lips, feel sore and raw. If you examine your genitals, you'll find that they may appear a bit redder than usual. The soreness and the redness usually disappear within a day or two.

But if a lesion or abrasion appears on your vaginal lips and doesn't go away after a couple of days, you should see your doctor. This is usually a sign of a sexually transmitted disease. If the lesions are painful and appear in small clusters, you may have gonorrhea or herpes. If the lesion looks like a wart, syphilis may be the cause.

Treatment

A sexually transmitted disease (STD) is a serious matter, because it can lead to permanent health problems. Gonorrhea, for instance, can lead to pelvic inflammatory disease, which is a major cause of sterility.

The treatment for any STD will be determined by your doctor according to the culture and type of lesion. The most important thing is to seek medical attention when you first suspect you may have an STD.

And, to prevent the spread of STDs, always use a condom.

VAGINAL MASS AND HEAVINESS, POSTMENOPAUSAL

Description and Possible Medical Problems

If it feels as though a mass of tissue has entered your vagina from your uterus and you've gone through menopause, it's possible that your uterus has fallen and is protruding into the vagina.

This condition, known as a prolapsed uterus, occurs in women who are not on estrogen replacement therapy because the lack of estrogen causes the uterus and other reproductive organs to lose their elasticity and tone. As a result, the uterus can "fall" into the vagina. Many women with a prolapsed uterus also have periodic urinary tract infections and/or urinary incontinence and even minor bleeding.

In severe cases, the uterus may even start to protrude outside of the vagina.

Treatment

If you have a fallen uterus, you will need surgery to correct it. Since mostly elderly women experience a fallen uterus, the uterus may be removed via the vagina to keep the risk of surgery, which increases with age, to a minimum.

The average hospitalization lasts about a week, but it varies greatly depending on other medical problems a woman may have. Even when an elderly woman has a fallen uterus, surgery is usually the best option. If, however, she is too frail for surgery, the doctor will insert a ring called a pessary that will help support the pelvic floor.

See also "Urinary Incontinence in Women over 50" above.

Chapter 15

FOR MEN ONLY: REPRODUCTIVE AND UROLOGICAL SYSTEMS

<table>
<tr><td colspan="2" align="center">BODY SIGNAL ALERT</td></tr>
<tr><td colspan="2">Call your doctor or urologist immediately if you experience any of the following symptoms:</td></tr>
<tr><td>SYMPTOM</td><td>POSSIBLE MEDICAL CONDITION</td></tr>
<tr><td>You see blood when you urinate</td><td>Urinary tract infection, prostate problem, bladder tumor</td></tr>
<tr><td>You notice that pus is coming from your penis</td><td>Sexually transmitted disease</td></tr>
<tr><td>You feel a hard lump in your testicle</td><td>Benign growth, cyst, cancer</td></tr>
<tr><td>You feel a severe pain in your testicle</td><td>Testicular torsion</td></tr>
<tr><td>You find it difficult or are unable to urinate</td><td>Prostate enlargement, acute urinary retention due to prostate enlargement</td></tr>
<tr><td>You notice that your chest has grown</td><td>Cancer, use of certain medications, use of steroids</td></tr>
</table>

HOW THE MALE REPRODUCTIVE
SYSTEM AGES

When it comes to how men regard the effects that aging has on their sexuality, I've seen three distinct groups of opinions: in one, a man believes the popular myth that his sexuality peaked years ago, when he was 18, so since then life's been all downhill. A man in the second group tends to deny that aging has any effect at all, even though his physiological signs tell him otherwise.

And then there's the group in between: At first, a man may rebel a little at the changes in his sexuality—which may be anything from needing more time to become fully erect to wanting to have sex less often—but he eventually accepts the changes and may even learn to use them as a way to make sexuality more exciting and challenging.

From the time a man is in his teens all the way to his 80s and 90s, his reproductive system ages slowly from one year to the next. For most men, sexuality continues to be a very important aspect of life throughout their lives. Sexual desire continues indefinitely, despite the popular image of an uninterested, grumpy old man. One problem an 80- or 90-year-old man may have is that he is ashamed of his sexuality, because he—along with a lot of other people of all ages—has bought into the myth that older people are not and should not be sexual. This myth about sexuality is particularly a problem if he is living in a nursing home or at home with his children, because if the people around him believe the myth, chances are he will, too.

Throughout life, illness and medication can have a significant impact on your sexuality; even acetaminophen and allergies can dampen a man's sexual desire. Though men do not experience a formal cessation of their reproductive ability such as women do when they enter menopause, the production both of sperm and testosterone decreases as a man ages. However, this usually has no bearing on his ability to father children; even 90-year-old men have become fathers.

As a man ages, it will take a bit longer to achieve an erection, and he'll notice that the erection will probably be less firm than when he was younger. After the age of 60, it may take a man 15 minutes to become fully erect, as compared to seconds for a young teenager. Ejaculation also takes longer and requires more stimulation, but all these changes might actually be advantageous to men who had problems with premature ejaculation in their early years, as well as to their partners.

The volume of a man's ejaculate decreases slightly, and he may not have an orgasm with every sexual encounter, which is probably a 180-degree turnaround from his youth. Regardless of these changes, however, sex can still remain a big part of his life.

Every man should have a yearly physical exam, including a prostate exam, starting at the age of 40. Your internist or family practitioner will feel for enlargement and asymmetry in the prostate gland. Some other tests may include a blood test for prostatic-specific antigen, or PSA, which is a good way to monitor prostate cancer if a diagnosis for cancer is positive. PSA levels may be elevated even if the prostate is enlarged and no cancer is present. However, I would not recommend a PSA as a sole screening test for prostate cancer. Another test, called prostatic acid phosphatase, is a blood test that will also show that the prostate is enlarged.

BODY SIGNAL ALERT

BREASTS, ENLARGED

Description and Possible Medical Problems

Among men who regularly work out with weights, firm, defined pectoral muscles are a sign of a well-exercised body. Some people think they're sexy, while others get turned off if they think they look too much like a woman's breasts.

However, no matter what your personal feelings are on the issue, if you notice that one or both of your breasts have grown larger recently, you need to see your doctor.

If both breasts feel fleshy and firm and the nipples are pointing slightly downward, you probably have a condition called gynecomastia, which is a frequent side effect of anabolic steroid use and heavy weight training. Sometimes, however, gynecomastia can occur if you have too much estrogen in your system. If your breasts suddenly get bigger and you're not currently taking anabolic steroids as a muscle enhancement or medication, then you should see your doctor.

Gynecomastia can also result from the presence of a benign or malignant tumor, although a tumor almost always affects just one breast, at least in the beginning. An enlargement will feel like a solid mass, while a tumor tends to be both smaller and harder. Especially in older men, when one breast grows larger, it may be a sign of a tumor.

But breast cancer—or any abnormality in the breast—is extremely rare in men, though it does occur. For every 100 women who get breast cancer, for instance, only 1 man will develop it. Since most men aren't aware that they can get breast cancer, they rarely check for it or even notice changes in their breasts. As a result, when breast cancer is diagnosed in a man, it's usually too late.

An underlying liver disease or endocrine disorder may also be responsible for your enlarged breasts. If you're exhibiting other signs of these diseases—such as jaundice and impotence in the case of liver disease, or sudden loss or gain of weight and fatigue in the case of endocrine disorders—see your doctor immediately. Another cause of gynecomastia in men is certain medications, particularly the drug cimetidine, which is commonly used to treat ulcers, and digoxin, which is prescribed for patients with heart arrhythmia.

Frequently, men who are overweight will develop lipomastia, a form of breast enlargement. In this case, larger breasts are due to an increased distribution of fat all over the body, with some of it settling in the breasts.

Treatment

If you're weight lifting and taking anabolic steroids, your breasts will remain enlarged until you stop both training and taking the medications.

The detection and diagnosis for a breast tumor in men is the same as for women. Sonography and/or mammography is used initially; if the mass appears to be suspicious, your doctor will do a biopsy to determine whether the cells are cancerous or not.

If you are taking either cimetidine or digoxin and you've noticed that your breasts have grown since you've begun the regimen, ask your doctor if he can switch you to another effective medication that won't give you these side effects. When you stop taking the drug, your breasts should return to their normal size.

If your breasts have grown because you've gained weight, the only treatment is a weight-reduction plan that includes exercise. Some men have actually undergone breast-reduction surgery to eliminate this embarrassing condition, but most either learn to live with it or reduce the prominence of their breasts by losing weight and building up the pectoral muscles that lie underneath.

BODY SIGNAL ALERT

DISCHARGE FROM PENIS WITH DIFFICULTY URINATING

Description and Possible Medical Problems

If you notice a discharge from your penis that looks like pus and you also find it difficult to urinate, see your doctor right away. These are the two major signs of a sexually transmitted disease, gonorrhea in particular. Because gonorrhea infects the urethra, which causes it to swell up, you may have trouble urinating.

Though it may seem as though sexually transmitted diseases have just now hit the newspapers and magazines, gonorrhea was actually a common disease back during World War II, when it reached epidemic proportions in some branches of the military. Today, even though AIDS has the spotlight when it comes to sexually transmitted disease, the incidence of gonorrhea has been slowly rising along with the spread of the HIV virus. In fact, some researchers believe that if you catch gonorrhea, you are more prone to contracting the HIV virus as well.

Treatment

If you think you have gonorrhea or another sexually transmitted disease, your doctor will take a sample of your discharge and have it analyzed in order to make a positive diagnosis. If you do have gonorrhea, he will prescribe a course of antibiotic for you to take, either doxycycline 100, twice a day for seven days, or erythromycin 500, which you should take four times a day for seven days. While you're taking the antibiotic, you should refrain from having sex to prevent the disease from spreading. Your doctor will also advise you that you should always use a condom whenever you're not totally sure of a partner's sexual history.

EJACULATION, PAIN ON, BLOOD IN THE SEMEN, ERECTION THAT DOESN'T SUBSIDE

Description and Possible Medical Problems

When you were in your early 20s, you would probably swear off sex for a year before you'd admit—to yourself or to anyone else—to having any problems with sex. Pain during intercourse? Hey, that was part of the learning experience. But it probably happened because you were so eager to get to it that you didn't think or care that your partner wasn't ready. And your partner was probably too shy to tell you.

How times have changed! You're older and presumably wiser and more willing to admit to those times when your body doesn't do what you expect it to do, which includes during sex. Some problems you may have are pain during intercourse; priapism, a very dangerous condition in which your erection doesn't subside; or blood in your semen. All are signs of potentially serious underlying health problems.

If you have blood in your semen, it's possible that you have prostatitis, which is an inflammation of the prostate; or perhaps a minor blood vessel has broken. Though it is rare, priapism is an emergency problem. Priapism may be a result of a clot that is preventing the blood from leaving the penis after sexual activity, or it could be due to a problem with your spinal cord.

Treatment

If you feel pain during intercourse, it may be because your partner isn't sufficiently lubricated. A lubricant such as K-Y Jelly will usually help.

If you have priapism, you need to treat it immediately by calling your doctor. Placing a cold compress on your penis will help while you drive to the emergency room. Your doctor may choose to perform bypass surgery to remove the clot or use medication to reduce your blood pressure to allow the blood to leave your engorged penis. If priapism is not treated within several hours of its onset, permanent erectile problems can result.

If you have prostatitis, your doctor may prescribe antibiotics and a combination of massage and sitz baths. He may also suggest that you just leave it alone to clear up on its own. With a broken blood vessel, the blood usually appears only once; the small blood vessels that are located around the male reproductive system usually heal within a day or so.

ERECTILE DYSFUNCTION WITH LOSS OF SEXUAL DESIRE

Description and Possible Medical Problems

Any man who tells me that he's never had a problem achieving and then maintaining an erection is lying. Whether it's due to stress, illness, fatigue, or medication, it's actually not unusual for a man to have trouble with getting and/or keeping his erection.

I define erectile dysfunction as the inability to achieve or maintain your erection 50% of the time. Impotence, on the other hand, I regard as the almost total absence of sexual activity because of the inability to maintain your erection all the time.

Once you have a problem achieving and/or maintaining an erection on even a single occasion, a vicious cycle can begin. For instance, one night your partner wants to have sex, but you don't because you're preoccupied with an argument you had at the office that day. But you try anyway because you want to make your partner happy. You get an erection, but you can't maintain it because your mind is a million miles away and, after all, you really didn't want to have sex in the first place. So you apologize and figure you'll make it up to your partner the next night.

When the next night rolls around, what frequently happens is that because you're so focused on doing everything right this time, it doesn't. If this happens a few more times, you may start to doubt your sexual ability and whether you are able to please your partner at all! Soon every sexual encounter is fraught with tension. You may even start to believe that your inability to maintain an erection is due to a physical problem.

Treatment

If you're having problems with your erection, the first step is to relax. If you're concerned that your inability to maintain your erection is because you physically can't, here's a strange but simple test. Since men almost always get an erection during REM sleep, take a strip of postage stamps and attach it around your penis before going to sleep. If you're like most men, in the morning the strip will be broken.

It's most likely, however, that you don't have a physical problem, so the next step is to address the stress or whatever else is responsible for your erectile dysfunction. Again, learning to relax may help. Letting your partner take the lead—which takes the responsibility off you—may also help. If, however, these techniques don't work, you may find it helpful to see a sex therapist. However, in most cases this is not necessary; when the stress clears up or you deal with your problem, your ability to maintain an erection will return.

IMPOTENCE

Description and Possible Medical Problems

Impotence is defined as a permanent inability to maintain an erection. As a result, sexual activity—including masturbation—reaches a near standstill. Sometimes impotence results because a man's sexuality changes with age: after the age of 50, his sexual activity can decline rapidly. One study shows that sexual activity in a man drops by 10% in his 50s, 20% in his 60s, 20% more when he's in his 70s, and 50% or more in his 80s.

But health problems and illness can also cause impotence. Stress can be one factor; heart disease may be another, since an erection occurs when the tissues in the penis fill with blood. If there is a problem with getting the blood to these tissues, an erection cannot occur. And high blood pressure can also cause impotence, as can prostate disease. After a man has prostate surgery, he may be in doubt about his sexuality; however, the surgery can also permanently alter his physical ability to achieve an erection.

Medications, such as drugs to control blood pressure like beta-blockers, can also be responsible. Smoking and alcohol both dilate the blood vessels, which again means there's less blood available to reach the penis. Depression is also a very common cause of impotence, and an underlying medical illness such as stroke or cancer can not only cause a man to lose all interest in sex but make him physically unable to have an erection.

Ask yourself the following questions:

1. Have I been depressed or ill lately?

2. Am I unable to have and maintain an erection at all? Or am I comparing it to the erections I had when I was 20 years old?

3. Have I become suddenly impotent, or has the condition developed more slowly?

4. Am I unable to achieve an erection all the time or only occasionally?

5. Are my legs cold or swollen?

6. Have my breasts or testicles become enlarged?

Treatment

If you think you are impotent, but you are not affected by any of the physical problems I've mentioned, the condition may be caused by stress, psychological problems, or anxiety that you've developed concerning sex. If, however, you believe your impotence is caused by a physical problem, see your doctor for advice and treatment. He will conduct a complete medical history and physical exam, as well as a number of tests, to determine the cause of your impotence. The exam will include a digital rectal exam, so he can check the prostate, and a manual exam of the testicles. He will also take your pulse in your abdomen and legs and perhaps do a sonogram, to check the amount of blood that is reaching your penis.

First, if you smoke or drink alcohol regularly, try cutting down or out completely to see if that affects your ability to achieve and maintain an erection. If your impotence has appeared suddenly, your physician may believe that a particular medication such as an antidepressant or antihypertensive is responsible; if this is the case, he will switch you over to another one that is just as effective but does not have the side effects. If you have become impotent over a period of time and your legs have felt cold and swollen lately, an underlying disease—most likely a vascular disease or diabetes mellitus—is responsible. And if you've noticed that your testicles or breasts have become larger, you may have an underlying endocrine disorder, such as thyroid disease. Treating a stroke, high blood pressure, heart disease, or cancer requires ongoing medication and lifestyle changes; once these are all in place, your impotence should disappear.

Some men may appear to be going through what has been called a male menopause when their testosterone levels drop below their normal range; this can result in impotence. In some cases, testosterone supplements have been used; however, they are rarely effective.

Some men who have had prostate surgery are permanently unable to achieve an erection on their own. However, there is a surgical technique in which an implant is placed in the penis to make it erect—all the time.

A man who wants more choice in the matter can use a pump device along with a surgically implanted sac in the penis. Whenever he wants to have an erection, a few squeezes of the hand pump, and bingo! instant erection: the sacs fill with fluid. Afterwards, he pumps again, and the fluid returns to a reservoir in the testicles. A man can also have an orgasm with this technique.

Does this sound too technical or make you squeamish? Another option is to inject the hormone prostaglandin directly into the urethra; this will provide an instant erection. The injection is easy to do and is not at all painful. Some of my patients have found it to be extremely satisfactory.

There is also a medication called yohimbine, which, when taken daily, seems to have the same effects as testosterone and will allow a man to achieve and then maintain an erection so that he can have an orgasm.

INCONTINENCE

Description and Possible Medical Problems

Even a bodybuilder discovers by the age of 50 that his muscles aren't as firm and toned as they were when he was in his 30s—or his 40s. With age, muscles lose their tone—even with regular exercise—and it takes longer for them to recover from exercise; for instance, instead of exercising one day and resting the next, you may need two days to recover. Needless to say, if muscles don't get any exercise at all, they become flabbier.

The muscles that control urination are no exception. However, even though incontinence is more of a problem in older women than in men due to their physiology, men can have the problem too, for many of the same reasons as women, such as a urinary tract infection, a common cause of urinary incontinence. Depression can also be a cause, as can certain medications such as stool softeners and antibiotics. When you suddenly become incontinent for no clear reason, this is known as urge incontinence; it can be caused by either a urinary tract infection or nerve damage to the bladder.

Once a urinary tract infection or stool impaction is ruled out, the most common cause of urinary incontinence is a condition called overflow incontinence. As the prostate enlarges, it constricts the urethra and therefore limits the flow of urine from the bladder. The bladder "overfills" because it never completely empties. As the bladder fills, there is so much urine in it that it overflows around the prostatic obstruction and drips out, usually without notice. Overflow incontinence can also develop in a frail elderly man or any man who has had prostate surgery.

Treatment

If an enlarged prostate is responsible for your incontinence, your urologist will start you on a treatment plan that may include a medication called Proscar to shrink the prostate, regular checkups, and possibly prostate resection surgery, which will relieve the pressure on the urethra.

See also "Urination, Difficulty in", below

BODY SIGNAL ALERT

TESTICLE, HARD LUMP IN

Description and Possible Medical Problems

In recent years, urologists have begun to recommend to their male patients that they get into the habit of checking their testicles each month for lumps and other growths they may find there, much as a gynecologist tells her patients to check their breasts each month.

Though problems occur more frequently in the prostate than in the testicles, it's still a good idea to get into the habit of checking your testicles since tumors that occur in the testicles frequently turn out to be malignant. And, as is true for women, any lump you find in its early stages is not likely to be painful until later, by which time treatment may not be effective.

Check your testicles one at a time, preferably after a shower. Feel the surface of the testicle through the scrotum and note any new growths on the surface, rolling the testicle between the index finger and thumb of both hands as you go. You should also compare the size of the testicle with the size it was in last month's exam. Is it harder or larger, or has it changed in any way? Once you've thoroughly checked one testicle, examine the other.

If you discover a lump on your testicle or notice any other changes, you should see your doctor or urologist right away. Although your risk of getting testicular cancer decreases as you get older, it's important to check your testicles every month.

The good news is that a lump or mass on the testicle is often due to another problem that is easily remedied. You may have a benign growth—which is usually the case if the growth appears within the scrotum and not on the testicle itself—or a painless cyst that appears on the epididymis, the tube that stores sperm next to the testicle.

Treatment

Anytime a patient notices a suspicious mass in his testicle, I suggest that he visit a urologist, who will do a sonogram of the mass to determine the exact site and whether the mass is hard or filled with fluid. If the urologist has any doubt, he will perform a biopsy. If the testicle is not cancerous—which is usually the case—it will be left in place.

If you have a cyst on the epididymis, your doctor will probably choose to leave it alone. If it continues to grow, however, it will eventually cause pain. At that point, your doctor will probably want to remove it surgically.

If the lump turns out to be cancerous, your doctor will need to treat it immediately by removing the entire testicle. This procedure is called an orchiectomy and is performed if the cancer has not spread beyond the testicle. Again, since only one testicle is usually affected, the other testicle will be left in place, meaning that your fertility will not be impaired. If your doctor feels that the cancer has spread, however, he will recommend that you also be treated with radiation or chemotherapy; this will result in sterility.

One of my patients is a 37-year-old man whom I diagnosed 10 years ago with testicular cancer; he was unmarried at the time. Before he was treated with surgery and radiation, he decided to have his sperm frozen so he would be able to father a child in the future, since the treatments would render him sterile. He also had a small testicular prosthesis placed into his testicular sac for cosmetic reasons.

Today, he's been cancer free since the surgery; he needs only an annual blood test and physical exam. He hasn't yet married, but his semen is intact if he needs it to become a father.

BODY SIGNAL ALERT

TESTICLE, SUDDEN PAIN IN

Description and Possible Medical Problems

If you're like most men, you know that a blow to your testicles can be excruciatingly painful, even if the same strike to another part of your body wouldn't even warrant a bruise. The pain usually lasts for no more than an hour, and no permanent damage is caused.

If, however, you feel a sudden, severe pain in one of your testicles and it hasn't been struck, you may have a condition known as testicular torsion, in which the spermatic cord—from which each testicle hangs—becomes twisted. This can happen either spontaneously or during physical activity. Testicular torsion can cut off the blood supply to the testicle, resulting in permanent damage if it's not treated right away with surgery.

An infection in the testicle is also common; it can be quite painful. In men over 35, the usual cause of testicular infection is bacteria that have spread from the urinary tract.

A sexually transmitted disease such as gonorrhea can also be the cause of an infection in the testicle.

Treatment

If you think you have testicular torsion, you should see your doctor or urologist immediately. He will first try to manually untwist the spermatic cord. It's likely, however, that even when he succeeds, he will also want to perform minor surgery by placing a few judiciously placed stitches that will prevent the cord from twisting again, which is a likely possibility. The surgical procedure to repair the torsion and prevent future episodes will require several days in the hospital and about a week of recuperation.

If the pain is caused by an infection in your testicle caused by bacteria in your urinary tract, the doctor will need to find out what particular bacterium is causing the infection. He will do a prostate exam through the rectum or massage the penis to extract a sample of discharge (if it exists) to send to the lab for a culture. An antibiotic will then be prescribed depending on the organism isolated. If the infection is caused by a sexually transmitted disease, your doctor will prescribe the antibiotic Floxin 300, which you will take twice a day for 10 days; your sexual partner or partners will also need to be treated.

THE PROSTATE

With the deaths of Frank Zappa, Telly Savalas, and Bill Bixby of prostate cancer, and with Senators Robert Dole and Alan Cranston going public with their own experiences with the disease, the spotlight has been thrown onto what has become the most common form of cancer in men. Up to 30% of all men over 50 show some degree of prostate cancer, and approximately 165,000 men are diagnosed with prostate cancer each year. Men start to become at risk for prostate cancer around age 40.

The prostate is a small gland in the pelvis just underneath the bladder that surrounds the urethra. After a man turns 40, his prostate begins to enlarge as a natural physiological response to aging. An enlarged prostate is called benign prostatic hyperplasia, or BPH. As the prostate grows, it can be more difficult to urinate, since an enlarged prostate constricts the urethra. However, medication such as Proscar or Hytrin can shrink the prostate to make urination easier. Urinary difficulties may also result from a condition known as acute urinary retention. This can be caused by over-the-counter cold preparations or prescription drugs, including antidepressants such as Elavil; calcium channel blockers such as verapamil, which are used to treat hypertension; and anticholenergics, or bowel, relaxants including Levsinex.

Though it may be easy for you to ignore your prostate, especially if you're not having trouble with it, I feel that every yearly physical should include an examination of your prostate. Most doctors agree. The issue surrounding surgery for prostate cancer, however, is more controversial; some physicians feel that removing the cancer when it first appears serves both as a curative and a preventive, while others take a more conservative position, feeling that a wait-and-see stance with regular checkups to monitor the progress of the cancer is important. Although most prostate cancers take years to develop, in some cases the cancer can develop within a matter of months.

If you have a family history of prostate cancer, get regular checkups and tests for BPH, including a digital exam of your prostate by your physician. The use of a screening test, such as a prostatic-specific antigen, or PSA, test, is still controversial, and its results are unproven.

Whenever I feel a hard nodule in a patient's prostate, I refer him to a urologist, even if he has no signs of urinary problems. The urologist will use a sonogram to check for cancer and will take a biopsy—which is a totally safe procedure—if he strongly suspects the presence of cancer. The biopsy is done either in the urologist's office or in the hospital on an outpatient basis.

If you have an enlarged prostate with no signs of cancer, taking 5 milligrams of Proscar once a day for at least six weeks can help keep your symptoms manageable. Also, your doctor may suggest that you take Hytrin, a mild antihypertensive medication that can have the immediate benefit of reducing the effect an enlarged prostate has on urinary retention. You'll usually start a regimen of Hytrin with a dosage of 1 milligram each day and slowly build it up to 5. Unlike with intestinal cancer or breast cancer, there's not much you can do to lower your risk of prostate cancer, such as changing your diet.

A great deal of evidence shows that men who have prostate cancer do extremely well, even when it has spread. The most common therapy uses the hormone estrogen; what's curious is that a form of cancer that only men get is treated with a female hormone, while breast cancer is typically treated with tamoxifen, a form of male hormone. The side effects of hormone treatment for prostate cancer include a loss of sexual desire and an increase in breast size.

In the meantime, take this test so you can get a clear idea of your risk for BPH:

Over the last month or so, how many times did you most typically get up to urinate from the time you went to bed at night until the time you got up in the morning?

0 1 2 3 4 5 or more times

0 = Not at all

1 = Less than 20%

2 = Less than 50%

3 = 50%

4 = More than 50%

5 = Almost always

Over the past month or so, how often have you had a sensation of not emptying your bladder completely after you finished urinating?

0 1 2 3 4 5

Over the past month or so, how often have you had to urinate again less than two hours after you finished urinating?

0 1 2 3 4 5

Over the past month or so, how often have you found that you stopped and started again several times when you urinated?

0 1 2 3 4 5

Over the past month or so, how often have you found it difficult to postpone urination?

0 1 2 3 4 5

Over the past month or so, how often have
you had a weak urinary stream?

                                                    0 1 2 3 4 5

Over the past month or so, how often have
you had to push or strain to begin urination?

                                                    0 1 2 3 4 5

Add up your answers.

If you scored from 1 to 7 points, you have a mild case of BPH.

If you scored from 8 to 19, you have a moderate case of BPH.

If you scored from 20 to 35, you have a severe case of BPH.

BODY SIGNAL ALERT

URINATION, DIFFICULTY IN

Description and Possible Medical Problems

If you frequently have trouble urinating and sometimes find that it's
almost impossible unless you turn on both faucets in the sink (plus the
shower), chances are you have a problem with your prostate (see sidebar: "The Prostate"). This is one of the most common diseases of men
over 50. Many times, however, the condition is temporary and caused by
cold medications or blood pressure pills.

Treatment

If you are having trouble urinating, you need to see your doctor or urologist. He will conduct a full physical exam, take blood tests, ask you if
your father had a severe case of prostate disease, and do a digital exam
to check the degree of the enlargement. In this procedure, the physician will insert a gloved finger into the rectum in order to feel the
prostate. He may also elect to do a sonogram to get an image of the
enlarged prostate and maybe even take a biopsy if he suspects cancer.

If you have an enlarged prostate, your doctor will prescribe Proscar, which will shrink your prostate and make it easier for you to urinate. If, however, you have prostate cancer, your doctor will take one of several different routes. He may decide to wait it out and regularly monitor the growth, or he may choose to perform a transurethral prostate resection, which, in effect, creates more room for the urethra by removing the part of the prostate that is constricting it. In rare cases, where the cancer is in an advanced stage, he may want to remove the prostate to prevent the cancer from spreading throughout your body.

Even though the idea of prostate cancer can be daunting, rest assured that the vast majority of men who have prostate cancer eventually die of another cause: old age.

Special Mention for the Elderly

A total inability to urinate usually affects men who are in their 70s and older. If an elderly male relative is unable to urinate and feels a pain in his groin, he should head for the emergency room immediately. This condition is called acute urinary retention and is most often caused when an enlarged prostate totally obstructs the bladder.

Your relative's doctor will first look for causes that are easily reversible, such as over-the-counter cold preparations, antihypertensive medication, antidepressants, or any new medication he's started taking recently. These are the most common causes of acute urinary retention; the prostate may already be enlarged, but other medications can make it even larger.

The first thing the physician will do is to place a thin rubber tube called a Foley catheter through the penis and into the bladder, which will bring immediate relief. The subsequent treatment will include a full prostate exam and the tests described previously. The Foley catheter will be removed after a day or so, when normal urination has resumed.

URINATION, FREQUENT

Description and Possible Medical Problems

Not only can an enlarged prostate make it more difficult to urinate, it can have the opposite effect, making you need to urinate more frequently. Since you're never able to empty your bladder fully, you'll prob-ably feel the urge to urinate more often because the signals that a full bladder sends to your brain remain the same.

Besides an enlarged prostate, also known as BPH (benign prostatic hyperplasia), another cause of more frequent urination can be diabetes; in fact, this is one of the first symptoms a person with adult onset dia-betes has.

Treatment

If you have a sensation of needing to urinate more frequently, see your doctor or urologist. He will take blood tests to rule out diabetes and perhaps check your prostate by examining it manually with a gloved fin-ger and perhaps a sonogram, which will allow him to determine the degree of enlargement.

If he suspects that diabetes is the cause, he will do a blood test to confirm the disease. If you do have diabetes, your doctor will design a program of diet and exercise and start you on insulin if he believes it is necessary.

BODY SIGNAL ALERT

URINE, BLOODY

Description and Possible Medical Problems

Anytime you notice blood suddenly appear in a place where you don't expect it, it can be startling. If it appears during urination, most of us would immediately call the doctor.

The fact is that when the blood appears in the urine stream can tell you what kind of problem you have. If you see blood when you first start to urinate, it's often a sign of a sore or infection in the penis, possibly caused by a sexually transmitted disease. If the blood shows up in the middle of urination, you may have a prostate problem. Or, if blood shows up as you're completing urination, it may mean that the problem is due to a bladder infection. Blood in the urine might be a sign of a bladder tumor or a symptom of an underlying urinary tract infection.

However, the most common cause of blood in the urine, no matter where it appears in the stream, is a kidney stone. The stone causes irritation in the urinary tract, which, in turn, causes bleeding. The amount of blood can be undetectable, or it may be obvious. Another sign of a kidney stone is a pain in the back that radiates into the groin and penis.

Treatment

If you have blood in your urine, regardless of where it appears, you'll need to see your doctor or urologist. He will do a blood test and take a urine sample to confirm the diagnosis based on your Body Signals. If he believes you have a sexually transmitted disease, he will check the secretion from the penis to make sure, then treat you with a round of antibiotics such as doxycycline or something else, as indicated. To treat a bladder or urinary tract infection, antibiotics are also necessary, though your doctor will also want to run additional tests to check for either a tumor in the bladder or a urinary tract infection. (Unlike women, though, men rarely get urinary tract infections.) To do this, he may want to refer you to a urologist, who will perform a cystoscopy, which will help him look directly at the inside of the bladder with a fiber-optic microscope, which will allow him to check for a tumor or infection. This procedure is usually performed on an outpatient basis, and you will need local anesthesia.

If, however, your doctor believes you have a bladder tumor, he will use a cystoscope to evaluate the cause of the bleeding. It might be a polyp, which can be removed surgically, or cancer, which is treated with a combination of anticoagulant therapy and chemotherapy.

One of my 49-year-old patients came to see me after noticing blood in his urine. After I ruled out an infection and kidney stone, the results of a cystoscopy revealed a small tumor in the bladder. My patient had the tumor removed in the hospital, during which time a tube was place in his bladder, via the penis, to keep the bladder clean and wash out any debris left over by the surgery. My patient didn't need any follow-up chemotherapy or radiation. Today—five years later—he sees his urologist yearly for routine checkups and an in-office cystoscopy and is doing terrific!

For prostate disease, your doctor will treat you with a medication such as Proscar and perhaps surgery.

See also sidebar: "The Prostate."

See also "Pain in One Side of Hip Running to Genitalia" in Chapter 10.

URINE, CHANGE IN STREAM OF

Description and Possible Medical Problems

One of the advantages men have over women when it comes to biology is the ability to urinate easily in inconvenient venues. Of course, there are some women who would disagree with me, who think this ability spoils men because there's no need for them to learn how to "hold it" on long car trips as women have to. Despite this argument, one clear advantage in my eyes is that it means that men are easily able to observe their urine stream; if it changes in some way, it can indicate an underlying illness.

For instance, the stream may split into two; this is often a sign of a kidney stone. Other symptoms may include pain in the groin and blood in the urine. A change in the urine stream can also be a sign of prostate problems; the number one symptom is needing more time than usual to urinate. As a doctor, one of the ways I check my prostate is at sporting events. When all of the men are lined up at the urinals, I'm always amazed how quick the young men are compared to the older men.

However, though a slower stream doesn't necessarily mean there's a problem, if you find you have urine dribbling from your penis after you thought you were through or you're unable to hold your urine for longer periods of time, you may have prostate disease. Sometimes, however, the fact that you make a great companion on long car trips because you don't have to stop every hour to find a patch of bushes may also be a sign of an enlarged prostate that's causing urinary retention.

See also sidebar: "The Prostate."

Treatment

Any change in your urine stream is a sign that you should see your doctor or urologist. If you have a kidney stone, your doctor will prescribe painkillers to help decrease the pain without interfering with or prolonging the process of passing the stone. He may also suggest a process called lithotripsy, which uses underwater ultrasound waves to break up the stone.

If you think you're having prostate problems with an enlarged prostate, you should make an appointment with a urologist, since early treatment of benign prostatic hyperplasia, or BPH, could prevent it from turning into prostate cancer down the road. To treat BPH, your doctor may take a wait-and-see attitude, but since you are already showing a symptom of BPH by a change in your urine stream, he may decide to begin treatment, first with the medication Proscar, which shrinks the prostate. If the medication does not have much effect, he may opt for a surgical procedure called a transurethral prostate resection, in which the parts of the prostate that are constricting the flow of urine are surgically removed to take the pressure off the urethra.

The resection is successful in most cases, but if the prostate continues to grow, there's a chance the operation may have to be repeated when urination again becomes difficult.

Chapter 16

LIMBS, JOINTS, AND MUSCLES

BODY SIGNAL ALERT

Call your doctor immediately if you experience any of the following symptoms:

SYMPTOM	POSSIBLE MEDICAL CONDITION
You suddenly lose the ability to move your arms	Stroke
Your shoulder is painful and you're unable to move it	Bursitis
You don't have enough strength to brush your hair, and you also have a feeling of malaise	Polymyalgia rheumatica
You experience pain in your shoulder during a walk or other exertion; the pain goes away on rest	Angina
You lose strength in your shoulders and hips, and a purple rash appears on your arms and wrists	Dermatomyositis
You suddenly lose the ability to move your legs	Stroke
Your calf becomes tender and painful	Deep-vein thrombosis
Your leg becomes red and inflamed	Cellulitis
You are unable to walk and have severe pain that starts in your back and radiates to your buttocks; you also lose some of the feeling in your legs	Sciatica
	Sciatica
You notice that the skin on your legs begins to break down	Vascular ulcer

---

HOW THE ARMS, LEGS,
AND MUSCLES AGE

As I talk with my midlife and older patients about how aging affects their bodies, I find that one of their most common complaints is how they find it increasingly difficult to keep pace with the busy lives they lead. In fact, the medical problems that bring patients into the office more often than any other illness involve limitations of movement and their concern that they're not able to run around as easily as before. The enormous sums of money that are spent on prescription medications, over-the-counter preparations, physical therapy, and surgery that promise to help us stay mobile attest to the frustration we feel when we can't move freely.

Many of these mobility problems are due to one of several kinds of arthritis—osteoarthritis and rheumatoid arthritis among them—and the related health problems that stem from these diseases. In fact, as many as 60 percent of the population over 55 report having a form of arthritis, whether it's mild or severe.

Arthritis is not the only disorder that affects our ability to stay mobile. Certain skin disorders and diseases of the heart, lungs, kidneys, and vascular system affect us as well, and aging affects the movements of our joints, ligaments, and muscles: the ligaments become less elastic, and the muscles lose some of their strength as a result of the decrease in muscle mass that is inevitable as we age—even in bodybuilders. No matter what, the best way to keep the joints, ligaments, and muscles in top working order, despite the effects of age, is to remain active and get some exercise every day.

A SPECIAL WORD ABOUT SYMPTOMS
AFFECTING YOUR ARMS AND LEGS

Whether you're having a problem with your arms or your legs, it's extremely important with any of the Body Signals in this chapter that you determine if the symptom appears equally on both sides of the body or affects only one side. When you're examining your symptoms, you should always notice the changes in size, temperature, color, and feeling that you're experiencing. As with any Body

Signal, your input can help your doctor arrive at the proper diagnosis and treatment.

The arms are not as prone to vascular diseases as the legs are. The most important question to ask is whether the problem is limited to a specific joint or occurring throughout the whole arm. For instance, numbness of the arm in one small area points to a different problem—the possibility of a compressed nerve, for example—than numbness of the entire arm, which is a sign of a stroke. It is essential to tell your doctor whether the problem is limited to one area or affects the entire limb.

The legs serve as the major support system for the body. As I've mentioned, a gradual decrease in muscle mass is normal with aging, but this decrease will not affect your ability to walk, except that you may need to slow down a little. However, the effects of chronic illnesses such as heart disease, arthritis, and neurological problems all seem to have a common denominator in that they gradually lead to an inability to use the legs. Therefore, one way to take care of your legs is to take care of your overall health, especially if you are prone to some of these illnesses.

As with the arms, in order to determine a diagnosis, you and your doctor need to know if the Body Signal is showing up in both legs or only one. You should also take care to notice any other changes in your mobility—for instance, if you suddenly find it more difficult to rise up out of a chair easily or it becomes more difficult to walk.

If one of your Body Signals is a swelling in the legs, there are three important things to consider. First, does the swelling appear in only one leg or in both? Second, when you push on the swollen area with your thumb, does an indentation remain when you remove your thumb? And third, has the swelling appeared suddenly, or has it been around for a long time?

If one leg begins to swell up, it may be a sign of phlebitis, in which a vein in the leg becomes blocked, or recurrence of an old case of deep-vein thrombosis, a condition in which a blood clot forms and can block a blood vessel. A swollen leg may also be a sign of a blockage in the abdominal cavity, such as a tumor that is pressing on the major vein. In addition, sometimes during a post-surgical period, especially after any kind of gynecological surgery, the lymphatic system can become blocked, which can cause a leg to swell up.

Sudden swelling of both legs can be an indication of either phlebitis or cellulitis, a skin infection. If, however, the swelling appears gradually, it may be a sign of an underlying kidney disease or the water accumulation that frequently occurs in cases of heart failure. In addition, if you have a history of phlebitis, the veins in your legs might have become damaged to the extent that body water begins to leak into the legs. This condition, which is known as postphlebitic syndrome, results in chronic swelling that is helped with the use of diuretics, surgical stockings, and elevation of the legs.

You should also compare the color and temperature of both of your legs and pay attention to whether old shoes or dress shoes that you don't wear very often are now tight. Also, look for obvious skin marks that are left by socks and shoes, since these can be an indication of water retention, which is often a sign of heart failure.

BODY SIGNAL ALERT

ARM, SUDDEN LOSS OF USE OF

Description and Possible Medical Problems

If you suddenly lose the ability to use your arms, it can be a scary thing. Most often, it is a sign of a stroke, which is caused when the blood supply to part of the brain is interrupted by a blockage or clot. Typically, a stroke affects only one side of the body, such as one arm, or an arm and leg on the same side, or even the face, arm, and leg.

Treatment

If you think you have had a stroke, you will need to see your doctor, who will do a complete medical history and physical exam and run some blood tests to check for problems that are easy to treat. These include blood sugar that is too high or too low, coronary disease, or a sodium-potassium imbalance, which frequently occurs in people who take diuretics.

This topic is covered in more detail in "Confusion, Acute" in Chapter 3.

ARMS, STIFFNESS AND PAIN IN, WORSENED BY USE, HELPED BY REST

See "Fingers, Change in Flexibility of" in Chapter 17.

CALF, BROWNISH DISCOLORATION OF

Description and Possible Medical Problems

Even though we know it's not good for us to bask in the sun, many people still strive to develop a deep, rich tan all over.

However, if you don't make a habit of sunbathing and your calves become brownish in color all on their own, it's probably a side effect of long-term heart failure. If this is the case, you probably experience chronic leg swelling and recurrent phlebitis. Due to the weakened blood vessels and poor circulation, blood slowly leaks out of the vessels, resulting in the brownish pigmentation of the skin.

Treatment

Although the brownish discoloration of the calves due to phlebitis or heart failure is not a health problem in itself and is essentially a cosmetic problem, there is no treatment for the condition besides wearing trousers or flesh-colored stockings.

CALF, CRAMP IN

Description and Possible Medical Problems

Your grandfather may have called it a charley horse, but you call it a painful cramp. Everyone has had a cramp in the calf appear suddenly and for no apparent reason. It may happen when you're sitting or driving and holding your foot on the accelerator for several hours, or it can wake you from a deep sleep. It can also appear during or after exercise; dehydration is a common cause.

No matter what the cause, the affected muscle will feel tight and hard, and though you know it will feel better to stretch, the cramp is so painful that you can barely move your leg.

Leg cramps frequently occur in pregnant women and in people who are taking diuretics, since these water pills frequently cause a loss of potassium from the body. (A low level of potassium in the body can also cause constipation, weakness, and an irregular heartbeat.)

Treatment

If you feel a cramp suddenly occur in your calf, you can try to stretch it out manually or by walking. If it's too painful to manage, try massaging your leg and the cramped area.

If your leg cramps frequently wake you in the middle of the night, you can try raising the foot of your bed or taking an over-the-counter medication such as Qval. If you are taking diuretics, you may want to take a potassium supplement to replace some of the potassium you're losing. These preparations come in pill, liquid, and powder form. However, since any potassium supplement can be potentially corrosive to the digestive system, some precautions are in order. I recommend that my patients use a coated potassium pill such as Slow-K or Micro-K or a granulated potassium supplement that is dissolved in orange juice. Your doctor will determine the best dosage for you, and you should never take all of your potassium pills at once if you have missed taking them for a day or so. Also, be sure to drink plenty of water each day, since dehydration can cause leg cramps in some people.

If cramps occur during exercise, it may help to stretch before and after each exercise session to loosen up the muscles and prevent them from tightening up.

BODY SIGNAL ALERT

CALF, SWOLLEN, PAINFUL WHEN WALKING

Description and Possible Medical Problems

Sometimes, after a hard workout, your calves will feel painful, but it's the kind of good ache that shows your muscles have been stressed so that they can become even stronger.

However, if your calf swells up and feels painful all over when walking and when you touch it, you may have a serious condition known as deep-vein thrombosis, which occurs when a blood clot forms in one of the main veins in the leg. Though such a clot is initially harmless, if it loosens from the side of the vein and begins to travel through the vein, it can eventually migrate to the lung and form a pulmonary embolus, which can block the flow of blood returning to the heart. People who are prone to developing a pulmonary embolus include those who are overweight and who smoke, as well as women who take hormonal birth control preparations.

Treatment

If your doctor thinks you have deep-vein thrombosis, she will first perform a physical exam to confirm that you do have the condition. She will also recommend that you be hospitalized so that a number of tests can be performed to determine the extent of the thrombosis. She will administer a Doppler test in addition to a test called a venogram, in which a special dye is injected into your foot before an X ray is done to check the location and size of the clot.

An anticoagulant medication such as heparin will be prescribed. This will be followed by a six-month regimen of another anticoagulant, Coumadin.

See also "Confusion, Acute" in Chapter 3.

ELBOW PAIN THAT IS SLOW TO HEAL

Description and Possible Medical Problems

You don't have to play tennis to get tennis elbow, a form of tendinitis in which you'll have a pain on the outside of your elbow that may run down your forearm. And you don't have to be a star pitcher to have pitcher's elbow, which is what you'll have when the pain appears on the inside of your elbow. In fact, many people today get tennis or pitcher's elbow from other activities, such as gardening and painting. The fact is that tennis elbow is a form of tendinitis called lateral epicondylitis and tends to appear when a repeated activity causes the tendons to become inflamed and microscopic tears to appear in them. Pitcher's elbow is known as medial epicondylitis.

Treatment

If you have tendinitis on either the inside or the outside of your elbow, you'll need to rest your arm for a few weeks and refrain from the activity or sport you believe caused the condition. Wearing an Ace bandage around your elbow will keep it stable and serve as a reminder to take it easy. Putting an ice pack on the area at night will also help reduce the inflammation.

Tendinitis takes a while to heal compared to other minor injuries, since it's difficult to immobilize the affected area totally. If the pain doesn't go away after a few weeks or gets worse, you should see your doctor, who will do an X ray to make sure you haven't sprained or fractured your elbow or forearm. She may decide to inject a corticosteroid medication like prednisone directly into the elbow for fast relief from the pain and swelling.

To prevent future problems with tendinitis in the elbow, some people find that wearing an elastic support wrap on the arm just below the elbow during activity will decrease the amount of strain on the tendons and therefore keep them from becoming inflamed again.

HEEL PAIN WHEN WALKING

Description and Possible Medical Problems

As you grow older, you've probably noticed the occasional slight aches and pains that seem to surface during the first few minutes of exercise and then fade away as your joints and muscles begin to move smoothly. Those same aches and pains may surface again the next morning as you get out of bed, but, once you start moving, they should go away.

However, if you have a pain in the back of your ankle at the heel that appears after you start to move or walk, it's probably not caused by the aches and pains of aging. Instead, you probably have Achilles tendinitis, an inflammation of the largest tendon in your body.

Achilles tendinitis is most common among people who are active; hard and regular exercise can cause small tears to form in the tendon, and these can be painful.

Treatment

If you think you have Achilles tendinitis, you'll need to stop exercising for at least a couple of weeks to allow the tendon to heal. Applying an ice pack to your heel can also ease the pain and inflammation; taking aspirin can also help. Your doctor will do an X ray of your foot and ask about your recent exercise habits. She may decide to inject a corticosteroid preparation such as prednisone directly into the area to reduce the pain and inflammation.

After the tendon has healed and you return to exercise, you'll need to adjust your habits to make sure the tendinitis doesn't return. Cutting down on the amount of exercise you get or switching from running to walking or swimming will also reduce your chances of reinjuring the tendon. Changing the kind of running shoes you wear or inserting an orthotic appliance into your shoe to elevate your heel and take some of the stress off your tendon is worth trying, too.

HIP PAIN

See "Fingers, Change in Flexibility of" in Chapter 17.
See "Shoulder, Pain in, with an Inability to Raise It" below.

BODY SIGNAL ALERT

INABILITY TO WALK WITH LOSS OF FEELING IN THE LEG

Description and Possible Medical Problems

Sciatica is a condition in which the sciatic nerve, which runs the length of the hamstring and through to the foot, becomes swollen and leads to pain and numbness in the leg. It is often due to a slipped disc, which occurs when one of the discs in your back that serve as cushions between the vertebrae either ruptures or bulges out and presses on one of the nerves that originate in the spine. This can occur due to age, overexertion, or a sudden twisting of your body.

Treatment

In many instances, a slipped disc that's responsible for sciatic pain may heal on its own. Doctors recommend bed rest, aspirin, and patience.

This topic is covered in more detail in "Pain in Lower Back with Numbness in Buttock and Leg" in Chapter 10.

KNEE, PAIN AND SWELLING IN, BECOMES WORSE AS DAY PROGRESSES

See "Fingers, Change in Flexibility of" in Chapter 17.

KNEE, PAIN IN, ESPECIALLY AFTER SPORTS ACTIVITY

Description and Possible Medical Problems

The knee may not be among the body parts that's injured most often, but it can be the most debilitating when it is.

To get an idea of all the things that can go awry with the knee, first consider its construction. The thighbone, or femur, joins with the shinbone, or tibia, at the kneecap, which is also known as the patella. In between the femur and tibia are two large discs of cartilage called the lateral meniscus and the medial meniscus. The femur fits into a groove in the kneecap and is quite content to move up and down within that groove, with the cartilage acting as a shock absorber. Content, that is, until something goes wrong.

The cartilage, specifically the meniscus, is the most often injured part of the body in sports, especially among women, since their naturally wider hips make them more susceptible to knee injuries. The thighbones of wider-hipped athletes connect to the knees at an angle, instead of lining up directly over the shins and feet, and that places added stress on the joint that can cause strain or damage.

In the less-than-ideal reality of participant sports, the kneecap is often jarred off its path, leading me to think of a bobsled run: sometimes it runs smoothly and easily, while at other times the "sled" goes from side to side and creates a lot of friction. In this condition, called patellofemoral dysfunction, the kneecap goes off center or even completely out of its groove at the end of the thighbone.

Treatment

Once a diagnosis is made regarding the knee's status, treatment can take one of many forms. Since the knee is an easily damaged joint, you should see your doctor, who will probably take an X ray of the knee and manually examine the knee as well as the way you're walking. She will tell you to rest the knee and take aspirin or Advil to ease the pain and inflammation.

If, however, your doctor determines that your X rays reveal a torn meniscus that requires surgery to remove, you will undergo arthroscopic surgery, which involves inserting a stainless steel surgical tube through a tiny incision at the side of the kneecap and suctioning the torn cartilage out. This popular operation has enabled people to indulge in their chosen sport within a week after surgery, if not the next day.

Tips and Precautions

Preventing knee injury consists of two components: warm-up and conditioning. Walking rapidly for five minutes will serve as a warm-up before your regular exercise session, and being in shape will give you sufficient strength to get through your workout. Injury occurs most often when you're tired or when you push past your energy reserves.

Stretching the hamstrings and other joints that surround the knee will also lessen the chance of injury to the knee. And if you strengthen the inside of the quadricep, or thigh muscle, with a combination of stretching and walking, it'll pave the way for smoothing the movement of the femur within the groove of the kneecap.

GOOD PAIN, BAD PAIN

Every amateur athlete—runner, cyclist, swimmer—knows about pain. Even those old-fashioned stalwarts who still subscribe to the "No pain, no gain" theory realize that pain comes in a variety of gradients and flavors. But to me there are only two kinds: good pain and bad pain.

Basically, the two kinds of pain can be categorized as muscle and joint—respectively, "good" and "bad." Muscle pain feels dull, like a strain, and can make any kind of activity uncomfortable. This kind of pain, which is "good," is the body's response to hard exercise, which the muscles need in order to get stronger. Often, with muscle pain, no single spot hurts; you'll simply feel an over-all ache. This is the only type of pain you should ever attempt to exercise through. Even then, you should proceed with caution.

Joint pain, on the other hand, is sharp and prevents you from achieving a full range of motion. Trying to exercise through joint pain is foolish and counterproductive. It will only worsen until you have no choice but to stop. Joint pain can be an indication of an underlying injury that without treatment—including rest—could well develop into a severe problem.

Some of the different kinds of pains runners get, for example, including shinsplints and tendinitis, can be ambiguous, and it's important to know how to approach such problems. A shinsplint, for instance, can be a warning of an impending stress fracture, a very serious injury. When in doubt, of course, it is better to be overly cautious.

There will also be times when you will be unable to diagnose your injury accurately because it combines, say, joint pain and tendinitis. In this case, you should see your doctor.

In the first place, people's individual perceptions of pain vary widely, and such variations can influence both training and treatment. For instance, one question that often gets asked is: Do men and women feel pain in different degrees? I believe that's a loaded question. For the most part, men and women feel the same degree of pain but may verbalize it differently because of individual past experiences of pain such as childbirth and cultural upbringing. There are some cultures that are more stoic than others vis a vis pain.

However, I do feel that perceptions can differ between novice exercisers and those who have been at it for years. Novices haven't suffered injuries before and haven't had to deal with rehabilitation and treatment, so they're more apt to be obsessed with the pain, while experienced athletes realize that pain goes with the turf; they're also more likely to give an injury time to heal.

The role of endorphins in combating pain has garnered a good deal of attention in the sports medicine community. One explanation for the role of endorphins has come to be known as the gate theory. Back in the early 1980s, two researchers from Canada and

London discovered that there are little "gates" in the brain that pass on the sensation of pain. However, according to the theory, if something else reaches them first, such as the endorphins produced by aerobic exercise, the gates will close and the pain messages won't reach the brain.

The gate theory is all very neat and logical, but some physicians believe that the concept of endorphins is totally overrated and that the gate theory is really just a framework to help us understand pain.

The lesson, then, is that while your chosen sport may hurt "so good," it should never hurt "so bad." The trick is to keep in touch with your body and to understand the often subtle differences in the signals it is sending you, because ignoring them can lead to disaster.

BODY SIGNAL ALERT

LACK OF STRENGTH IN ARMS WITH FEELING OF MALAISE

Description and Possible Medical Problems

If you feel as though you've lost most of the strength in your arms and you feel a sense of malaise, you may have a condition known as polymyalgia rheumatica, a disease that occurs when the blood vessels in the musculoskeletal system become inflamed. Polymyalgia rheumatica affects mostly women over the age of 50. In addition to the muscular ache and weakness, you may also have a low-grade fever and weight loss.

Treatment

If you have these symptoms, you should see your doctor. If she determines that you do have polymyalgia rheumatica, she will probably prescribe the corticosteroid prednisone to help reduce pain and inflammation.

This topic is covered in more detail in "Backache with Weakness" in Chapter 10.

BODY SIGNAL ALERT

LACK OF STRENGTH IN SHOULDERS AND HIPS WITH DEEP RED RASH ON ARMS AND WRISTS

Description and Possible Medical Problems

Muscle ache that's accompanied by weakness is a common occurrence. But if you have a constant dull ache in the muscles around your shoulders and/or the backs of your hips and you don't have the strength you once did, you may have a rare, progressive disease called polymyositis. This disorder is a variation of dermatomyositis, in which the muscle pain and lack of strength are frequently accompanied by a rash, which is a deep red and may be scaly. The rash most often appears around the eyes and on the neck, chest, hands, and elbows.

Both polymyositis and dermatomyositis are arthritic disorders, but they primarily affect the muscles, which become inflamed and swollen in both diseases, and not the joints, as other forms of arthritis do. Doctors believe that polymyositis and dermatomyositis are caused by a defect in the immune system.

Treatment

If your doctor discovers you have polymyositis, dermatomyositis, or polymyalgia rheumatica, he will probably prescribe the corticosteroid prednisone to help reduce pain and inflammation. Prednisone will also help lessen the rash and inflammation that accompany dermatomyositis. Prednisone works by increasing the body's tolerance to the inflammation in the blood vessels and tissues, thus alleviating the symptoms.

This is covered in more detail in "Backache with Weakness" in Chapter 10.

BODY SIGNAL ALERT

LEG, PAINFUL, SWOLLEN, AND RED

Description and Possible Medical Problems

If you've ever had a skin infection, you know what to look for: red, broken skin, perhaps with some discharge. Cellulitis is a condition in which an infection appears underneath the skin; your calf will become swollen and red with shiny skin that is painful to the touch. You may also have a fever.

Cellulitis can form in response to an insect bite or as a result of poor circulation, which is a sign of heart failure.

Treatment

If you think you have cellulitis, you should see your doctor, who will perform a physical examination with a particular eye toward ruling out deep-vein thrombosis, which is a serious medical condition (see "Calf, Swollen, Painful When Walking" above for more details).

To treat cellulitis, you will need to be hospitalized for about a week. You will be treated with warm soaks and an intravenous antibiotic, either penicillin or oxacillin. You will also need to rest during your stay in the hospital as well as for a week or two after you return home. You will probably also continue to take antibiotics while you are recuperating.

BODY SIGNAL ALERT

LEG, SUDDEN LOSS OF USE OF

See "Arm, Sudden Loss of Use of" above.

BODY SIGNAL ALERT

LEG ULCER (OPEN SORE)

Description and Possible Medical Problems

You're probably familiar with ulcers in your stomach. But did you know that you can also develop an ulcer on your leg, where the skin actually begins to break down? This is called a vascular ulcer.

People who have chronic heart failure, vascular failure due to arteriosclerosis, or diabetes are prone to developing an ulcer on the leg, since these diseases reduce the flow of blood to the legs, eventually causing the skin to break. This can cause the retained water that is common to these diseases to ooze out of the leg, forming an ulcer. If the ulcerated skin becomes infected, cellulitis, a serious skin disorder, can develop.

Treatment

If you think you have a leg ulcer, you should see your doctor, who will conduct a complete history and physical exam. This may also include a vascular test of the legs to test your circulation.

Treatment for a leg ulcer will be for the underlying disease as well as the ulcer itself. To help the ulcer heal, your doctor may prescribe antibiotics, frequent meticulous cleaning, special dressings, and special boots called Una boots. Your doctor may also recommend that you have an arteriogram done to help determine if you can improve the blood flow to your legs, which will reduce your chances of additional ulcers forming.

LEGS, SWOLLEN, WITH PROMINENT VEINS, USUALLY NOT PAINFUL

Description and Possible Medical Problems

Out of all the changes the aging process incurs on the body, the one many women fear most is the appearance of varicose veins: prominent, enlarged veins that appear in the legs. Though people in their 20s can have varicose veins, the condition is more common among midlife and older adults, particularly women. In addition, people who spend a lot of hours on their feet are more prone to developing varicose veins.

Varicose veins are the result of faulty valves in the veins in the legs. The valves typically help to send blood back to the heart from the legs. However, when the valves become strained or stretched or damaged in some way, the blood flows back down into the vein, where it collects and builds up pressure. The vein, in turn, becomes distended and twisted, making it visible through the skin.

Since varicose veins are more of a cosmetic annoyance than a real health problem, many people learn to live with them. Usually, varicose veins are painless. Sometimes, however, an ulcer will form in the vein near the ankle or on the skin because of the great decrease in circulation. This results in an undernourished vein or patch of skin where an ulcer can form.

They may also swell up. The vein itself may become painful, the skin on the ankle near the valve may begin to itch, and your entire leg may become swollen. Most women with varicose veins find they experience these severe symptoms a few days before their periods; the rest of the time, they're not particularly bothered by their varicose veins.

Treatment

If you have varicose veins, it's a good idea to stay off your feet as much as you can, in order to reduce the pressure in your veins and keep them from becoming more prominent. When you do have to stand for a long period of time, it's a good idea to wear elastic support stockings, which will help compress the veins and prevent excess blood from collecting in them, as well as provide extra pressure to help pump the blood back into the vein toward the heart. As much as possible, keep your legs elevated to reduce the work your veins have to do as well as the pressure in the veins.

When the varicose veins become very prominent and painful and ulcers may form, your doctor may suggest you undergo surgery to remove them from your legs, a procedure commonly called stripping the veins. The circulation in your legs will not be affected, since the smaller remaining veins will quickly grow in size in order to assume the responsibility of the vein that was removed, supplying the leg with blood before sending it back to the heart.

The recovery period after the operation will be about six weeks. During recuperation and after, your doctor will recommend that you walk as much as possible to circulate the blood through the legs and wear support stockings.

BODY SIGNAL ALERT

SHOULDER, PAIN IN DURING EXERCISE, DISAPPEARS WITH REST

Description and Possible Medical Problems

If you're not accustomed to regular exercise, on those occasions when you do exert yourself, such as walking up a flight of stairs, you may feel a generalized pressure in your shoulder that passes when you sit down and catch your breath again. You may decide it's probably due to your sedentary ways.

This is a classic symptom of angina pectoris, a sign of arteriosclerosis.

Treatment

If you think you have angina pectoris, you should see your doctor. He will give you a physical exam and ask you questions about the nature and frequency of the pressure in your chest. If the pressure and your other symptoms have been occurring frequently, he may recommend that you be hospitalized to prevent an impending heart attack.

This is covered in more detail in "Chest Pressure When Walking, with Sweating or Shortness of Breath" in Chapter 11.

BODY SIGNAL ALERT

SHOULDER, PAIN IN, WITH AN INABILITY TO RAISE THE ARM

Description and Possible Medical Problems

Okay, the weekend's here, and now it's time to make up for five whole days of relative inactivity. Racquetball after work Friday night, touch football on Saturday morning, and you promised to clean off those high shelves in the basement in the afternoon—when suddenly you're sidelined. Halfway through your list of activities, to your dismay, you find you cannot raise your arm because every time you try, you feel a sharp pain in your shoulder.

Secretly, you may be pleased—you really didn't want to spend part of your weekend cleaning out the basement—but it also means that your fishing trip on Sunday is impossible. So you start thinking of quick ways to heal your shoulder.

Not so fast. It sounds as though you have a classic case of bursitis, a condition in which the bursa, a sac filled with a small amount of fluid that helps cushion your joints, becomes inflamed and totally fills with fluid. Because the sac is inflamed, anytime a joint moves near it, you'll feel a sharp pain. Also, because the inflamed sac takes up more room than usual, it is difficult to move your arm or shoulder.

Bursitis is most often caused by an injury to the area or sudden overuse of the joint. Though it is commonly referred to the shoulder, bursitis can also appear in the knee, hip, elbow, or anywhere there is a bursa to minimize the friction between joints. For example, when the bursa that surrounds your elbow becomes inflamed and fills with fluid, the condition is called olecranon bursitis.

Because bursitis is common in certain occupations, some interesting names for bursitis have cropped up, depending on the area of the body. For instance, there's housemaid's knee and miner's elbow, as well as weaver's bottom, which is actually a form of bursitis in the hip.

Treatment

If you think you have bursitis, try taking aspirin or Advil to relieve the pain and reduce the swelling of the bursa. Ice packs can also help reduce the swelling. Also, try to rest your shoulder until you are able to move it through your full range of motion. The bursitis will usually clear up in a week with these treatment methods. However, if your shoulder is still painful and your range of motion is still limited after a week, you should see your doctor, who will examine your shoulder and check your range of motion. She will probably inject a corticosteroid medication directly into the bursa to relieve the pain and decrease the swelling instantly.

Once you've had a bout with bursitis in your shoulder, you may find that if you repeat the same patterns of overuse, the bursitis will probably come back. The best way to prevent future problems with bursitis is not to be so gung ho with weekend activities, rather to ease into them instead. Better yet, make it a point to exercise regularly during the week, and your bursitis will probably be a thing of the past.

A person who needs to limit the movement of the elbow while a bout of olecranon bursitis clears up, may find that an Ace bandage works well. If you've limited your activity and your elbow still hurts, you should see your doctor, who will drain the excess fluid from the bursa at the tip of your elbow.

BODY SIGNAL ALERT

VARICOSE VEIN THAT BECOMES TENDER AND PAINFUL

Description and Possible Medical Problems

If you have surface varicose veins that become tender and painful, you probably have a condition known as superficial phlebitis, more commonly known as phlebitis. Phlebitis may occur because of a vein in the leg becoming inflamed due to injury or a clot, being inactive for more than several weeks, sitting in an airplane seat for hours, or taking estrogen.

In addition to the pain and tenderness, the entire length of the vein may become hard and the skin around the vein may be itchy.

Treatment

Many people confuse superficial phlebitis with deep-vein thrombosis. The truth is that superficial phlebitis usually appears in a vein near the surface of the skin, while deep-vein thrombosis occurs in veins deep in the legs or abdomen and is a potentially life-threatening illness in which a blood clot forms within a blood vessel.

There are several things you can do to treat the pain of phlebitrs. Taking aspirin or Advil will help relieve the pain and reduce the swelling. You should also try to elevate your legs whenever you're sitting or lying down. Some people find that applying moist heat to the legs or soaking in a warm tub helps.

A mild case of phlebitis will usually disappear within a week. However, you should see your doctor to rule out deep-vein thrombosis.

VEINS, SMALL AND BLUISH

See "Small, Red Spider Veins" in Chapter 4.

Chapter 17

HANDS AND FEET

BODY SIGNAL ALERT

Call your doctor immediately if you experience any of the following symptoms:

SYMPTOM	POSSIBLE MEDICAL CONDITION
Your knuckles are painful, stiff, and swollen	*Rheumatoid arthritis*
You notice a change in the flexibility of your hand	*Tenosynovitis or osteoarthritis*
Your hand becomes contracted and you are unable to extend your ring finger and pinky	*Dupuytren's contracture*
Your hands become swollen and red, especially after a puncture wound	*Cellulitis*
Your hands are painful and swollen, and the skin becomes tight and shiny	*Scleroderma*
Your hands become numb	*Carpal tunnel syndrome*
The first joint of your big toe or another single joint is painful, swollen, and red	*Gout*
You have pain and stiffness in several of your joints	*Osteoarthritis*

HOW THE HANDS AND FEET AGE

The effects the aging process has on your hands are usually a giveaway to your age. Other parts of the body that show maturity can easily be altered with a face-lift or tummy tuck, but the telltale signs of age are always right there in your hands, not only in appearance but in their capabilities. Hands that are nimble in youth eventually become hands that may be unable to perform even simple tasks. However, arthritis is not necessarily a part of growing older, and I've seen many aging artisans who can still use their hands with great precision and skill.

Typically, as the hand ages, the skin becomes thinner and the muscles on the back of the hand begin to lose some of their tone. The veins and bones become more prominent, and the area between the thumb and first finger is especially prone to losing muscle. On the whole, muscular strength in the hand may decrease, but the decrease is gradual enough that, for most of us, our hands can function effectively well into our 80s and 90s.

Like the hand, the nails are a part of the body that provides a clue to the general health of the rest of your body. Many times, the first signs of an underlying medical illness, such as cancer or cardiovascular disease, show up in the nails. For instance, the nails of lung cancer patients begin to spoon, while the nails of people who have vascular disease frequently thicken or turn blue underneath. Many women use nail polish and other adornments as a cosmetic and a form of expression. Unfortunately, nail polish can mask possible medical problems that are evident in the nails and even create new ones.

Starting in your 50s, the aging nail may start to become brittle and gray. Polishes and nail treatments made with alcohol and formaldehyde can cause the nails to dry out even more. And artificial nails and many layers of polish can lead to a fungal infection in the real nails.

Even though your nails become drier and more brittle, you can preserve them by keeping them clean and well groomed. I've also seen many cases where nails have become stronger with intake of gelatin and vitamins, especially the B vitamins.

Feet don't normally show the signs of aging as hands do, since they spend most of their time covered up and protected from the elements and sun. As a result, many of us tend to take our feet for granted. Indeed, the foot is often the part of the body that is least examined in the course of a regular medical exam. As a result, many people suffer from foot problems that are never diagnosed, such as warts and corns. Foot care is especially important for diabetics, because their poor circulation leaves them more prone to infections that can develop into a serious skin infection called cellulitis. It is also important for elderly people, since proper foot care can help prevent falls.

BODY SIGNAL ALERT

ARTHRITIS, RHEUMATOID

A positive diagnosis of rheumatoid arthritis requires four of the following seven criteria. Critera 1 through 4 must be present for at least six weeks.

1. Morning stiffness that lasts for at least one hour before it slowly begins to improve

2. Three joints or more inflamed, with wrists and elbows also possibly involved

3. Involvement of at least one hand joint

4. The same joint of the body on both the left and right sides involved at once

5. Rheumatoid nodules, body growths under the skin near joints or in the hands or ankles (extensor surfaces); these can be found under the surface of the arm under the skin or near the protrusion from the elbow

6. Blood test showing rheumatoid factor

7. X-ray changes that are typical for osteoarthritis

Many times, rheumatoid arthritis can be detected in the blood and is a symmetrical disorder of the joints accompanied by deformity and morning stiffness. The patient may also have:

Skin nodules

Lung involvement

Dryness in mouth and eyes

Skin eruption (vasculitis)

Carpal tunnel syndrome

FEET, PAINFUL GROWTHS
ON SOLES OF

Description and Possible Medical Problems

As we grow older, we become attuned to the little aches and pains that, although they may not totally restrict our movement are nevertheless there—and they weren't before. A creak in the knee during a walk or a knuckle that begins to swell the second you type for more than a certain number of minutes—these things are annoying, but we can still carry on.

When a pain occurs on the bottom of your foot, however, and makes it difficult to walk, it's probably not just any old ache or pain but a plantar wart, also called a verruca plantaris. A plantar wart is caused by the same virus that's responsible for the warts that appear on your hands, and it has a characteristic dark spot in the middle. One way in which it differs from the wart on your finger is that it is usually level with the surface of skin because of the pressure of walking, which makes it recede into the skin.

Treatment

You can usually let an ordinary wart clear up by itself or use an over-the-counter preparation to freeze it so it falls off. With a plantar wart, however, you usually don't have the luxury of time, since it hurts with every step.

If you have a plantar wart, you should see your doctor. He will use cryotherapy to freeze it off, lasers to burn it off, or topical medication such as an aspirin derivative or a mild acid, which will cause the wart to eventually dry up and fall off. Whatever removal method is used, it is not painful, and the wart should fall off in about four days.

FINGERS, BENT AND TURNING
AWAY FROM THUMB

See "Knuckles, Painful, Stiff, and Swollen" below.

BODY SIGNAL ALERT

FINGERS, CHANGE IN FLEXIBILITY OF

Description and Possible Medical Problems

It may occur suddenly or over the course of several months. But a change in the flexibility of the fingers happens to everyone with aging, in varying degrees and for various reasons.

One cause may be a condition called tenosynovitis, in which the sheaths that surround each of the tendons in your hands become inflamed. Because the sheaths swell up in a space that's tiny to begin with, your tendons can become constricted and cause a loss of movement in your fingers. Tenosynovitis can be caused by either overuse or a bacterial infection. Osteoarthritis is another possible reason why your fingers become less flexible. This is a condition in which the cartilage that protects the ends of your bones and also acts as a shock absorber begins to wear down after decades of constant use. Without the cartilage, the bones lack the ability to absorb shock and therefore become stiff and more difficult and painful to use. People who use their fingers and hands a lot are more prone to developing osteoarthritis, due to the resulting wear and tear on their fingers.

Treatment

If you think you have tenosynovitis, you should see your doctor. The most likely prescription you'll receive is a suggestion to rest your hand for as long as a week and take aspirin or another over-the-counter painkiller as often as you need until you are able to move your fingers freely again. Once you return to the activity that caused the tenosynovitis, you should seek the advice of a physical therapist so that the condition does not recur. If your doctor believes the condition is caused by a bacterial infection, he will also prescribe an antibiotic such as penicillin.

If, however, you have osteoarthritis, some lifestyle changes will be necessary. Osteoarthritis can be quite fickle: some days you'll be fine, while on others you'll find it's difficult to accomplish anything because of the pain. Aspirin and other over-the-counter preparations can help reduce the pain and inflammation so you can work. You should also ask your doctor about doing exercises to strengthen your hands, since toning the muscles around the joints can help prevent flare-ups. In some cases, a heating pad or a device that provides moist heat to the joints also helps. When the pain is especially severe, your doctor may suggest an injection of a corticosteroid medication directly into the hand for immediate relief. However, most of the time, it's better in the long run to rely on less intrusive ways of dealing with osteoarthritis.

FINGERS, REDNESS UNDER RING

See "Neck With Red 'Necklace,'" in Chapter 8.

FINGERS, SWOLLEN, UNABLE TO MOVE

See "Fingers, Change in Flexibility of" above.

BODY SIGNAL ALERT

HANDS BECOME TIGHT AND SHINY

Description and Possible Medical Problems

If you've ever waxed your legs at home and you decided to leave the wax on for a while so you could see what it felt like to walk around encased in wax, you already have a pretty good idea of what the disease scleroderma feels like.

Scleroderma is a rare disease that is characterized by tight, shiny skin that severely cuts down on the amount of flexibility you have. The skin may also be swollen and painful. Scleroderma is often associated with arthritis since it is a disease of the connective tissue and advances slowly; it can take two years to develop fully.

Scleroderma occurs when the collagen in the connective tissue starts to harden. The cause of scleroderma, however, is not known, although a defect in the immune system has been postulated.

Besides your fingers and hands, scleroderma can affect the feet and face, as well as the esophagus, which can make swallowing difficult. More women than men are affected by scleroderma.

Treatment

If you think you have scleroderma, you should see your doctor, who will do a blood test and possibly a biopsy of your skin to help confirm the diagnosis. He will also check your ability to swallow; if it isn't affected, he will want to check regularly to see if it deteriorates. If swallowing becomes difficult, you should see an ear, nose, and throat specialist and/or a speech pathologist. Together, the two will advise you on the best foods and best way to eat.

Along with painkillers or aspirin, your doctor may prescribe antibiotics to reduce the swelling. You may also require regular sessions with a physical therapist in order to maintain your flexibility.

Although the disease takes a couple of years to develop fully, the good news is that that your skin won't get any worse after that.

BODY SIGNAL ALERT

HANDS, NUMB

Description and Possible Medical Problems

What do hard-playing athletes have in common with computer users, carpenters, butchers, factory workers, and do-it-yourselfers? Increasingly these days, the answer is carpal tunnel syndrome.

If you use your hands a lot in any way, you're at risk for carpal tunnel syndrome. The signature symptoms include numbness, tingling, and weakness in the hand. The symptoms typically are distributed over the first three fingers and are especially common at night.

Carpal tunnel syndrome occurs when the median nerve of the wrist becomes compressed by the flexor tendons, which pass through a tunnel in the wrist called the carpal ligament. A variety of activities and conditions, including repetitive wrist movements, can cause the tendons to swell, leading to excessive pressure on the nerve.

Treatment

If you think you have carpal tunnel syndrome, I recommend a conservative initial treatment, including rest, splinting, hot soaks, and anti-inflammatory medication. If these initial methods don't work, injections of corticosteroids will help relieve the swelling of the flexor tendons.

Too many people—and doctors—opt for surgery for carpal tunnel syndrome, but I feel this should be viewed as a last resort. Surgery should generally be reserved for cases that fail to respond to conservative measures. The standard operation involves cutting the transverse carpal ligament, which creates more room in the tunnel for the tendons and median nerve that pass through it. Some surgeons go for a synovectomy, which opens up the sheath that surrounds the nerve, though I think it's unnecessary. Opening up the transverse carpal ligament is usually enough to relieve the pressure on the nerve.

Tips and Precautions

As carpal tunnel syndrome has received a lot of attention in the last few years, so has the study of ergonomics, which helps people find ways to work and play that fit more naturally with the way their bodies are built. If, for instance, you spend a lot of time at a computer and find that the angle of the keyboard causes your wrists to ache and your hands turn numb, you can buy a keyboard that is more user friendly. With such a keyboard you hold your hands above and parallel to the keyboard, instead of flexing them up from the wrist and resting them on the edge. In fact, manufacturers are now making everything from scissors to wooden mixing spoons that are ergonomically correct.

HANDS, RED, SCALY,
AND ITCHY

See "Scalp, Itchy" in Chapter 4.

BODY SIGNAL ALERT

HANDS, SWOLLEN AND RED, ESPECIALLY AFTER A PUNCTURE WOUND

Description and Possible Medical Problems

Remember Madge, the manicurist in the TV ad who recommended that her clients soak their hands in dishwashing liquid to soften them? After they reacted with shock, Madge reassured them, and they gamely put their hands back into the solution.

Most of us know better and would prefer real moisturizer, just to make sure. After all, washing dishes—a common activity even in these days of automatic dishwashers—still tends to leave your hands red and swollen for about 30 minutes after you finish no matter what you do.

If, however, you have red, swollen hands that don't clear up and if you've recently injured your hand in some way, you may have a condition called cellulitis, which is a skin infection. Cellulitis occurs when streptococcus bacteria enter the body, usually through broken skin. Besides red, swollen hands, you may notice that small red lines appear on your skin in a weblike design and your skin feels hot to the touch. You may also have a fever.

Treatment

If you think you have cellulitis, you should see your doctor. You'll need to soak your hands in warm water for 10 minutes three or four times daily. The best course of treatment is Tylenol, though in severe cases I'll also prescribe a course of an antibiotic such as penicillin or erythromycin, taken four times a day for at least two weeks. When the cellulitis is severe, hospitalization is necessary for intravenous antibiotic therapy.

HEEL, PAIN IN WHILE STANDING OR WALKING

Description and Possible Medical Problems

Of the countless medical conditions throughout the years, some can be avoided completely if you use a little common sense. For instance, most of the foot problems I see won't occur if you wear shoes that fit properly.

This includes heel pain. The tough pad that comprises your heel serves as a shock absorber for your entire foot as well as the rest of your body. If you feel a pain in your heel every time you take a step, the pad of your heel is probably inflamed, which may be caused by absorbing too much shock. Though some people may call your condition a heel spur, this is a misnomer, since a heel spur is a problem with the bone of the heel, in which part of it becomes calcified. A heel spur is excruciatingly painful, since a bone is digging directly into your skin.

Heel pain is usually due—again!—to wearing shoes that don't fit properly or pounding on your heel while walking or running. Women are also prone to heel pain when they switch from high heels to flat shoes. High heels force you to walk on your toes, whereas if you start to wear flats, there will be more weight on your heel than it's accustomed to.

Treatment

If you think you have an inflamed heel pad, try changing the shoes you wear to comfortable, flat shoes that have a lot of padding in the heel. While the pain remains, however, you can take aspirin and apply ice to reduce the swelling. This is all most people need. Others, however, will need to see their doctor, who may decide to inject corticosteroids into the heel for instant relief.

BODY SIGNAL ALERT

JOINTS, STIFFNESS AND PAIN IN

Description and Possible Medical Problems

As you get older, you've probably discovered that you just can't do everything as easily and smoothly as you once could. While you used to bounce out of bed in the morning, it may take you longer to get up and about, and your joints may become stiff and painful as the day wears on; you may also sometimes feel as though you have sand in your joints because any movement can make them feel gritty.

These are all signs of osteoarthritis, a condition in which the cartilage that absorbs the shock of the bone begins to break down from years of use. Fingers, wrists, back, hips, and knees—every joint can be affected. The stiffness usually doesn't appear when you first wake up but tends to increase as the day goes on. The joints can also become deformed, since fluid can accumulate in them; this can make them tender to the touch.

By the age of 45, osteoarthritis starts to appear, and by the age of 75, almost everyone shows some degree of osteoarthritis.

Treatment

Unlike rheumatoid arthritis, there is no blood test that will positively diagnose osteoarthritis. An X ray or MRI, however, can show the degree to which the cartilage of each joint has worn away.

Osteoarthritis hates activity, but you'll love it because regular exercise will help to decrease the pain and stiffness in your joints. That's why you should move your joints as much as you can for as long as possible; it's a good idea to walk at least twenty minutes a day, every day.

When the pain of osteoarthritis flares up, you can take either aspirin or Advil, two or three times a day. Aspirin and Advil are anti-inflammatory medications that help reduce the pain as well as the inflammation, while Tylenol will only help relieve the pain.

If aspirin or Advil doesn't help relieve your pain, your doctor may suggest that you take one of the stronger non-steroidal anti-inflammatory medications such as Naprosyn, Feldene, Clinoril, Motrin, or Indocin. The entire class of medications that are used to treat osteoarthritis, including aspirin and Advil—but not Tylenol—are known as nonsteroidal anti-inflammatories, or NSAIDs.

Several words of caution, however: NSAIDs can cause ulcers. Your doctor might prescribe a medication such as Carafate or another antiulcer medication to take with the NSAID to protect your stomach. As a greater precaution, NSAIDs should always be taken with food.

NSAIDs can also cause bloating, water retention, and intestinal upset. If you have hypertension, it's probably not a good idea to take them since they can increase your blood pressure even more. And NSAIDs can cause headaches, skin rashes, and kidney problems. In people who are prone to wheezing, they can aggravate the condition, and they can also make abnormalities show up on liver and blood tests.

Because of all these side effects, it's important that your doctor monitor you regularly if you decide to take an NSAID to treat your osteoarthritis or rheumatoid arthritis. However, you must take it regularly and it may take up to a week to start to ease your pain.

BODY SIGNAL ALERT

KNUCKLES, PAINFUL, STIFF, AND SWOLLEN

Description and Possible Medical Problems

If the knuckles of your hands swell up and you think you have arthritis, stop a moment. Arthritis is a general term that is used in combination with other words such as "rheumatoid" and "osteo-" to describe your medical condition more fully.

If a part of your hand such as the palm or wrist or your knuckles begins to swell up and ache, and the pain and stiffness seem to be at their worst when you first wake up in the morning but are there one day and gone the next, chances are you have rheumatoid arthritis. Osteoarthritis, on the other hand, generally results from wear and tear of the synovium by the bones on the joints (see also "Joints, Stiffness and Pain in" above). Rheumatoid arthritis is caused by a defect in the immune system that affects the synovium, the thin sheath that surrounds the joints, to break down while rheumatoid arthritis may make your fingers turn away from your thumb at about a 45-degree angle. Rheumatoid arthritis can also affect other organs in the body, including the cardiovascular system and the lungs, which can become inflamed from the disease.

Rheumatoid arthritis has an unpredictable nature. It may flare up without warning and be a constant problem for several years before disappearing completely. This can be the disease's most frustrating aspect, since just as the symptoms have subsided for a while and you think you're over them, they can appear again without warning.

Treatment

Rheumatoid arthritis is manageable to a certain extent. If you think you have rheumatoid arthritis, you should see your doctor, who will do a blood test to determine if you have an antibody called rheumatoid factor in your system.

If you do have rheumatoid arthritis, your doctor will work with you to

design ways of coping with the disease. The best program for rheumatoid arthritis includes rest and non-weight-bearing exercise such as
walking, as well as certain medications you can take when the pain
becomes severe. This medication may include aspirin, which reduces
the inflammation and eases the pain, and corticosteroid drugs such as
prednisone.

In rare cases, your doctor may suggest cytotoxic drugs, which are
used to treat cancer, or a procedure called plasmapheresis, in which a
pint or so of your blood is taken out and put through a centrifuge to
separate the plasma from the blood cells. The cells are then combined
with new plasma and returned to your circulatory system. The purpose
is to give the immune system an extra boost at a time when it may
really need it.

The most important thing to do, however, is to learn to accept the
disease and to do whatever's necessary to treat your symptoms when
the disease does flare up.

NAILS, DEFORMITY IN, WITH DISCOLORATION AND THICKENING

Description and Possible Medical Problems

If you're a woman who enjoys wearing polish on your nails, you probably
think that your nails look ugly, even a bit anemic, when they're bare.
There may be a few spots here and there, some discolored parts, and
even a thickened area or two. Thank goodness for nail polish, you may
say, since you can cover up those ugly spots.

If you notice spots, discolorations, or areas that have thickened on
your nails, you actually shouldn't be wearing polish at all. You may have
a fungal infection, which, in some cases, is caused by wearing nail polish, since the nail isn't able to breathe. One tiny fungus spore can attach
to the keratin—the protein your nail is made from—of your nail when
it's uncovered, and from there multiply and eat away at your nail until
the entire nail is affected. If you polish over the fungal spore, it doesn't
die but, in essence, becomes trapped with all of that lovely keratin from
which it can make an excellent meal!

Treatment

If you think you have a fungal infection of a nail, you need to see your doctor. Although there are many over-the-counter topical preparations available, they are not usually very effective because they don't penetrate the nail. Instead, they contain the infection in the nail and prevent it from spreading to the skin around the nail. Fungal infections are extremely difficult to treat.

Your doctor can prescribe a treatment called Spornox, an oral medication taken once a day that will destroy the fungus. Treatment may last for at least three months. In the meantime, while the infection clears up—which may take as long as nine months, or the amount of time it takes your nail to grow out—don't wear nail polish, and wear gloves whenever you immerse your hands in water, since water may cause the fungus to spread, as it thrives in a warm, moist environment.

NAILS, GROOVES ACROSS THE

Description and Possible Medical Problems

Our nails reveal a lot about our health. It's not uncommon for the nail to become affected by a serious disease. In fact, a good medical detective will be able to tell when you become sick and for how long you've been suffering just by looking at your nails.

When horizontal grooves appear across your nails, it's a common sign that a person is recovering from a severe illness. You see, when a person is sick for an extended period of time, the body seems to cut down on the amount of nutrients it sends to nonvital areas such as nails so that it can put its resources into boosting the immune system and/or ridding the body of the illness. And so the growth of the nails slows down, which results in the grooves.

Treatment

If grooves appear across your nails, you don't have to do a thing. When you recover from your illness and your nails begin to grow again, the grooves will disappear, though it may take several months for the nail to grow out.

BODY SIGNAL ALERT

PAIN AND SWELLING IN A SINGLE JOINT

Description and Possible Medical Problems

Gout is one of those diseases that sounds old-fashioned, like something your grandmother used to complain about to your grandfather: "Now, Harry, don't eat that pastrami, or your gout will act up." At least, that's the way it used to go in my grandparents' house.

Gout is actually a sign that the kidneys are not functioning well. The kidneys produce uric acid, which is normally excreted through your kidneys in your urine. If, however, for some reason your body produces more uric acid than your kidneys are able to process, it stays in the body. It typically gravitates toward the joints, collecting in the form of uric acid crystals. Collection sites commonly include the first joint of the big toe, but the crystals can also collect in the wrists, elbows, and knees, causing pain and swelling in these joints as well.

Gout is similar to rheumatoid arthritis, since it strikes with great unpredictability. After an initial experience of gout, you may not have to worry about it anymore, since some people have only one attack and that's it. Others, however, will suffer from regular attacks. Unfortunately, the more frequent the attacks, the more likely the gout will spread to other joints.

Some people are genetically prone to gout, although drinking alcohol, taking antibiotics, or eating rich foods—as my grandfather did—is more often the cause since it can cause the body to produce more than the usual amount of uric acid.

Treatment

If you think you're having an attack of gout, contact your doctor. Unlike other painful joint disorders, it's not a good idea to self-medicate it with aspirin, since aspirin can delay the amount of time it takes your body to rid itself of the excess uric acid.

Your doctor will ask you if you've had previous problems with gout, and he'll do blood and urine tests to confirm that you have a high amount of uric acid in your system. Though after your first attack you may not have any more problems with gout, it's still important to do what you can to prevent future attacks. Drinking lots of water is one of the best preventive measures there is for this illness.

If, however, your attacks continue, your doctor will prescribe an anti-inflammatory drug such as Indocin 25 for you to take three or four times a day whenever you feel an attack coming on. He may also recommend you take a prescription painkiller such as Tylenol with codeine to keep your discomfort to a minimum.

Though gout can be painful, if you take action at its onset, it's very easy to control it. However, you'll probably still have to lay off the pastrami, as my grandfather did.

BODY SIGNAL ALERT

RING FINGER AND PINKY CONTRACTING INTO PALM

Description and Possible Medical Problems

One of my patients recently told me a story about the time he first became aware of a rare but puzzling disorder of the ring finger and pinky called Dupuytren's contracture.

"I was about 11, and I was at one of those tacky country fairs with my family. My sister had already won a couple of prizes at the wheel of fortune and the goldfish bowls, but so far I wasn't having any luck.

"Until we got to the ring toss. Instead of a mere stick pointing towards the sky, there were all these fake hands with everything but the index finger pointing up. In fact, I remember looking up to see what they were all pointing at.

"I bought a few rings for a quarter and managed to hook one out of three. I wanted to try again for the second tier of prizes, but my parents were ready to go. The prize I won was this cut-off rubber hand with red paint smeared all over the wrist. I flopped it around at my sister, who grabbed the hand and tried to make it give me 'the finger' behind my parents' backs.

"All she could manage was to fold in the ring finger and pinky. She was only seven, so she didn't know which was the correct obscene gesture. But at the instant I saw the ring finger and pinky folded in, I thought that it looked just like my father's hand."

Indeed, this condition, called Dupuytren's contracture, is genetic and is most prevalent in men in their 40s. This was precisely the case with my patient. Dupuytren's contracture occurs when the tissue located in the palm of your hand becomes thick and actually starts to shrink, pulling the fingers into the palm. The cause of Dupuytren's contracture is not known, but in addition to being a genetic condition, it also frequently appears in epileptics and alcoholics. Dupuytren's contracture is usually not painful; however, it can make any work that involves your hands difficult and even impossible.

Treatment

Surgery is often recommended in order to regain the full use of your hand. The process involves removing the shrunken tissue; in many cases, this will be enough to free up movement. Some people, however, will need skin grafts to the area in order to regain the full range of motion. In both cases, however, you will need to work with a hand therapist or physical therapist to totally regain the use of your hand.

SKIN, CRACKED, RED, AND DRY ON HANDS AND FINGERS

Description and Possible Medical Problems

Advertisements for hand creams and moisturizers make a big deal out of the great things these products will do for your hands. You've seen the before-and-after pictures: the red, scaly skin in the "before" shots; the baby-soft, smooth skin that looks almost too good to be true in the "after." Oh, yes, and the smile.

Sometimes the advertisement mentions in tiny print that the photos were not retouched; of course you can assume that all the other ads that don't mention this fact do play around with the photos to make the hands in the "after" picture look almost too good to be true.

Your hands probably start to become dry and cracked in late fall and then stay that way for the rest of the winter, due to the dry air and cold.

Though they don't reflect on the state of your health, dry, cracked hands can be painful.

Treatment

When your hands become dry, red, and cracked, you probably wish someone would come along and retouch your hands the way it's done in the before-and-after pictures. In the real world, of course, it's not as easy as that, but it does come close.

Most people slather on hand cream when their hands become dry. And that's good—but you can go one better by putting moisturizer on your hands after you wash them, while they're still damp. This will help keep your hands moisturized by sealing the water into your skin and forming a protective layer between your hands and the elements. Some people also wear gloves whenever they go out, which is another way to protect your hands.

TOENAIL, PAINFUL

Description and Possible Medical Problems

We've all been guilty of cutting our toenails the way the experts say we're not supposed to: too short and rounded, and not square. You know who you are! If you're the type who's determined to always get every last bit of everything, whether it means clearing your plate or cutting your toenails, sooner or later you're going to have a problem with an ingrown toenail.

An ingrown toenail occurs when the nail starts to grow into the skin. Though usually it is just painful, it may become infected. Although cutting your toenail incorrectly can cause an ingrown toenail, shoes that are too tight and press the nail into the skin can be a factor as well.

Treatment

If you have an ingrown toenail, you should trim it carefully so that the nail is no longer digging into the skin; soaking it first will help soften it and make it easier to cut. You may also want to treat it with an antiseptic such as Bactine. To prevent future ingrown toenails, clip your nails straight across and wear shoes that don't restrict your toes.

TOES, RED, ITCHY, WITH PAIN BETWEEN

Description and Possible Medical Problems

Athlete's foot is such a common condition that the moment your feet start to itch and become red and the skin between your toes cracks, you probably already know what the problem is.

In fact, athlete's foot is such a common condition that an entire industry of powders and lotions seems to have been built around it. Some other products also use the issue of athlete's foot prevention— "Use our special sandals in the shower at the gym and avoid athlete's foot forever!"—to sell their own products.

When it comes right down to it, athlete's foot is a fungal infection that is easy to catch but also easy to treat. The best growing conditions for athlete's foot include a moist environment such as a shower that other people use, like in a locker room, and shoes and socks that don't allow your feet to breathe. In addition to redness, itching, and cracks between the toes, the skin may be flaky and will smell foul.

Treatment

To treat athlete's foot, the best thing you can do is to keep your feet as dry as possible with talcum powder or an antifungal powder for athlete's foot such as Tinactin. It's also a good idea to wear shoes and socks that breathe—such as cotton socks and leather shoes—and sandals or other open-toed shoes as often as possible.

Usually these techniques will clear up athlete's foot within a few days. If they don't work or your athlete's foot gets worse, see your doctor. You may need a prescription antifungal powder or cream or an antifungal medication.

TOES WITH HARD AND PAINFUL NODULES

Description and Possible Medical Problems

When I was a kid and my aunts used to sit around complaining about their corns, I always thought of that old Bugs Bunny cartoon where an ear of corn sprang full blown from somebody's foot. I looked at my aunts' clunky orthopedic shoes, but they didn't look as though they could hold something that big.

After 4 years of medical school and 20 years of practice, I know a little bit more about corns. A corn usually appears on a toe where the skin has become thickened, usually by the pressure and/or friction of shoes that don't fit right. A callus is a close, thick-skinned relative of a corn— except that it usually appears on the sole of the foot and over a wider area.

Though corns and calluses are annoying and corns are sometimes painful, they probably won't prevent you from staying on your feet.

Treatment

If you get a corn or callus, you should first soak it in warm water for about 10 minutes. Then you can rub it away with a pumice stone or use a special over-the-counter cream that softens the skin. There are also special corn pads you can buy that will reduce the friction between your shoe and your foot.

But the best way to treat a corn as well as to prevent it in the future is wearing shoes that fit properly. It might also help to choose shoes with a leather upper that will easily mold to your feet instead of fighting against them.

WRIST, BUMP ON

Description and Possible Medical Problems

It seems that we've been trained from birth to regard any new lumps or bumps that appear on our bodies with a suspicious eye and a brain trained to think of the "C word": cancer. Therefore, whenever a lump or bump turns out to be something else and is actually harmless, the relief is usually palpable.

This is the good news if you notice a lump or bump that appears on the back of your wrist, called a ganglion cyst. It's usually painless and occurs when a gellike material escapes from a joint or a synovium, a tendon sheath in your wrist. It collects in one spot, causing the area to swell up, and may be either soft or hard.

Treatment

If you think you have a ganglion cyst, you should see your doctor. Though you're probably reading your Body Signals correctly, the chance does exist that the growth is a tumor or a malignant growth. Your doctor will do an X ray and/or a sonogram to help determine the status of the growth. If, as in most cases, he does discover a ganglion cyst, he will drain it with a needle while applying pressure to it, to make sure none of the gel remains.

Chapter 18

WHEN YOUR WHOLE BODY FEELS LOUSY: HIDDEN BODY SIGNALS AND THE TESTS THAT REVEAL THEM

BODY SIGNAL ALERT

Call your doctor immediately if you experience any of the following:

SYMPTOM	POSSIBLE MEDICAL CONDITION
You've recently lost weight and are experiencing increased urination, thirst, and malaise; a blood test shows an elevation of your glucose levels	*Diabetes mellitus*
You're diabetic and are experiencing heart palpitations, sweating, and confusion	*Hypoglycemic reaction*
You've recently lost weight without trying	*Depression, thyroid problems, cancer*
You've noticed a change in your emotional state and have become increasingly confused	*Fever, delirium*

WHAT'S A HIDDEN BODY SIGNAL?

In my 20 years of practice, I've discovered that the human body is a marvelous model of cause and effect. This is underscored in Chapters 3 through 17: when you have a specific physical complaint, you can look it up and immediately know whether you should wait it out or call the doctor. It's these obvious Body Signals that make my job as a physician much easier: I make a diagnosis based on a patient's symptoms and then order a treatment that's designed to help.

This same human body, however, can also be extremely frustrating, mysterious, and stubborn when it refuses to yield up specific symptoms and instead prefers to spread them throughout the body. As the practice of medicine gets more technical, I find that these instances of generalized symptoms and complaints and overall malaise are increasing. It's as if the body is teasing both me and my patients: "Ha! Just when you think you've got me all figured out, I'll just throw a little wrench into the works just to keep you in your place!"

Today, the biggest challenges in medicine concern patients who complain that their whole body feels lousy. Unfortunately, most of us simply dismiss this general feeling of "unwell-being" and only after some sort of medical catastrophe—such as a heart attack or diabetes—occurs do we look back and realize we saw "it" coming all along. Actually, these "hidden Body Signals," as I call them, were there all along. It is these often confusing, often exasperating, nonspecific signs and symptoms that we'll tackle now.

This chapter discusses two types of hidden Body Signals:

1. Those you can feel and that affect the entire body, such as *fever, chills, night sweats,* and *malaise.* These types of symptoms are considered "hidden Body Signals" because they can hide more serious illnesses that you'd never suspect unless you saw your physician.

2. Those you cannot feel and that can be revealed only by physical examination, blood tests, and other diagnostic tools. For example, one of the most common hidden Body Signals is high blood pressure: it's "hidden" because you can't see or feel it. It can be detected only when a trained medical professional actually measures your blood pressure. In this chapter, I describe the Body Signals that are revealed by various medical tests and discuss what to do about them.

You should note that each of the entries follows the format of the previous chapters.

BLOOD COUNT TESTS, ABNORMAL

Description and Possible Medical Problems

If you feel more tired and look paler than you usually do, there are a number of causes your doctor will look for, but it's likely that the first one he will check will prove to be the cause. Fortunately, it is also the easiest to treat.

Anemia is a medical condition in which the red blood cells contain less hemoglobin than is normal for a healthy, well-functioning circulatory system. Hemoglobin is composed mostly of iron, which is why all the commercials for dietary iron supplements stress that without their products you'll be more prone to developing anemia.

On the surface this is true, but in actuality it's not that simple. While anemia is frequently caused by a lack of iron in the diet, it can also be due to a defect within the digestive system. Anemia can also be the result of a deficiency of another nutrient, including vitamin B_{12} or folic acid.

Because the symptoms of the different causes of anemia are similar, your doctor may want to conduct further blood tests to determine the kind of anemia you have in addition to testing for other possible reasons for your fatigue and pallor.

The first test your doctor will conduct is called a complete blood cell count. This will provide the doctor with a clear picture of the composition of your blood by counting the number of each type of blood cell— red, white, and platelets—and comparing it to that of nonanemic blood. Red blood cells should make up 40% to 45% of the blood's composition in women and 45% to 50% in men. If the numbers from your blood test fall below these figures, you probably have anemia.

In addition to a reduced blood cell count, the test will also reveal an elevated blood cell count, typically when the body is producing a surplus of white blood cells, the condition known as leukemia. Interestingly, the symptoms for anemia and leukemia are similar.

Treatment

Whether the results of an abnormal complete blood cell count show reduced or elevated blood counts, your doctor is the best person to recommend the proper course of treatment. If you have anemia, your doctor will suggest you take iron supplements as well as increase the amount of iron-rich foods in your diet. Though leukemia is the more serious disease, it can be treated successfully with customized chemotherapy regimens, especially if it's caught early.

BLOOD PRESSURE, ELEVATED
(HYPERTENSION)

Description and Possible Medical Problems

In some social circles, it may seem at times as if the primary topic of conversation is blood pressure, most often that it's too high. But high blood pressure really is a major health problem in America because it can lead to a number of other serious diseases. Simply put, high blood pressure is a condition in which blood moves through your arteries at a pressure that is too high for good health.

If you are diagnosed with high blood pressure, your doctor will want to determine the length of time your pressure has been elevated, to get an idea of its severity. The signs your doctor will look for include changes in the blood vessels of the eye, which may affect your vision, an enlarged heart, and an elevated blood urea nitrogen (BUN) level, which shows that the kidney has been damaged due to the elevated pressure. A routine blood test will also detect the other serious risk factors that aggravate high blood pressure, such as elevated cholesterol and blood sugar levels.

Treatment

More often than not, the cause of your elevated blood pressure will not be obvious. The next step, then, is to treat the elevated blood pressure itself. It's important to keep in mind that, when treating high blood pressure, the doctor and patient are also working together to prevent a future heart attack or stroke. Therefore, it's essential to find a treatment plan that can be implemented and managed well over time with relative ease.

The usual treatment for this condition is a course of medication, lasting sometimes months or even years. However, since most people resist this approach unless it is absolutely necessary, doctors can forestall the use of medication, at least in the beginning. I and many of my colleagues believe in a logical, proven plan of treatment that begins—simply enough—with patient education.

Diet is the first part of your treatment, since salt affects kidney function, which in turn causes the blood pressure to rise. Don't add table salt to your food, and stay away from foods that are salty, including pickles, pretzels, popcorn, and other salty snacks. Get into the habit of reading food labels, and resist fried fast foods and restaurants that normally use large quantities of salt in their food, such as Chinese and other ethnic cuisines. Low-fat milk and dairy products are good foods if you have hypertension, since some research suggests that a diet low in calcium may encourage the development of high blood pressure.

As for exercise, I feel that walking briskly for twenty minutes a day is the best activity for anybody, regardless of the state of one's health, since it lowers one's stress level and increases physical conditioning. For some people, a low-salt, low-fat diet with a daily brisk walk is all they need to control their blood pressure. However, if you wish to pursue more strenuous activities, it's important that you get a go-ahead from your physician first. If you haven't been active for a long time, he may ask you to take a stress test so he's sure your heart can withstand the additional effort. Relaxation techniques and exercises such as biofeedback and yoga are also helpful in reducing your blood pressure, so ask your doctor for advice on how to use these methods as well.

If changing your diet and exercise routine and learning to relax fail to lower your blood pressure, only then do I recommend that you take medication. Once you start on medication, however, it's important that you continue with your diet and exercise program so that you can keep your medication to a minimum.

The good news is that there are a wide variety of medications available to help lower blood pressure. My goal as a physician is to find the perfect medication for each person. Sometimes this is an easy process, but often it is a frustrating challenge.

As I've mentioned, the major problem with high blood pressure is that most of the time you won't have any symptoms. Unfortunately, once you start taking medication to treat your condition, you may experience adverse reactions such as headaches and dizziness, until your doctor finds the medication right for you. At this point, many people stop taking the medication before it even has a chance to work. Or else, you may want to start taking other medications to treat your side effects, which in turn can cause more side effects. Before you know it, you can spend a significant part of your day opening bottles and swallowing pills. That's why when I first start a person on blood pressure medication, I strongly recommend that in the beginning she visit me in my office at least once a week so I can assess the effectiveness of the medication and her adverse reactions, if any. It's important for you, as a patient, to feel like an integral part of the medical treatment team with whom you are working.

Here's a brief overview of the most commonly prescribed medications to treat high blood pressure, along with their side effects.

- Diuretics such as HydroDIURIL, hydrochlorothiazide, Lasix, furosemide, and Bumex have been used for many years to treat high blood pressure. They help remove body water and therefore reduce pressure within the circulatory system. Side effects of diuretics can include dehydration, potassium depletion, weakness, and elevated cholesterol levels. Your doctor may also recommend you take a potassium supplement. In addition, people who are taking diuretics need to reduce their intake of salt, since increased sodium levels can also deplete the body's stores of potassium.

- Beta-blockers slow the heart rate and the metabolic rate, help ing to reduce the buildup of pressure in the circulatory system. They include medications such as Inderal (propranolol), Corgard, Tenormin, and Lopressor. Some side effects of beta-blockers include coldness in the extremities, a slowed heart rate, and elevated cholesterol levels. Beta-blockers can also cause wheezing in asthmatics and people who have emphysema. If you must stop taking beta-blockers, it's important that you be weaned from them gradually; since beta-blockers slow the heart rate, if you stop taking them, your heart rate will suddenly increase, causing an increase in the amount of oxygen that is delivered to the heart. This added stress can lead to angina or a heart attack.

- Calcium channel blockers are a large class of medication that includes Procardia (nifedipine), verapamil, and Cardizem (diltiazem). They work by dilating the blood vessels, which takes some of the stress off the heart. These drugs produce relatively few side effects, but when they do occur they include either a rapid or slowed heart rate, swollen ankles, and intestinal upset.

- ACE inhibitors include Zestril, Prinivil, and Monopril. These are strong medications that work by altering the action of an enzyme that regulates blood pressure. ACE inhibitors are also routinely prescribed to preserve kidney functions in diabetics. Side effects can include an upset stomach and a chronic cough.

- Another medication is Hytrin, an alpha-blocker, which is used to lower blood pressure and also has the bonus of reducing the size of the prostate in men, which will help cut down on the problem of prostate enlargement later on in life (see Chapter 15, "For Men Only"). There is also a medication called Catapres, which comes in the form of a patch that can be worn for a full week and administers a slow, constant flow of medication to lower blood pressure.

- Other medications, such as Aldomet, have been around for decades and were once routinely prescribed by doctors but are not used today unless other medications have failed to lower blood pressure, since Aldomet produces many side effects, including liver and blood abnormalities. Another side effect of high blood pressure medications for men is impotence. Understandably, some men are reluctant to bring up the subject with their physicians, but your physician's response will be strictly tempered by his medical viewpoint, and he'll simply ask when you first noticed the problem. He'll then suggest that you try another kind of blood pressure medication that won't interfere with your sexuality.

Treating high blood pressure with medication presents a real challenge to physicians today. But many times, all that is necessary is to prescribe one or two types of medication that will bring the elevated blood pressure down to a normal level, combined with sensible diet and exercise and relaxation techniques. At other times, however, you will need to experiment with multiple drug regimens before you and your doctor arrive at the right combination of medication with the smallest number of side effects. You need to be patient, and don't stop taking your medication without first discussing it with your doctor.

As long as we're on the subject of medication for high blood pressure, remember to take your medications as prescribed whenever you visit your doctor for follow-up checkups, unless your doctor tells you otherwise. It's also a good idea to order your prescriptions in small amounts at first. At the beginning of your treatment plan, you and your doctor will be experimenting with different medications to find the right one for you. This can be costly. Either ask your doctor to prescribe small amounts or ask your pharmacist to halve your prescription.

Special Mention for the Elderly

If you have an elderly relative who has high blood pressure and is also quite frail, it's important to weigh the risks of taking the medication against the potential benefits. Lowering the blood pressure too drastically can cause further weakness, falls, and confusion and can ultimately be as harmful to her health as the high blood pressure. Ideally, the doctor, patient, and family should decide together about ways to control your loved one's blood pressure without the side effects that may have a negative impact on the quality of her life.

ALL ABOUT BLOOD PRESSURE READINGS

An elevated blood pressure level is a hidden signal that can be detected only by actually measuring the blood pressure, preferably by a medical professional who has expertise and experience. In spite of all the high-tech equipment used today, I recommend that it be taken the old-fashioned way with a stethoscope and mercury sphygmomanometer, which employs a cuff and pressure gauge that uses mercury to measure the pressure. Though it's important to get a blood pressure reading that is as accurate as possible, there are many factors that can give an inaccurate reading, among them a cuff that is applied incorrectly—for instance, over clothes—or one that is too small, which is common in a person who has large arms. The cuff should be the correct size and fit snugly. I've also seen cases when the person who is taking the reading doesn't really know how to interpret the sounds she is hearing through the stethoscope. When in doubt, ask a trained medical professional to take the reading.

The blood pressure reading should be taken while you are sitting or standing and on several different occasions, to correct for inaccuracies as well as for any nervousness on your part. For instance, if you have the well-known "white coat syndrome," you may suddenly become very nervous in the presence of a doctor or nurse, even if you've known the person for years. This anxiety will naturally send your blood pressure level skyrocketing. If you have one elevated reading, don't be alarmed. This could be due not only to the stress of the office visit but also to other stresses in your life. Likewise, that high-fat fast-food lunch you ate an hour before your appointment can also cause a higher-than-normal blood pressure reading. If you have a high reading during the first few visits, your doctor may decide to take separate readings on both arms.

However, I believe that having you rest and lie down before a blood pressure reading doesn't provide for an accurate reading, either, because it doesn't reflect the true state of your health. After all, how many of us are that relaxed in the course of a normal day? The many stresses of modern life, including poor diet and lack of exercise, are, after all, the major causes of high blood pressure. In fact, I always have a patient come back to the office at least twice before I start her on any medication, unless that first blood pressure reading is dangerously high.

Even though most people view having their blood pressure taken as a routine procedure during a checkup, they remain surprisingly unfamiliar with the numbers of their reading and what they mean. There are two numbers that are used to measure your blood pressure. The upper, or larger, number is called the systolic pressure, and it refers to the pressure your blood is exerting on the arteries whenever your heart beats. In a healthy person, the systolic pressure should not be above 140. The lower number is called the diastolic blood pressure, and refers to the pressure that is exerted on your arteries between heartbeats. This number should not be above 90. A normal reading is considered to be 120 over 80. A borderline reading is 140 to 150 over 90 to 100. If, however, your blood pressure is 150/100, I view it as a serious risk that you will need to address immediately with a combination of diet, drugs, and relaxation techniques.

For years, the medical establishment has believed that the critical number is the diastolic number. We do know that this number is the most important indicator of good health in men and women up to about the age of 60. As a patient becomes older, however, the more critical number becomes the systolic number.

High blood pressure that goes undetected and untreated increases your risk factor for developing other cardiovascular diseases such as premature aging of the blood vessels and arteriosclerosis, in which plaque deposits accumulate in the blood vessels. This causes the vessels to narrow and can lead to an interruption of blood flow in the body. If this occurs in the brain, it can lead to a stroke; in a major artery or blood vessel, it can cause angina pectoris or a heart attack. Kidney deterioration or an intestinal stroke can also occur as a result of high blood pressure. The condition tends to be more common in women and African Americans. Needless to say, an elevated cholesterol level and a history of cigarette smoking will make high blood pressure worse.

I feel that even if you have no family history or past personal history of high blood pressure, it's still a good idea to have your blood pressure taken by an experienced medical professional at least once a year.

A WORD ABOUT ELEVATED CHOLESTEROL LEVELS

Cholesterol. It's one of those words everyone automatically labels as bad while, in fact, the jury is still out deliberating. Somewhere along the line, you've probably noticed that less ink is being spilled in books and magazines on the word diet and more on heart disease and cholesterol.

Frequently connected with the topic of cholesterol are words such as monounsaturated and polyunsaturated fats, lipoproteins, HDL, LDL, and triglycerides. No matter how many times we hear them, many people are forever confused. What do they all mean, and what relationship do they have to the health of your heart and cardiovascular system?

Let's start with the easy part, the definitions. Cholesterol is a waxlike, fatty substance that is natural to all animals. It is necessary to the working of our bodies, which make and use it, for example, to manufacture substances in our cell membranes and nerves. We ingest cholesterol by eating food products obtained from animals. The cholesterol we eat is called dietary cholesterol. The cholesterol in our blood is called serum cholesterol. When you are tested for cholesterol, your serum cholesterol will be measured and you will be given a number that represents a certain number of milligrams of cholesterol per 100 milliliters of blood. Anything under 200 is considered to be healthy. From 200 to 240 is considered to be borderline high, 240 to 300 is high risk, and over 300 is dangerous.

Though cholesterol is a natural and necessary component of our bodies, too much serum cholesterol is dangerous. It clogs up the bloodstream by sticking to the walls of the arteries. As cholesterol clings to the arterial walls, it eventually becomes hardened with calcium. This condition is called arteriosclerosis. Arteriosclerosis clogs arteries everywhere: the carotid arteries feeding the brain, the coronary arteries supplying the heart, the femoral arteries supplying the legs—you get the picture. Arteriosclerosis is one of the causes of stroke, heart attack, and the advanced form of poor circulation called peripheral vascular disease. If arteriosclerosis becomes severe enough, it is treated surgically with a bypass operation in which the surgeon creates a tubular pathway for blood to flow around the clogged obstruction or, sometimes, scrapes the clot out of the artery. A bypass operation improves a deteriorating situation when someone is having a heart attack or losing a limb, but nothing works as well as prevention.

That's why everyone is taking a mean look at cholesterol, which is turning out to be the buzzword of health in the 90s. You can significantly decrease the likelihood of developing arteriosclerosis by monitoring your serum cholesterol and keeping it within a healthy range by eating the right foods and participating in a regular exercise program.

Sounds easy, but it's not. The American Heart Association recommends that to keep our cholesterol down we reduce our total fat intake to 30% or less of our daily calorie intake. We should also avoid foods high in cholesterol such as lard, butter, and eggs.

Fats come in a variety of styles: saturated, monounsaturated, polyunsaturated, cholesterol, and fish oils. Some are called good fats, some are called bad fats. The ones that get the worst press are saturated fats and cholesterol, because they are considered most at fault in causing arteriosclerosis. Cholesterol comes only from animals or foods that come from animals, such as milk and eggs. Plants never contain cholesterol. However, although a food such as a coconut contains no cholesterol, its high in saturated fat, which can raise your serum cholesterol. To control your cholesterol level, you should lower your intake of both cholesterol and saturated fat. For example, butter has cholesterol and saturated fat while margarine contains saturated fat but no cholesterol. Therefore, if you eat a lot of margarine, it's likely that your serum cholesterol levels will rise. Except for coconut oil and palm oil (typically found in commercially prepared cookies and cakes and in some "imitation" dairy products), most saturated fats and cholesterol come from animal sources. It was generally believed in the past that vegetable fats—the monounsaturated and polyunsaturated varieties—are easier for the body to process and cause less disease.

For some people, decreasing dietary cholesterol does not sufficiently lower their serum cholesterol. Some studies indicate that high serum cholesterol is associated with diets high in fats, period, regardless of whether they're the good unsaturated types or not. A low-cholesterol diet that contains more than 30% fat can stimulate an increase in serum cholesterol by triggering the body's own cholesterol-making mechanisms. So it makes sense that the easiest way to control your cholesterol level is to watch your intake of total fat, since cholesterol can be produced in the body even by salad oil and peanut butter.

Here are some more definitions. HDL stands for high-density lipoprotein, LDL stands for low-density lipoprotein. A lipoprotein is a molecule that carries cholesterol in the blood. High-density lipoproteins carry cholesterol in a fashion the body can utilize; they allow the cholesterol to break off when it is needed. Low-density lipoproteins carry cholesterol into the bloodstream but do not allow the body to use it. Therefore, much of the low-density lipoproteins end up as cholesterol plaque deposits on the walls of arteries. The good news is that HDLs are stimulated into action by regular exercise.

And then there are triglycerides. When the body digests either saturated and unsaturated fat, it breaks it down into molecular chains. These chains then bind together in a triplet form called triglycerides. Triglycerides flow from the intestines through the lymphatic system and then into the bloodstream. The greater the amount of triglycerides in the bloodstream, the thicker the blood. This causes a strain on the heart, since it has to pump a thicker liquid through the blood vessels. If this condition is compounded by a narrowing blood vessel system due to arteriosclerosis, the thickened blood may have a difficult time getting through the smaller vessels and some of the body may be deprived of oxygen and nutrients. This is not a healthy scenario for the heart or any other body part. High triglycerides in the blood can usually be brought down by cutting concentrated sweets from the diet.

Then there's the genetic factor. Maybe we can control outside factors to improve our health, but some of us are simply genetically predisposed to heart disease. Surprisingly, some people who have low blood cholesterol levels still have heart attacks. No one knows why. Researchers are attempting to determine which genes are responsible for preventing or delaying heart disease, either on their own or in combination with diet and/or drugs.

Until they know the answers, however, my best advice is to follow the advice of the American Heart Association, which says the best thing to do is to control your blood cholesterol levels through diet, exercise, and weight control.

CHOLESTEROL LEVEL ABOVE 200

Description and Possible Medical Problems

There have been hundreds of books written on this topic, and it's likely that hundreds more will be written in the years to come. Then why is the public still generally confused about cholesterol and what—if anything—should be done to bring down an elevated cholesterol level?

These are the facts: A normal cholesterol reading will be 200 milligrams or less. If your cholesterol tests above 200, it's necessary to check all of your blood lipid levels with a series of blood tests, taken after fasting at least six hours.

I feel a cholesterol test should be performed by a reputable lab and interpreted by your physician. The result of a test done with a finger prick at work or at home should be used only as a screening. If the number is elevated, you should then make an appointment with your doctor.

The spotlight has turned on cholesterol because even in people of normal weight, an elevated cholesterol level increases the risk for developing premature aging of the blood vessels, which leads to heart and kidney disease, cerebral stroke, and other vascular diseases. Diabetes, some forms of liver disease, and some of the medications that are used to treat acne and high blood pressure can also cause your cholesterol levels to go up. Elevated cholesterol levels may also be due to genetics, but most often it's due to the high amounts of cholesterol and saturated fat people include in their diets.

Treatment

In many cases, a low-fat diet and exercise program and significant weight reduction will reduce an elevated cholesterol level. If they don't, medication may be prescribed. The problem is that you may feel you can return to your previous diet and sedentary lifestyle since you're taking medication. Unfortunately, this will only increase your cholesterol levels as well as your need for higher doses of medication. Since most cholesterol-lowering medications have some side effects, your physician will need to monitor you closely by testing your liver function and vision. He may also order other diagnostic tests according to the type of medication prescribed. As always, both the doctor and the patient should consider both the benefits and the risks before considering any medication program.

In my opinion, the total cholesterol consumption for one day should not be more than 200 milligram, an amount many fast-food meals easily exceed. The total diet should certainly not have more than 30% of its calories in fat. There are many excellent books on this topic that will help you learn how to decrease your intake of fat, including my own, *Dr. Bruce Lowell's Fat Percentage Finder* (published by Perigee Books).

You should keep in mind that your cholesterol level should not be taken as a simple number by itself. You should ask your doctor about the components of your total cholesterol reading, since a high total cholesterol reading could mean high LDL and low HDL cholesterol levels, which is a healthy balance to strive for.

FEVER, CHILLS, NIGHT SWEATS

Description and Possible Medical Problems

Whenever a patient tells me he has a fever or chills, the first thing I need to know is if he is in the 40s or 50s or over the age of 80.

Because fever occurs less frequently as a person ages, a high fever in an elderly person is often an indication of a serious health problem. When an elderly person has a high fever, she may become delirious, which will increase her chance of falling and breaking a hip or even becoming unconscious.

A high fever may be caused by a simple virus, such as a bacterial infection in the sinuses, bowels, or lungs, or by a more serious infection in the bloodstream called sepsis.

My feeling is that if you have any fever that's above 100 or 101 degrees F. for more than 24 hours, you should seek medical attention—sooner if confusion or delirium starts to set in.

If you have a fever, here are some questions to ask yourself that will help your doctor narrow down the cause:

1. Besides the fever, what other symptoms do I have, such as a cough, nasal stuffiness, muscular aches and pains, diarrhea, and/or pain when urinating?

2. How long have I had these symptoms: a day, a week, or longer?

3. Do I have night sweats or chills?

4. Is my fever getting better or worse? Is it accompanied by weakness and a general feeling of malaise?

If an elderly relative is feverish, ask yourself the following questions:

1. Has the weather been hot lately ? If so, does she have an air conditioner and does she use it?

2. Have you noticed any recent changes in his mental state? Has he become increasingly confused?

3. Have there been any changes in her appetite?

4. Has he been acting listless lately?

Treatment

If your fever is mild, 100 or 101 degrees F., you should take two aspirin or Tylenol every four hours and get plenty of rest. For most people, this is all that's necessary.

If, however, despite this self-treatment, the fever doesn't break or gets worse after six hours, you should see your doctor, who will take your complete medical history and conduct a physical exam as well as any diagnostic tests.

For midlife patients, treatment is usually performed on an outpatient basis. An elderly person, however, might need to be hospitalized and treated with intravenous fluids as well as antibiotics. An elderly person rarely gets a high fever. Therefore, a fever of 101 or higher in an elderly man or woman should be taken quite seriously, and you should seek medical attention immediately.

The most important thing to do is monitor your temperature and your general state of health and call your doctor if you start to feel worse.

BODY SIGNAL ALERT

GLUCOSE LEVEL, ELEVATED

Description and Possible Medical Problems

Though you've probably heard that the primary symptoms of diabetes are an increase in thirst and urination and fatigue, sometimes a simple blood test that shows an elevation in glucose level is the first indication of this initially hidden disease.

A normal blood sugar level is 60 to 120. Often when the blood sugar level is only slightly elevated—above 120—there are few apparent side effects, if any. Even in extreme cases, when people are obese and sedentary, their complaints may consist of vague symptoms such as weakness and nausea. Sometimes people also develop double or blurred vision due to an abnormal sugar level; in more severe cases, weight loss, thirst, and increased urination can be the major symptoms. If you have these Body Signals, it is important that your doctor know if anyone in your family has ever had diabetes and especially if your mother had diabetes when she was pregnant. You should also tell your doctor about any recent weight gain or loss.

If an elevated blood sugar level goes undetected and untreated, full-blown diabetes can eventually develop. Besides the necessity of daily insulin medication, I've seen many other diabetic problems that can affect the quality of a person's life. These can include numbness, which appears most often in the feet and hands, vaginal yeast infections, skin rashes that form in the folds of body fat and on the anus and penis, and even bladder infections. Usually, it's these annoying symptoms that bring patients to the doctor, and they don't have a clue that they have diabetes until a blood sugar test confirms it. I see this occur most often in people who are in their 40s. In fact, the typical case that I regularly see is a 50-year-old who gradually develops high blood sugar levels because of the lethal combination of obesity, a high-fat diet, and a sedentary lifestyle. Diabetes results because there is not enough insulin in the systems to treat the unusually high glucose levels in the body.

Diabetes is a disease in which there is not enough insulin to process the blood sugar, which can often lead to heart and kidney disease—many diabetics also have elevated cholesterol levels—as well as disorders of the peripheral nervous system and vision. These complications are why it's important to catch and treat the disease early.

Diabetes can make its appearance in a number of different ways. The disease may form slowly and become more apparent over a long period of time, or symptoms may suddenly appear over the course of a few weeks. Usually, however, the person will have an elevated blood sugar level for at least several months to a year, and then the level will rise to a point where it is abnormal, which will cause the first symptoms of diabetes to appear.

Sometimes, if you're taking a corticosteroid such as prednisone, the medication will elevate your blood sugar level. If you are taking steroids, your physician will ask you to schedule regular office visits to detect and treat elevated blood sugar levels before diabetes occurs.

Though diabetes occurs primarily in people who are overweight and sedentary, some people get diabetes because their bodies don't produce enough insulin, not because their blood sugar levels are high. Often, these diabetics are thin, and they usually know they have the disease by the time they are 30 years old.

If your blood sugar test shows evidence of an elevated glucose level, you should ask yourself the following questions:

1. Do I have a family history of diabetes?

2. Did my mother have an elevated blood sugar level during her pregnancy?

3. Am I taking steroids or diuretics?

4. Have I recently gained or lost weight?

Treatment

The primary treatment for diabetes, regardless of the cause or the patient's age, is reducing the sugar in the diet and increasing the amount of exercise. Only if a patient fails to modify his lifestyle will I recommend medication to control the disease. Oral agents in the form of tablets such as Glucotrol, DiaBeta, and Micronase, taken by mouth once or twice a day in dosages of 5 to 10 milligrams, are very effective in controlling the disease when combined with diet and exercise. If, however, the patient fails to control the disease with diet, exercise, and oral medication, insulin injections, which are usually done once a day in the morning, will become necessary.

Because it is both difficult and extremely important to treat diabetes correctly, it is essential that you and your physician approach this illness as a team. In fact, in the beginning, your doctor might suggest that you consult a dietician who regularly works with diabetics as well as an endocrinologist to help you monitor your illness and determine the various steps you need to take in order to control it. Today, there are many home monitoring devices such as blood glucose meters and urinalysis strips that will help you check your blood sugar daily, as well as a variety of insulin regimens. Many hospitals have specialized centers that work with diabetics to help them understand their illness and assist their physicians to ensure the best possible treatment: recommended diet and exercise programs, insulin, oral medication, and emotional support groups are some of the services provided. You should contact your local diabetes society for information about the center nearest you.

Special Mention for the Elderly

In my experience, I've seen that elderly diabetics tend not to control their disease as well as younger people do, due to constant fluctuations in the availability and quality of food, frequently missed meals, and forgetting to take their medication. This can cause two separate problems. (1) Low blood sugar, which can occur in a person who has missed a few meals, can cause a hypoglycemic episode, which can result in falling and confusion. In the long term, this can result in permanent confusion. (2) When blood sugar gets too high, a life-threatening diabetic coma may result. That is why, when I have an elderly diabetic patient, I try to have her install a medical alert call system in case of an emergency.

HDL CHOLESTEROL LEVEL BELOW 40

Description and Possible Medical Problems

The HDL part of the total cholesterol level is believed to be the primary protector against heart disease. It tends to be lower in men than in women and seems to be a problem especially in people who lead a sedentary lifestyle.

The HDL is the healthy cholesterol, and it should be high—that's the "H" in HDL. Usually, a low HDL level is in itself very serious because when the HDL is low, the LDL tends to be high, resulting in a total cholesterol level that can be dangerously high.

Treatment

A low HDL level can be treated in the same way as a cholesterol level over 200: with diet, exercise, and perhaps medication. In older women, the use of an estrogen replacement therapy might be beneficial. In men, it's particularly important to use exercise to help raise the HDL level. For both men and women, a low-fat, low-cholesterol lifestyle is imperative, since there is no medication that can raise the HDL to an acceptably high level.

See also "Cholesterol Level Above 200" above.

KIDNEY TEST, ABNORMAL

Description and Possible Medical Problems

Your two kidneys are workhouse organs that work in tandem with the urinary system to remove fluid and waste products from your tissues and blood. When they begin to malfunction in some way, it's frequently due to an underlying illness such as high blood pressure, diabetes, heart failure, primary kidney disease, or a side effect of a particular medication.

Treatment

To diagnose a kidney ailment positively, your doctor will administer a number of tests, including a urinalysis to test the composition of the urine, a blood test to determine the amount of urea and nitrogen that is excreted through the kidneys (also called a BUN test), and perhaps an X ray or an intravenous pyelogram (IVP), which provides a clear picture of the kidneys on an X ray.

Because any abnormalities in the kidneys can cause permanent damage to the organs if they're not treated, your physician will want to begin treatment right away. And since the kidneys often begin to malfunction because of a medical problem elsewhere in the body, your doctor's recommended course of treatment will depend on what she determines to be the primary cause.

LDL CHOLESTEROL
LEVEL ABOVE 120

Description and Possible Medical Problems

LDL stands for "low-density lipoprotein." I like to think of this cholesterol as the "lethal" cholesterol, and the numbers in a cholesterol test should be low, under 120.

Treatment

See "Cholesterol Level Above 200" above

LIVER FUNCTION TEST, ABNORMAL

Description and Possible Medical Problems

Since the primary function of the liver is to detoxify the blood, if the liver fails to do its job properly, the problem will immediately become evident through a routine blood test. An abnormal liver function test can be caused by many diseases, including hepatitis, viral inflammation of the liver, an injury to the liver, such as cancer or alcohol abuse, gallbladder disease, and certain medications, such as Cognex and Mevacor.

Treatment

Since each specific liver disease requires its own individual treatment, if your doctor discovers a problem with your liver, he will immediately order a regimen for you. This may include medication such as corticosteroids to reduce inflammation, a diet that's restricted in protein, fat, and alcohol, and rest. Some liver diseases, such as viral hepatitis, can be highly contagious, so your doctor may recommend that your family members receive immune globulins against hepatitis.

MALAISE

Description and Possible Medical Problems

Over the course of a year, I'll see 5,000 or more patients who come to me for treatment. Of all the symptoms my patients tell me they have, malaise, or a general sense that they're not feeling as well as they could, is one of the most common complaints I hear. Unfortunately, whenever a patient tells me she is feeling weak and unwell, it opens the door to the possibility of every single medical problem on earth. This can be frustrating and overwhelming to the physician as well as to the patient, so if she simply says she doesn't feel quite right, I ask her to be as specific with her complaints as she can. It's important to keep in mind that age and activity levels have a lot to do with how people define malaise. For instance, the malaise of a 20-year-old athlete who cannot run 10 miles every day because of an injury is much different from the 50-year-old executive who can't seem to find the energy to go to work or the 65-year-old grandmother who just feels too tired to do chores around the house.

If you have been feeling weak and out of sorts lately, answering the following questions will help your physician zero in on the possible causes:

1. How long have I been feeling unwell? A week, a month, or longer?

2. Has there been a change in my appetite or thirst? In my urination or bowel habits?

3. Have I gained or lost a significant amount of weight in the last few weeks or months?

4. For women, if I am still menstruating, has my cycle or flow, or both, changed recently?

5. Have I recently had a fever, night sweats, or a physical intolerance to hot or cold temperatures?

6. Have I recently traveled abroad or to a different region of the country?

7. Do I have a symptom such as a rash, arthritic pain, or swollen glands?

8. Do I think I might have been bitten by a tick recently?

9. Have I been undergoing problems in my personal life lately?

10. Do I have a past history of a serious illness that was cured or went into remission? Have I begun to take a new form of medication recently?

11. Has my urine darkened in color recently?

12. Do I have a history of blood transfusion, sharing a hypodermic needle, drug abuse, or even one unsafe sexual encounter?

13. Do I feel a general ache in my bones?

Treatment

Your answers to the above questions will determine the form of treatment your physician will advise, since treatment will depend largely on what is causing your malaise. For instance, if you have recently lost weight and noticed that your bowel habits have changed, the cause could be the fact that you're worrying about one of your children who recently moved across the country to take a new job. At worst, you could be suffering from cancer or bleeding in the gastrointestinal tract, but this is a very rare cause of malaise. The more specific you are in narrowing down your symptoms and your recent health history, the better your physician can treat you.

If you've lost weight and are frequently thirsty, it's a clear sign of diabetes. And if you've recently traveled to an area where deer roam freely and you feel tired and under the weather, you may have been bitten by a deer tick; a rash will help alert your physician to a possible diagnosis of

Lyme disease. There is also always the chance that your discomfort is caused by menstrual changes that are leading you toward the onset of menopause. Then again, a general feeling of malaise may simply be due to physical deconditioning if you have recently adopted a more sedentary lifestyle.

Your age, of course, will have some bearing on your physician's final diagnosis. If an elderly person complains of malaise, her doctor will be looking for signs of cancer, a blood disorder, or lymphoma. For people in their 40s, 50s, and 60s who are feeling unwell, a physician will probably investigate certain infectious diseases first.

You should keep in mind that the above are only a handful of the possible causes of malaise; there are, in fact, many different illnesses in which this symptom is present. Because of this, make sure your doctor has as much information as possible so she can prescribe the most effective and fastest-acting treatment possible. I feel that an investigation of both your recent and lifelong medical history is vital to ensure proper diagnosis and course of healing.

Special Mention for the Elderly

In an elderly person, other factors may be causing malaise. These can include thyroid disease, a rheumatological disorder such as temporal arteritis, polymyalgia rheumatica, heart disease, and interaction among several of the medications she is taking. Again, making sure she is as specific as possible about recent changes in her health will help guide her treatment.

BODY SIGNAL ALERT

PALPITATIONS, CONFUSION, SWEATING IN A DIABETIC

Description and Possible Medical Problems

If you see a person who is visibly confused and sweating and is suffering from heart palpitations, and if you know for a fact that he is diabetic, you should call 911 for assistance right away. The cause is probably hypoglycemia, or a blood sugar level that is too low. If the level gets even lower or is not treated immediately, it can lead to a loss of consciousness.

If you're not sure the person has diabetes, check for an ID bracelet or a dog tag that identifies her as a diabetic.

Treatment

Ask for advice from the emergency dispatch operator. He may tell you that if the person can sit up slightly and is able to swallow liquid without choking, you can try to give her some sips of orange juice or a sugary syrup while you wait for the paramedics to arrive. There are some diabetics who keep an emergency supply of glycogen ready for just such an emergency.

SKIN, PALE

See "Skin, Pale" in Chapter 9.

SKIN, YELLOW, WITH DARK URINE

See "Skin, Yellow, with Dark Urine" in Chapter 9.

TRIGLYCERIDE LEVEL ABOVE 150

Description and Possible Medical Problems

The triglyceride level is nothing more than the amount of fat that is found in the bloodstream. A test to determine your triglyceride level will be included as part of a cholesterol test; triglycerides alone pose very little risk to your health. I feel the value should be 150 or less. Currently, there is a lot of controversy in the medical establishment over whether an elevated triglyceride level alone increases the risk of heart disease. Even though I believe that for good health the triglyceride level should be at 150 or less, an elevated triglyceride level will be treated only if it is extremely high, in excess of 800 milligrams/100cc, which is an indication of a pancreatic problem or advancing arteriosclerosis. Elevated triglycerides are often caused by heredity, but, like the HDL and LDL cholesterol levels, more often than not they're a result of a high-fat diet, uncontrolled diabetes, and heavy smoking—particularly in women.

Treatment

The primary treatment for a high triglyceride level is medication, but again, only if the level is above 800. Your doctor will also prescribe a low-fat diet and moderate exercise program for you to follow. However, an underlying condition, such as diabetes, must also be treated in order to bring the triglycerides down to a normal level. I've found that in some rare cases a triglyceride level above 200 is caused by taking a medication such as Accutane, which is used to treat acne. In this case, discontinuing the medication will lower the triglyceride level to its previous state.

WEIGHT GAIN

Description and Possible Medical Problems

Americans treat weight gain as a modern-day blasphemy of sorts, no matter whether they're talking about 5 pounds or 50. I feel far too many men and women are totally obsessed with a process that I view as pure physics most of the time: weight gain is the body's natural reaction when a person takes in more calories than his body needs. Most of the time, it's as simple as that. Excess weight is one of the major contributors to America's health problems and is so common because of the high-fat, high-calorie, sedentary life many people lead. When a person weighs more than 20% above his ideal weight, he automatically becomes more prone to developing high blood pressure, increased cholesterol levels, diabetes, and arthritis, as well as the psychosocial problems that go along with carrying extra weight, such as low self-esteem and emotional isolation.

As a physician, I become very concerned when one of my patients gains a lot of weight in a short period of time and/or morbid obesity develops.

However, the aging process works in such a way that a weight gain might actually be due not to an increase in body fat, but rather to an increase in the amount of water the body retains. This excess water can be the result of kidney, heart, or liver failure, and it accumulates most often in the abdomen or in the legs. Weight gain that results in fat and occurs without a corresponding increase in caloric intake can be a side effect of corticosteroid preparations such as prednisone, which are prescribed to treat arthritis or asthma. The face will commonly take on a round, moonlike look, and a hump may develop on the upper back. Prednisone can also raise blood sugar levels and aggravate an existing case of osteoporosis. However, the good news is that these symptoms and the weight gain will develop only in people who take high doses of the steroid for more than three or four months. Many times, however, an inactive thyroid is the first condition your doctor will check for. This can be diagnosed with a physical exam and a simple blood test.

Treatment

A complete medical history and physical exam as well as a series of specific diagnostic tests will help your doctor determine the necessary treatment for your unexplained weight gain.

As with any medical treatment, the risks must be weighed against the benefits when you and your doctor decide about your specific treatment. If your doctor has prescribed steroids to treat another medical condition, you should realize that the short-term use of steroids for a week or even up to a month has not been found to cause any permanent weight or health problems. You'll lose the extra pounds once you stop taking the steroids.

Water pills, or diuretics, can help reduce a weight gain of a few pounds that comes before menstruation and is caused by water retention—if they're used judiciously. However, they do not help reduce the body's stores of fat and are dangerous to use on a reduced-calorie diet since they can cause potassium depletion and dehydration.

Since most cases of weight gain are caused by eating too much and/or moving too little, what I'm going to say next is going to sound boring, but I'm going to say it anyway. If your weight gain is the direct result of too many calories and not enough exercise, you're going to have to change your lifestyle if you want to lose weight. A sensible weight-reduction plan should include a low-fat, low-calorie diet and regular physical exercise. Your doctor is the best person to advise you about the best course of action for you.

Special Mention for the Elderly

Weight gain in an elderly person can be a sign of water accumulation, especially if it's accompanied by shortness of breath, an inability to lie flat at night, and swollen ankles. An increase in weight in an elderly person can lead to heart failure. I tell elderly patients who have had heart failure in the past to weigh themselves in the early morning after they urinate. I also tell them that if their weight is up two or three pounds over the course of several days and they have some of the other signs of heart failure I've mentioned, they should call me so I can advise them on proper treatment. Sometimes, if their other signs aren't serious, I'll tell them just to take another water pill; other times, however, I'll ask them to come in to see me.

In addition, weight loss that's due to body water can be an indication of heart problems, and I give my patients with weight loss these same guidelines.

BODY SIGNAL ALERT

WEIGHT LOSS

Description and Possible Medical Problems

Since, like many Americans, you may have been fighting excess body weight for most of your life, you may be heartened to discover that weight loss is a common part of the aging process. However, this weight loss begins when people reach their mid to late 60s, and it usually amounts to only a few pounds a year, if that. Even though your scale says you weigh less, any pounds that are lost due to the aging process are mostly lean body mass or muscle mass, not fat. This leaves most people with less strength than they had just a few years before. Since the process is usually slow, the weight loss usually goes unnoticed except for when they are weighed in at their annual checkup or observe a change in their physical stature.

The time you and your doctor should become concerned about weight loss, however, is when both your weight and your general health rapidly deteriorate over a short period of time. If you have lost 10% of your weight over a period of a month or two, I usually become quite concerned, and the younger my patient, the more concerned I become.

If a person who is quite overweight loses a couple of pounds without trying, the loss might not initially seem serious, but this too can be the sign of a medical problem.

As with the case of malaise, weight loss can occur because of either the normal physiological changes of aging or a more serious illness.

That's why a complete medical history and physical exam with the necessary diagnostic tests are extremely important in any instance of unexplained weight loss. Thyroid problems may cause you to feel overheated, while cancer or a hidden infection may be responsible for a fever or night sweats. If you are coughing or feel short of breath, you may have emphysema or lung cancer. There is also the possibility that if weight loss is accompanied by a cough, swollen glands, a fever, and/or a general feeling of malaise, you might have been exposed to the HIV virus, which can lead to the development of AIDS.

If you have recently lost weight without trying, either a few pounds or 10 or more, you should ask yourself the following questions:

1. Over how long a time has the weight loss occurred?

2. Have I also experienced a change in my appetite or bowel habits?

3. Do I suffer from heat intolerance, nervousness, or heart palpitations?

4. Do I have night sweats, occasional fevers, or newly enlarged glands?

5. Am I coughing a lot lately? Do I suffer from shortness of breath?

6. Do I have a prior history of a serious illness?

7. Do I regularly use alcohol or tobacco?

8. Have I ever had an unsafe sexual encounter, shared a hypodermic needle, or had a blood transfusions?

Treatment

If your doctor determines that the loss of a few pounds is due to the aging process, he will probably recommend that you do nothing. Of course, many people who have struggled with their weight their entire lives will be thrilled at the fact that the pounds have seemingly come off effortlessly. If this continues, however, and is accompanied by weakness and malaise, your doctor may recommend that you increase your caloric intake with nutritious foods—not high-fat, high-calorie junk foods—and that you also step up your exercise program. The reason? Muscle weighs more than fat, and exercise serves the dual purpose of reducing fat stores and building up lean muscle mass, which will ultimately increase your strength.

If the aging process is not the culprit, your doctor will tailor your treatment to whatever underlying medical problem is responsible. Again, as with malaise, it's important for you to be as specific as you can when you describe your symptoms to your physician, since this is what will ultimately help him to determine your treatment.

I want to tell you a story about a patient I once had who was about 60 years old and who had spent her entire life fighting and losing her battle with chronic obesity. She had been on numerous diets without success. Unfortunately, she ended up developing breast cancer—which can be more common in women who are overweight—and she subsequently underwent radiation and chemotherapy. In the process, she lost 50 pounds. At the end of her treatment, she was heartened to find that her cancer had been totally eradicated. She was healthy and doing quite well, so after her treatment stopped, she decided to continue to lose weight until she had lost a total of 60 pounds. To lose the extra weight, she followed the advice of her oncologist, who had recommended a low-fat, low-calorie diet to prevent a recurrence of her cancer.

All was well until she suddenly became concerned that the real reason why she was losing weight was that her cancer had returned. She became scared and returned to her old eating habits; she promptly gained back 30 pounds. She told me she was afraid to lose any more weight because everyone thought her weight loss was due to her cancer; therefore, she felt that as long as she gained weight, she was cancer free. She did remain cancer free, but her weight went up and down for many years. The moral of this story is: Despite past health conditions, if you lose weight and feel healthy, listen to your body. It's telling you everything is working as it should.

Special Mention for the Elderly

In an elderly person, weight loss can have certain causes a doctor would never consider to be a problem in a younger person. For one, your elderly aunt may not be able to obtain nutritious food because she's unable to make it out of the house to go shopping and there's no one else around to do it for her. Poorly fitting dentures can make it uncomfortable for her to eat, or she may be experiencing increasing senility due to Alzheimer's disease, cancer, or an underlying infection and has lost her appetite.

As with younger people, I consider weight loss in an elderly person to be serious if she loses more than 10% of her body weight over the course of a month or two. If this happens, I'll order a blood test to determine if there is evidence of malnutrition. Lower serum protein levels, albumin levels, and lymphocyte counts are all signs that the immune system is beginning to deteriorate, making an elderly person more prone to infections, bedsores, falls, and other health problems. These can depress the appetite even more.

The treatment for your elderly relative will depend on the cause. Using Meals on Wheels, taking food supplements, and getting new dentures, as well as possibly going into a nursing home are some of the steps that might be considered by the doctor and the patient's family.

WEIGHT LOSS WITH INCREASED THIRST AND URINATION

See "Glucose Level, Elevated" above.

Appendix A

ROUTINE TESTS AND PROCEDURES

The following lists include the routine exams and procedures physicians generally recommend for adults age 40–64 and 65 and older every 1–3 years. Obviously, they are not exhaustive, and much depends on a person's medical history and other individual circumstances. However, the information presented will serve as a good guide to the typical periodic checkup.

AGES 40–64

Screening

Physical Exam

High-risk groups. Complete skin exam for persons with a family or personal history of skin cancer, frequent occupational or recreational exposure to sunlight, or clinical evidence of premalignant lesions.

Complete oral cavity exam for persons who use tobacco or drink excessive amounts of alcohol or those with suspicious symptoms or lesions detected through self-examination.

Palpitation for thyroid nodules for persons with a history of upper-body radiation therapy.

Auscultation for carotid bruits for persons who have risk factors for cerebrovascular or cardiovascular disease (e.g., hypertension, smoking, coronary artery disease, atrial fibrillation, diabetes), neurological symptoms, or a history of cerebrovascular disease.

Laboratory/Diagnostic Procedures

High-risk groups. Fasting plasma glucose for the markedly obese, persons with a family history of diabetes, or women with a history of gestational diabetes.

Syphillis test VDRL or RPR for prostitutes, persons who engage in sex with multiple partners in areas in which syphilis is prevalent, or have contacts with persons with active syphilis.

Urinalysis for bacteriuria for persons with diabetes.

Chlamydial testing for persons who attend clinics for sexually transmitted diseases, attend other high-risk health care facilities (e.g., adolescent and family planning clinics), or have other risk factors for chlamydial infection (e.g., multiple sexual partners or a sexual partner with multiple sexual contacts).

Gonorrhea culture for prostitutes, persons who have multiple sexual partners or a sexual partner who has multiple contacts, sexual contacts of persons with culture-proven gonorrhea, or persons who have a history of repeated episodes of gonorrhea.

Counseling and testing for HIV for persons seeking treatment for sexually transmitted diseases; homosexual and bisexual men; past or present intravenous drug users; persons with a history of prostitution or multiple sexual contact; women whose past or present sexual partners were HIV-infected, bisexual or IV drug users; persons with long-term residence or birth in an area with a high prevalence of HIV infection; or persons who had a blood transfusion between 1978 and 1985.

Tuberculin skin test (PPD) for household members of persons with tuberculosis or others at risk for close contact with the disease (e.g., staff of tuberculosis clinics, shelters for the homeless, nursing homes, substance abuse treatment clinics, dialysis units, correctional institutions); recent immigrants or refugees from countries in which tuberculosis is common (e.g., Asia, Africa, Central and South America, Pacific Islands); migrant workers; residents of nursing homes, correctional institutions, or homeless shelters; or persons with certain underlying medical disorders (e.g., HIV infection).

Electrocardiogram for men with two or more cardiac risk factors (high blood cholesterol, hypertension, cigarette smoking, diabetes mellitus, family history of coronary artery disease); people who would endanger public safety were they to experience a sudden cardiac event (e.g., commercial airline pilots); or sedentary or high-risk males planning to begin a vigorous exercise program.

Hearing test for persons frequently exposed to excessive noise.

Fecal occult blood sigmoidoscopy for persons aged 50 and older who have first-degree relatives with colorectal cancer; a personal history of endometrial, ovarian, or breast cancer; or a previous diagnosis of inflammatory bowel disease, adenomatous polyps, or colorectal cancer.

Fecal occult blood colonoscopy for persons who have a family history of familial polyposis coli or cancer-family syndrome.

Bone mineral content for perimenopausal women who have an increased risk for osteoporosis (e.g., Caucasian race, bilateral ovary removal before menopause, slender build) and for whom estrogen replacement therapy is not recommended.

Counseling

Diet and Exercise

Fat (especially saturated fat), cholesterol, complex carbohydrates, fiber, sodium, calcium.
Caloric balance.
Selection of exercise program.

Substance Use

Tobacco cessation.
Alcohol and other drugs.
Limiting alcohol consumption.
Driving/other dangerous activities while under the influence.
Treatment for abuse.

High-risk groups. Intravenous drug users who share or use unsterilized needles and syringes.

Sexual Practices

Sexually transmitted diseases: partner selection, condoms, anal intercourse.
Unintended pregnancy and contraceptive options.

Injury Prevention

Safety belts.
Safety helmets.
Smoke detectors.
Smoking near bedding or upholstery.

High-risk groups. Back-conditioning exercises for persons at increased risk for low-back injury because of past history, body configuration, or types of activities.

Prevention of childhood injuries for persons with children in the home or automobile.

Falls by the elderly for persons with older adults in the home.

Dental Health

Regular tooth brushing, flossing, dental visits.

Other Primary Preventive Measures

High-risk groups. Skin protection from ultraviolet light for persons with frequent exposure to sunlight.

Discussion of aspirin therapy for men who have risk factors for myocardial infarction (e.g., high blood cholesterol, smoking, diabetes mellitus, family history of early-onset coronary artery disease) and who lack a family history of gastrointestinal or other bleeding problems or other risk factors for bleeding or cerebral hemorrhage.

Discussion of estrogen replacement therapy for perimenopausal women who have an increased risk for osteoporosis (e.g., Caucasian, low bone mineral content, bilateral ovary removal before menopause, early menopause, slender build) and who are without known contraindications (e.g., history of undiagnosed vaginal bleeding, active liver disease, thromboembolic disorders, hormone-dependent cancer).

Immuni\zations

Tetanus-diphtheria (TD) booster.

High-risk groups. Hepatitis B vaccine for homosexually active men, intravenous drug users, recipients of some blood products, or people in health-related jobs who are frequently exposed to blood or blood products.

Pneumococcal vaccine for persons who have medical conditions that increase the risk of pneumococcal infection (e.g., chronic cardiac or pulmonary disease, sickle-cell disease, nephrotic syndrome, Hodgkin's disease, asplenia, diabetes mellitus, alcoholism, cirrhosis, multiple myeloma, renal disease, conditions associated with immunosuppression).

Influenza vaccine for residents of chronic care facilities and persons suffering from chronic cardiopulmonary disorders, metabolic diseases (including diabetes mellitus), hemoglobinopathies, immunosuppression, or renal dysfunction.

This list of preventive measures is not exhaustive. It reflects only those topics reviewed by the U.S. Preventive Services Task Force. Your doctor may wish to add other preventive measures on a routine basis,

after considering your medical history and other individual circumstances. Examples of conditions not specifically examined by the Task
Force include:

Chronic obstructive pulmonary disease.

Hepatobility disease.

Bladder cancer.

Endometrial disease.

Travel-related illness.

Prescription drug abuse.

Occupational illness and injuries.

Be Alert for:

Depressive symptoms.

Suicide risk factors: recent divorce, separation, unemployment,
depression, alcohol or other drug abuse, serious medical illnesses, living
alone, or recent bereavement.

Abnormal bereavement.

Signs of physical abuse or neglect.

Malignant skin lesions.

Peripheral arterial disease for persons over age 50, smokers, and persons with diabetes mellitus.

Tooth decay, gingivitis, loose teeth

The recommended schedule for the above exams and procedures
applies only to the periodic visit itself. The frequency of the individual
preventive services listed in this section is left to the clinician's discretion as dictated by past medical and family history.

AGES 65 AND OVER

Schedule: Every Year
Leading causes of death:
Heart disease
Cerebrovascular disease
Obstructive lung disease
Pneumonia/influenza
Lung cancer
Colorectal cancer

Screening

History

> Prior symptoms of transient ischemic attack.
> Dietary intake.
> Physical activity.
> Tobacco/alcohol/drug use.
> Functional status at home.
> Physical exam.
> Height and weight.
> Blood pressure.
> Visual acuity.
> Hearing and hearing aids.
> Clinical breast exam.

High-risk groups. Auscultation for carotid bruits for persons who have risk factors for cerebrovascular or cardiovascular disease (e.g., hypertension, smoking, coronary artery disease, atrial fibrillation, diabetes), neurological symptoms (e.g., transient ischemic attacks), or a history of cerebrovascular disease.

Complete skin exam for persons with a family or personal history of skin cancer, frequent occupational or recreational exposure to sunlight, or clinical evidence of precursor lesions (e.g., dysplastic nevi, certain congenital nevi).

Complete oral cavity exam for persons who use tobacco or drink excessive amounts of alcohol or those with suspicious symptoms or lesions detected through self-examination.

Palpitation for thyroid nodules for persons with a history of upper-body radiation therapy when they were a child, for an increased thymus gland, or previous history of thyroid nodules.

Laboratory/Diagnostic Procedures

> Nonfasting total blood cholesterol.
> Dipstick urinalysis.
> Mammogram.
> Thyroid function tests.

High-risk groups. Fasting plasma glucose for the markedly obese, persons with a family history of diabetes, or women with a history of gestational diabetes.

Tuberculin skin test (PPD) for household members of persons with tuberculosis or others at risk for close contact with the disease (e.g., staff of tuberculosis clinics, shelters for the homeless, nursing homes, substance abuse treatment clinics, dialysis units, correctional institutions); recent immigrants or refugees from countries in which tuberculosis is common (e.g., Asia, Africa, Central and South America, Pacific Islands); migrant workers; residents of nursing homes, correctional institutions, or homeless shelters; or persons with certain underlying medical disorders (e.g., HIV infection.)

Electrocardiogram for men with two or more cardiac risk factors (high blood cholesterol, hypertension, cigarette smoking, diabetes mellitus, family history of coronary artery disease); persons who would endanger public safety were they to experience sudden cardiac events (e.g., commercial airline pilots); or sedentary or high-risk males planning to begin a vigorous exercise program.

Pap smear for women who have not had previous documented screenings in which Pap smears have been consistently negative.

Fecal occult blood sigmoidoscopy for persons who have first-degree relatives with colorectal cancer; a personal history of endometrial, ovarian, or breast cancer; or a previous diagnosis of inflammatory bowel disease, adenomatous polyps, or colorectal cancer.

Fecal occult blood colonoscopy for persons with a family history of familial polyposis coli or cancer-family syndrome.

Counseling

Diet and Exercise

Fat (especially saturated fat), cholesterol, complex carbohydrates, fiber, sodium, calcium.

Caloric balance.

Selection of exercise program.

Substance Use

Tobacco cessation.

Alcohol and other drugs.

Limiting alcohol consumption.

Driving/other dangerous activities while under the influence.

Treatment for abuse.

Injury Prevention

Prevention of falls.
Safety belts.
Smoke detectors.
Smoking near bedding or upholstery.
Hot-water heater temperature.
Safety helmets.

High-risk groups. Prevention of childhood injuries for persons with children in the home or automobile.

Dental Health

Regular dental visits, tooth brushing, flossing.

Other Primary Preventive Measures

Glaucoma testing by eye specialist.

High-risk groups. Discussion of estrogen replacement therapy for women who have an increased risk for osteoporosis (e.g., Caucasian, low bone mineral content, bilateral ovary removal before menopause, early menopause, slender build) and who are without known contraindications (e.g., history of undiagnosed vaginal bleeding, active liver disease, thromboembolic disorders, hormone-dependent cancer).

Discussion of aspirin therapy for men who have risk factors for myocardial infarction (e.g., high blood cholesterol, smoking, diabetes mellitus, family history of early-onset coronary artery disease) and who lack a family history of gastrointestinal or other bleeding problems or other risk factors for bleeding or cerebral hemorrhage.

Skin protection from ultraviolet light for persons with frequent exposure to sunlight.

Immunizations

Tetanus-diphtheria (TD) booster.
Influenza vaccine.
Pneumococcal vaccine.

High-risk groups. Hepatitis B vaccine for homosexually active men, intravenous drug users, recipients of some blood products, or persons in health-related jobs who are frequently exposed to blood or blood products.

This list of preventive measures is not exhaustive. It reflects only those topics reviewed by the U.S. Preventive Services Task Force. Your doctor may wish to add other preventive measures on a routine basis, after considering your medical history and other individual circumstances. Examples of conditions not specifically examined by the Task Force include:

Chronic obstructive pulmonary disease.

Hepatobility disease.

Bladder cancer.

Endometrial disease.

Travel-related illness.

Prescription drug abuse.

Occupational illness and injuries.

Be Alert for:

Depressive symptoms.

Suicide risk factors: recent divorce, separation, unemployment, depression, alcohol or other drug abuse, serious medical illnesses, living alone, or recent bereavement.

Abnormal bereavement.

Changes in cognitive function.

Medications that increase the risk of falls.

Signs of physical abuse or neglect.

Malignant skin lesions.

Peripheral arterial disease.

Tooth decay, gingivitis, loose teeth.

The recommended schedule for the above exams and procedures applies only to the periodic visit itself. The frequency of the individual preventive services listed in this section is left to the clinician's discretion, except as indicated in other footnotes.

Appendix B

MET LIFE HEIGHT
AND WEIGHT TABLES

Men

Height	Small Frame	Medium Frame	Large Frame
5'2"	128–134	131–141	138–150
5'3"	130–138	133–143	140–153
5'4"	132–138	135–145	142–156
5'5"	134–140	137–148	144–160
5'6"	136–142	139–151	146–164
5'7"	138–145	142–154	149–168
5'8"	140–148	145–157	152–172
5'9"	142–151	148–160	155–176
5'10"	144–154	151–163	157–180
5'11"	146–157	154–166	161–184
6'0"	148–160	157–170	164–188
6'1"	152–164	160–174	168–192
6'2"	155–168	164–178	172–197
6'3"	158–172	167–182	176–202
6'4"	162–176	171–187	181–207

Women

Height	Small Frame	Medium Frame	Large Frame
4'10"	102–111	109–121	118–131
4'11"	103–113	111–123	120–134
5'0"	104–115	113–128	122–137
5'1"	106–118	115–129	125–140
5'2"	108–121	118–132	128–143
5'3"	111–124	121–135	131–147
5'4"	114–127	124–138	134–151
5'5"	117–130	127–141	137–155
5'6"	120–133	130–144	140–159
5'7"	123–136	133–147	143–163
5'8"	126–138	136–150	146–167
5'9"	129–142	139–153	149–170
5'10"	132–145	142–158	152–173
5'11"	135–148	145–159	155–176
6'0"	138–151	148–162	158–179

INDEX

NORMANDALE COMMUNITY COLLEGE
9700 FRANCE AVENUE SOUTH
BLOOMINGTON MN 55431-4399